CRASH COURSE
Obstetrics and Gynecology

Other Titles in the Crash Course Series

There are 23 books in the Crash Course series in two ranges: Basic Science and Clinical. Each book follows the same format, with concise text, clear illustrations and helpful learning features including access to online USMLE test questions.

Basic Science titles
Pathology
Nervous System
Renal and Urinary Systems
Gastrointestinal System
Respiratory System
Endocrine and Reproductive Systems
Metabolism and Nutrition
Pharmacology
Immunology
Musculoskeletal System
Cardiovascular System
Cell Biology and Genetics
Anatomy

Clinical titles
Surgery
Cardiology
History and Examination
Internal Medicine
Neurology
Gastroenterology
OBGYN

Forthcoming:
Psychiatry
Imaging
Pediatrics

Obstetrics and Gynecology

Naureen Alam, MD
Department of Obstetrics and Gynecology
Pennsylvania Hospital
Philadelphia, Pennsylvania

UK edition authors:
Nick Panay, Ruma Dutta, Audrey Ryan, J.A. Mark Broadbent

UK Series editor:
Daniel Horton-Szar

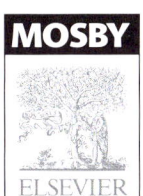

MOSBY
ELSEVIER

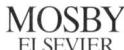

1600 John F. Kennedy Blvd.
Suite 1800
Philadelphia, PA 19103-2899

CRASH COURSE: OBSTETRICS AND GYNECOLOGY   ISBN-13: 978-1-4160-2958-8
Copyright 2007 by Mosby, Inc., an affiliate of Elsevier, Inc.   ISBN-10: 1-4160-2958-3

All rights reserved. No part of this publication may be reproduced or transmitted in any form or by any means, electronic or mechanical, including photocopying, recording, or any information storage and retrieval system, without permission in writing from the publisher. Permissions may be sought directly from Elsevier's Health Sciences Rights Department in Philadelphia, PA, USA: phone: (+1) 215 239 3804, fax: (+1) 215 239 3805, e-mail: healthpermissions@elsevier.com. You may also complete your request on-line via the Elsevier homepage (http://www.elsevier.com), by selecting "Customer Support" and then "Obtaining Permission".

Notice

Knowledge and best practice in this field are constantly changing. As new research and experience broaden our knowledge, changes in practice, treatment and drug therapy may become necessary or appropriate. Readers are advised to check the most current information provided (i) on procedures featured or (ii) by the manufacturer of each product to be administered, to verify the recommended dose or formula, the method and duration of administration, and contraindications. It is the responsibility of the practitioner, relying on their own experience and knowledge of the patient, to make diagnoses, to determine dosages and the best treatment for each individual patient, and to take all appropriate safety precautions. To the fullest extent of the law, neither the Publisher nor the Author assumes any liability for any injury and/or damage to persons or property arising out of or related to any use of the material contained in this book.

Adapted from Crash Course Obstetrics and Gynaecology by Nick Panay, Ruma Dutta, Audrey Ryan, and J.A. Mark Broadbent, ISBN: 0-7234-3151-5. Copyright © 2004.

The rights of Nick Panay, Ruma Dutta, Audrey Ryan, and J.A. Mark Broadbent to be identified as the authors of this work have been asserted by them in accordance with the Copyright, Designs and Patents Act, 1988.

Library of Congress Cataloging-in-Publication Data

Alam, Naureen.
  Crash course : obstetrics and gynecology / Naureen Alam. – 1st American ed.
    p. ; cm. – (Crash course)
  Rev. ed. of: Obstetrics and gynaecology / Nick Panay . . . {et al.}. 1st ed. Edinburgh ; New York : Mosby, 2004.
  Includes bibliographical references and index.
  ISBN 1-4160-2958-3
    1. Obstetrics—Outlines, syllabi, etc. 2. Gynecology—Outlines, syllabi, etc. I. Obstetrics and gynaecology. II. Title. III. Title: Obstetrics and gynecology. IV. Series.
  {DNLM: 1. Genital Diseases, Female-diagnosis. 2. Medical History Taking—methods. 3. Physical Examination—methods. 4. Pregnancy Complications—diagnosis. WP 141 A318c 2007}
  RG112.O732 2007
  618—dc22
                                                                          2006044951

Acquisitions Editor: Alex Stibbe
Project Development Manager: Stan Ward
Publishing Services Manager: David Saltzberg
Designer: Andy Chapman
Cover Design: Antbits Illustration
Illustration Manager: Mick Ruddy

Printed in China

Last digit is the print number:
9 8 7 6 5 4 3 2 1

Working together to grow libraries in developing countries

www.elsevier.com | www.bookaid.org | www.sabre.org

ELSEVIER   BOOK AID International   Sabre Foundation

Preface

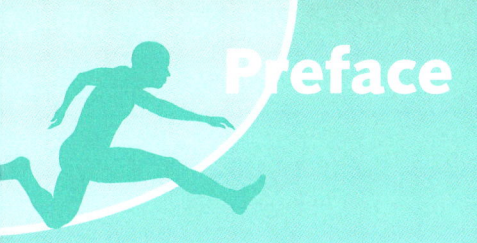

Crash Course: Obstetrics and Gynecology is meant to prepare the medical student rotating through his/her clinical clerkship for the uncomplicated obstetric and/or gynecologic patient as well as the diverse pathology that may arise. Furthermore, the book contains the relevant information that will help students prepare for all steps of the USMLE and COMLEX examinations, including recent research, updated pharmacologic and disease management information, and clarifying figures and tables.

Obstetrics and gynecology is a truly unique specialty, in which the physician cares for a woman throughout her entire life. From the birth process through puberty, reproductive health, and ultimately menopause, obstetrics and gynecology provides a very rewarding and fulfilling profession. It was a great delight to write this book in the hopes to inspire medical students to embrace the challenge of obstetrics and gynecology and to consider it as a career choice.

Naureen Alam, MD

Acknowledgments

My thanks to the original UK authors, Nick Panay, Ruma Dutta, Audrey Ryan, and J.A. Mark Broadbent, who took the specialty of obstetrics and gynecology and made a succinct and practical text that allows students to learn the information needed to pass the shelf exam confidently.

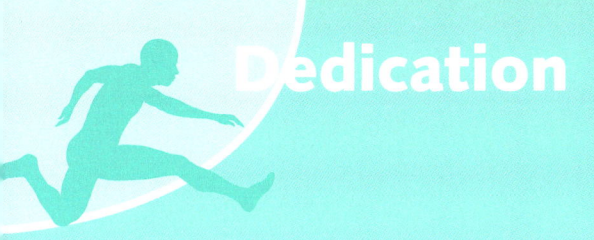

Dedication

To Rammy, whose unconditional love and support provided me the strength and motivation to complete this book.

To my parents, whose excitement about my "first book" and seeing my name in print has been inspiring.

To Jafar and Rabia, who have always been there for me and have seen me through all my milestones.

To all my friends and family, for your infinite love and support.

To my colleagues, physicians, and nurses alike, and especially to my patients, thank you for the inspiration to continue taking care of women.

Contents

Preface v
Acknowledgments vii
Dedication ix

Part I The Patient Presents with 1

1. **Abnormal Bleeding** 3
   Absent periods 3
   Heavy periods 6
   Intermenstrual and postcoital
      bleeding 7
   Painful periods 7
   Postmenopausal bleeding 9

2. **Pelvic Pain and Dyspareunia** 11
   Differential diagnosis 11
   Relevant history 11
   Physical exam 13
   Appropriate work-up 14

3. **Vaginal Discharge** 17
   Differential diagnosis 17
   Relevant history 17
   Physical exam 18
   Appropriate work-up 19

4. **Vulvar Symptoms** 21
   History 21
   Examination 22
   Appropriate work-up 23

5. **Urinary Incontinence** 25
   History 25
   Physical exam 26
   Laboratory studies 26

6. **Prolapse** 29
   Differential diagnosis 29
   Relevant history 29
   Physical exam 30
   Appropriate work-up 31

7. **Bleeding and/or Pain in Early
   Pregnancy** 33
   Relevant history 33
   Physical exam 34

   Appropriate work-up 35
   Recurrent miscarriage 35
   Trophoblastic disease 37

8. **Infertility** 39
   Taking the history 39
   Physical exam 41
   Work-up of infertility 41

9. **Menopause** 45
   Presentation and differential
      diagnosis 45
   Bleeding disturbances 45
   Vasomotor symptoms 45
   Psychologic symptoms 45
   Systemic menopausal symptoms 46
   Long-term symptoms of menopause 46

10. **Bleeding in the Second and Third
    Trimesters of Pregnancy** 49
    Differential diagnosis of bleeding 49
    Relevant history 49
    Physical exam 50
    Appropriate work-up 50
    Management 51

11. **Large- or Small-for-Dates** 53
    Differential diagnosis 53
    Relevant history 53
    Examination of the patient with an
       S > D or S < D uterus 54
    Investigation of the patient with an
       S > D or S < D uterus 54

12. **Abdominal Pain in the Second and
    Third Trimesters of Pregnancy** 57
    Differential diagnosis 57
    Relevant history 57
    Physical exam 58
    Appropriate work-up 59
    Management 60

13. **Hypertension in Pregnancy** 61
    Differential diagnosis 61
    History 61

xi

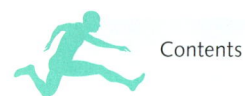

Contents

    Physical exam 61
    Work-up 62

14. **Stillbirth** 65
    History 65
    Physical exam 66
    Work-up 66
    Management of stillbirth 67
    Follow-up 67

15. **Failure to Progress in Labor** 69
    Relevant history 69
    Physical exam 70
    Work-up 71
    Management 72

16. **Abnormal Fetal Heart Rate
    Tracing in Labor** 73
    Features of the fetal heart rate
        tracing 73
    Physiology 75
    Monitoring uterine contractions 75
    History of the patient who
        presents with an abnormal fetal
        heart rate tracing in labor 76
    Examination of the patient who
        presents with an abnormal fetal
        heart rate tracing in labor 76
    Investigating the abnormal fetal
        heart rate tracing 77

17. **Bleeding after Delivery** 79
    Postpartum hemorrhage 79
    History to focus on the differential
        diagnosis 79
    Examination 80
    Appropriate work-up 81

18. **Maternal Collapse** 83
    Hemorrhage 83
    Amniotic fluid embolism 84
    Acute myocardial infarction 84
    Eclampsia 84
    Diabetic emergency 84
    Drug toxicity 86
    Puerperal sepsis 86
    Thromboembolism 87

Part II Diseases and Disorders 89

19. **Abnormal Uterine Bleeding** 91
    Amenorrhea 91
    Menorrhagia 94
    Postmenopausal bleeding 100
    Further reading 102

20. **Fibroids** 103
    Symptoms of uterine fibroids 103
    Complications 103
    Clinical evaluation 104
    Indications for treatment 104
    Medical therapy 104
    Surgical treatment 105
    Advances in fibroid treatment 105
    Further reading 105

21. **Endometriosis** 107
    Etiology 107
    Sites of endometriosis 108
    Symptoms 108
    Infertility 108
    Clinical evaluation 110
    Differential diagnosis 110
    Treatment 110
    Further reading 112

22. **Benign Ovarian Tumors** 113
    Incidence 113
    Etiology 113
    Diagnosis 114
    Examination 114
    Work-up 115
    Management of a benign ovarian
        tumor 115
    Further reading 116

23. **Gynecologic Malignancy** 117
    Ovarian malignancy 117
    Uterine endometrial tumors 119
    Uterine sarcoma 120
    Cervix 120
    Cervical carcinoma 123
    Vulvar tumors 124
    Vaginal tumors 126
    Further reading 127

24. **Vulvar Disease** 129
    Histology of the vulva 129
    Vulvar dystrophies 129
    Neoplasia 129
    Dermatologic conditions 132
    Further reading 132

Contents

25. Pelvic Inflammatory Disease 133
- Definition 133
- Incidence 133
- Etiology 133
- Diagnosis 133
- History 133
- Examination 133
- Work-up.......................134
- Complications..................134
- Treatment.....................135
- Prevention 135
- Further reading................135

26. Urinary Incontinence 137
- Incidence 137
- Etiology 137
- Appropriate work-up 139
- Complications..................139
- Treatment.....................139
- Further reading................141

27. Pelvic Organ Prolapse 143
- Definition 143
- Incidence 144
- Pelvic anatomy.................144
- Etiology 145
- Clinical features 145
- Management 146
- Further reading................148

28. Infertility 149
- Anovulation 149
- Uterine and pelvic problems.....149
- Tubal problems.................149
- Male infertility 150
- Unexplained infertility..........151
- Ovarian hyperstimulation syndrome....151
- Prognosis for the infertile couple 152
- Further reading................152

29. Early Pregnancy Failure 153
- Miscarriage....................153
- Recurrent miscarriage..........154
- Ectopic pregnancy 155
- Trophoblastic disease 157
- Further reading................159

30. Menopause 161
- Definitions 161
- Pathophysiology................161
- Clinical features of menopause........161
- Management 163
- Further reading................165

31. Contraception, Sterilization, and Unwanted Pregnancy 167
- Introduction 167
- Natural family planning methods 167
- Barrier methods 167
- Hormonal contraception........168
- Intrauterine devices 169
- Female sterilization............170
- Male sterilization 171
- Termination of pregnancy 171
- Further reading................171

32. Gynecologic Endocrinology 173
- Amenorrhea: primary and secondary ...173
- Hirsutism and virilism 173
- Further reading................178

33. Prenatal Diagnosis.................179
- Who is offered prenatal diagnosis?....179
- Techniques for prenatal diagnosis......179
- Further reading................182

34. Multiple Pregnancy 183
- Incidence of multiple pregnancy.......183
- Diagnosis of multiple pregnancy.......183
- Etiology of multiple pregnancy........183
- Complications of multiple pregnancy ...186
- Intrapartum management of a twin pregnancy..................187
- Higher order multiple pregnancies 188
- Further reading................188

35. Hypertension in Pregnancy 189
- Nonproteinuric hypertension in pregnancy.....................189
- Pre-eclampsia 190
- Eclampsia 191
- Further reading................193

36. Medical Disorders in Pregnancy 195
- Anemia.......................195
- Asthma.......................195
- Diabetes......................195
- Epilepsy 198
- Human immunodeficiency virus 199
- Liver disorders 200

xiii

Multiple sclerosis 201
Psychiatric disorders 201
Drug and alcohol dependence 203
Thromboembolism 203
Thyroid disorders 205
Further reading 206

37. Antepartum Hemorrhage 207
Definition 207
Incidence 207
Etiology 207
Placenta previa 207
Placental abruption 208
Vasa previa 210
Circumvallate placenta 210
Unexplained antepartum
   hemorrhage 210
Further reading 211

38. Premature Labor 213
Incidence 213
Clinical evaluation and investigation
   of women in preterm labor 214
Treatment of women presenting in
   preterm labor 215
Management of future pregnancies ... 217
Further reading 217

39. Malpresentation and Malpositions
of the Occiput 219
Malpresentation 219
Malposition 228
Further reading 230

40. Labor 231
Onset of labor 231
Progress in labor 231
Mechanisms of normal delivery:
   action of the uterus 235
Delivery of the fetus 235
Management of the first stage
   of labor 235
Management of the second stage
   of labor 239
Management of the third stage
   of labor 239
Induction of labor 240
Failure to progress in labor 241
Further reading 243

41. Operative Intervention in Obstetrics ... 245
Episiotomy 245
Perineal repair 246
Vacuum delivery 246
Forceps delivery 247
Cesarean section 248
Further reading 250

42. Complications of the Third Stage
of Labor and the Puerperium 251
Postpartum hemorrhage 251
Early postpartum hemorrhage 251
Placenta accreta 253
Uterine inversion 253
Uterine rupture 253
Late postpartum hemorrhage 253
Lactation 253
Postpartum infection 254
Postpartum mental illness 254
Thromboembolic disease 256
Further reading 256

43. Maternal Death 257
Pregnancy mortality surveillance
   system 257
Causes of maternal death 257
Further reading 260

Part III History and Examination 261

44. Taking a History 263
Patient details 263
Chief complaint 263
History of presenting illness 263
Past gynecologic history 264
Past obstetric history 264
Past medical history 265
Review of systems 265
Drug history 265
Family history 265
Social history 265
Allergies 265

45. Prenatal Care 271
The history 271
Examination 275
Laboratory studies 275
Planning prenatal care 277
Education at initial visit 277

Contents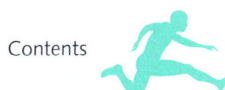

46. Examination 279
    General examination. 279
    Abdominal examination 279

47. Common Investigations 293
    Imaging techniques 293
    Laparoscopy 295

Hysteroscopy 295
Cervical cytology/colposcopy 295
Urodynamics. 297

Glossary. 299
Index. 301

XV

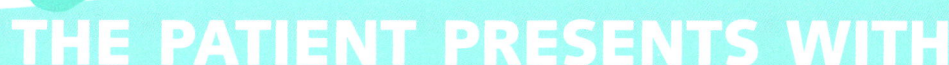

THE PATIENT PRESENTS WITH

1.	Abnormal Bleeding	3
2.	Pelvic Pain and Dyspareunia	11
3.	Vaginal Discharge	17
4.	Vulvar Symptoms	21
5.	Urinary Incontinence	25
6.	Prolapse	29
7.	Bleeding and/or Pain in Early Pregnancy	33
8.	Infertility	39
9.	Menopause	45
10.	Bleeding in the Second and Third Trimesters of Pregnancy	49
11.	Large- or Small-for-Dates	53
12.	Abdominal Pain in the Second and Third Trimesters of Pregnancy	57
13.	Hypertension in Pregnancy	61
14.	Stillbirth	65
15.	Failure to Progress in Labor	69
16.	Abnormal Fetal Heart Rate Tracing in Labor	73
17.	Bleeding After Delivery	79
18.	Maternal Collapse	83

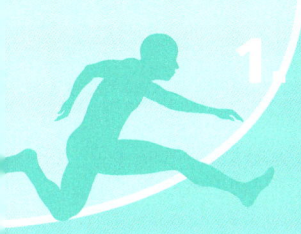

1. Abnormal Bleeding

Absent periods

The absence of periods is called amenorrhea and can be either:
- Primary, when menstruation has never occurred, or
- Secondary, when menstruation has occurred but not for at least 6 months.

The causes can be broken down into the following five major categories, which are shown in greater detail in Fig. 1.1:
- Central nervous system (CNS).
- Gonadal dysfunction.
- Genital tract disorders.
- Endocrine disorders.
- Drug therapy.

A history of post-pill amenorrhea is usually the result of pre-existing pathology that has been masked by the oral contraceptive pill (OCP).

History

There are so many causes of amenorrhea that it is important to focus the history onto the relevant systems. These can be broadly grouped into five main areas:
- Gynecologic.
- CNS.
- General health.
- Endocrine disorders.
- Drugs.

Gynecologic
A full gynecologic history is mandatory. By definition, menarche will not have occurred in women with primary amenorrhea. In women with secondary amenorrhea, the timing of menarche and pubertal development will establish whether this is normal, precocious, or delayed (see Chapter 32).

The duration of amenorrhea and the presence of symptoms of pregnancy or menopause should be noted (see Chapter 30).

Menstrual irregularity, or oligomenorrhea, from the time of menarche can suggest polycystic ovary syndrome, especially if associated with obesity and hirsutism. Cyclical pain might indicate congenital or acquired outflow obstruction to menstrual fluid.

Pituitary failure can occur after massive postpartum hemorrhage (PPH; Sheehan's syndrome), and so a full obstetric history should be taken. This should include early pregnancy loss with subsequent uterine curettage, which can lead to Ashermann's syndrome. Relevant gynecologic surgery includes cervical surgery, which can cause stenosis and, more obviously, oophorectomy and hysterectomy.

Central nervous system
A past history of head injury or more recent symptoms of CNS tumor, such as headache and vomiting, should be elicited. Visual-field disturbance might indicate an expanding pituitary tumor and galactorrhea could indicate hyperprolactinemia.

General health
The general health of the patient should be assessed. Emotional stress, from any cause, can precipitate amenorrhea, as can weight loss from dieting, anorexia nervosa, or severe systemic illness. The reduced peripheral fat stores and body mass index (BMI) that are commonly seen in female athletes can cause amenorrhea even though these women are fit and well.

Endocrine disorders
Thyroid disease and diabetes mellitus can present with amenorrhea, and symptoms of these disorders should be elicited. Hirsutism and virilism can be caused by congenital adrenal hyperplasia (CAH), polycystic ovary syndrome (PCOS), or an androgen-secreting tumor of the ovary or adrenal (see Chapter 32).

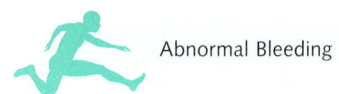

Abnormal Bleeding

Fig. 1.1 Causes of primary and secondary amenorrhea.

Causes of primary and secondary amenorrhea	
Primary	**Secondary**
Central nervous system	*Central nervous system*
Hypothalamus: 　Kallmann syndrome 　tumor/trauma 　hypothalamic amenorrhea 　weight loss 　stress 　athleticism	Hypothalamus: 　Kallmann syndrome 　tumor/trauma 　hypothalamic amenorrhea 　weight loss 　stress 　athleticism
Pituitary: 　tumor necrosis (Sheehan syndrome) 　hyperprolactinemia 　prolactin-secreting tumor< >　hypothyroidism 　drugs	Pituitary: 　tumor necrosis (Sheehan syndrome) 　hyperprolactinemia 　prolactin-secreting tumor 　hypothyroidism 　drugs
Gonads	*Gonads*
Streak gonads	Streak gonads (rarely)
Polycystic ovary syndrome	Polycystic ovary syndrome
Hormone-secreting tumors of ovary	Hormone-secreting tumors of ovary
Androgen insensitivity	Androgen insensitivity
Cervix	
Postsurgical stenosis	
Vagina	
Congenital absence	
Imperforate hymen	
Endocrine	*Endocrine*
Diabetes	Diabetes
Thyroid disease	Thyroid disease
Adrenal disease	Adrenal disease
Drugs	*Drugs*
Phenothiazines	Phenothiazines

Drugs

Many prescribed drugs can cause amenorrhea by producing either hyperprolactinemia or ovarian failure, and a detailed drug history should be taken (see Chapter 32 for more details).

Examination

A general examination should be performed, with particular emphasis on signs of thyroid disease and diabetes mellitus. The BMI should be calculated (kg divided by m^2). Anosmia (absent sense of smell) is associated with Kallmann's syndrome. The typical appearance of Turner's syndrome should be apparent: short stature, webbing of the neck, increased carrying angle at the elbow, and coarctation of the aorta. The presence of galactorrhea should be noted.

A full gynecologic examination is mandatory. Assessment of development of secondary sexual development must be made and Tanner's system can be used for this (see Fig. 1.2). Absent secondary sexual characteristics might constitute delayed

Absent periods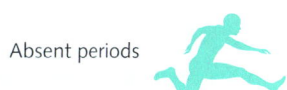

Tanner staging of puberty

Stage	I	II	III	IV	V
Breast	Pre-pubertal	Budding	Small adult breast	Areola and papilla form secondary mound	Adult breast
Pubic hair	Pre-pubertal	Sparse growth of slightly pigmented hair	Darker, coarser, beginning to curl and spread over the symphysis	Hair has adult characteristics but not adult distribution	Adult

Fig. 1.2 Tanner staging of puberty.

puberty (see Chapter 32). Incongruous pubertal development might also suggest underlying pathology. For example, normal breast development in the presence of absent pubic or axillary hair is often found in women with androgen insensitivity. Poor breast development with normal pubic and axillary hair or hirsutism, virilism, and obesity can be signs of raised circulating androgens secondary to PCOS, CAH, adrenal tumors, or androgen-secreting ovarian tumors.

Pelvic examination should assess the patency of the vagina. If a hematocolpos is present it often causes a blue-colored bulge at the introitus. An enlarged uterus might represent a pregnancy, and ovarian masses might be palpable.

Work-up
The following group of studies should be performed as indicated:
- Chromosomal analysis.
- Hormone profiles.
- Imaging studies.

Chromosomal analysis
Chromosomal analysis should be performed on women with primary amenorrhea where a chromosomal abnormality is suspected. Buccal smears or blood samples can be taken for this purpose.

Hormone profiles
The first hormone test to be performed is a urinary pregnancy test. This detects the presence of β-human chorionic gonadotrophin (hCG) and can be performed quickly in the outpatient setting.

Serum gonadotrophin levels are important. Levels of follicle-stimulating hormone (FSH) and luteinizing hormone (LH) are raised with ovarian failure, and in "hypothalamic" or hypogonadotrophic amenorrhea the levels will be at the lower limits of normal (see Chapter 32 for more details on hypogonadotrophic hypogonadism). In PCOS, the LH:FSH ratio is usually greater than 2.5.

Serum prolactin levels should be checked to exclude hyperprolactinemia. Thyroid-stimulating hormone (TSH) and free thyroxine levels should be tested if there is clinical suspicion of thyroid dysfunction or if hyperprolactinemia is confirmed.

Serum testosterone levels might be normal or raised with PCOS, although free testosterone is usually raised. If serum testosterone levels are high, then an androgen-secreting tumor of the ovary or adrenal should be suspected.

Imaging studies
An ultrasound scan of the pelvis should be performed. This will identify the typical ultrasound appearances of polycystic ovaries (enlarged ovaries with increased central stroma associated with multiple peripherally sited follicles). The presence of an intrauterine pregnancy, hematometra (blood within the endometrial cavity) or hematocolpos (an accumulation of menstrual blood in the vagina) should also be identified.

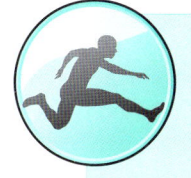 A pelvic ultrasound scan (preferably performed vaginally) is virtually mandatory in the investigation of abnormal bleeding.

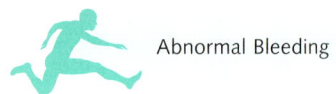

Abnormal Bleeding

CNS tumors can be excluded by performing computed tomography (CT) or magnetic resonance imaging (MRI) scans of the head, and a lateral skull X-ray will identify pituitary fossa changes associated with an enlarging pituitary tumor.

Heavy periods

Heavy periods are a common gynecologic complaint. The average blood loss during a typical menstrual cycle is approximately 30 mL. Only about half of women complaining of heavy periods actually have menorrhagia, which is defined as more than 80 mL of menstrual blood loss (MBL) per period. Both local and systemic conditions can cause menorrhagia (Fig. 1.3).

History
A full gynecologic history should be taken. Particular emphasis should be made as to the pattern of menstruation: irregular menstruation implies the possibility of anovulation. Subjective assessment of menstrual flow does not correlate well with objective menstrual loss. However, the presence of clots and excessive flow, wearing double protection (internal and external), nocturnal soiling, and interference with work or social events all imply increased menstrual loss. Symptoms of iron-deficiency anemia might be present, including lethargy and shortness of breath.

Causes of menorrhagia	
Types of cause	Specific of cause of menorrhagia
Systemic disorders	Thyroid disease
	Clotting disorders
Local causes	Fibroids
	Endometrial polyps
	Endometrial carcinoma
	Endometriosis/adenomyosis
	Pelvic inflammatory disease (PID)
	Dysfunctional uterine bleeding
Iatrogenic causes	Intrauterine devices (IUDs)
	Oral anticoagulants

Fig. 1.3 Causes of menorrhagia.

Dysmenorrhea, or painful periods, is often associated with menorrhagia and it is usually experienced when the flow is heaviest. Premenstrual pain can indicate endometriosis, which is discussed further in Chapter 21. (Dsymenorrhea is discussed in more detail later in this chapter.)

A variety of medical illnesses may lead to menorrhagia. Furthermore, a history of PCOS increases the risk of endometrial hyperplasia and carcinoma. Symptoms of thyroid disease or clotting disorders can indicate a systemic cause of menorrhagia. Clotting disorders presenting with menorrhagia usually do so in the teenage years.

A contraceptive history is important. Recent cessation of OCPs might indicate menstrual intolerance (the return of normal periods that appear heavier than the withdrawal bleeds associated with the OCP). Symptoms of heavy or painful periods dating from the insertion of an IUD would suggest that this is the cause.

Examination
General examination should be aimed at identifying signs of iron-deficiency anemia, thyroid disorders, or clotting disorders. Abdominal examination might reveal a mass arising from the pelvis.

Speculum examination could reveal vaginal discharge and cervical pathology, including cervicitis or frank malignancy. Occasionally, endometrial polyps or pedunculated fibroids will be seen prolapsing through the cervical os. Bimanual examination might reveal an enlarged uterus due to fibroids, pelvic tenderness associated with endometriosis or PID and any adnexal masses.

Work-up
Work-up is aimed at excluding the systemic and local causes of menorrhagia and includes:
- Blood tests.
- Ultrasound.
- Hysteroscopy.

A complete blood count (CBC) should be performed in all cases. Thyroid function and clotting studies should only be performed if clinically indicated.

A pelvic ultrasound will identify uterine enlargement caused by fibroids and adnexal masses. Endometrial polyps or submucous fibroids should be suspected if the endometrial thickness is excessive.

An endometrial biopsy should be performed, either in the outpatient clinic or at the same time as hysteroscopy. This might show endometrium inappropriate to the menstrual cycle secondary to anovulation, endometrial hyperplasia, or carcinoma. A Pap smear should be performed if indicated.

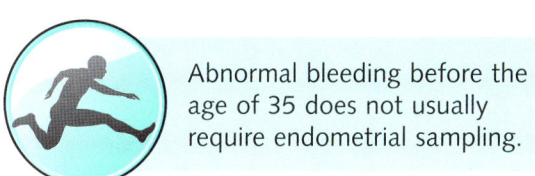

Abnormal bleeding before the age of 35 does not usually require endometrial sampling.

The most effective way of excluding intrauterine pathology is by diagnostic hysteroscopy. This can be performed in the outpatient setting with minimal analgesia and will identify endometrial polyps and submucous fibroids.

Intermenstrual and postcoital bleeding

Intermenstrual and postcoital bleeding are common symptoms that can indicate serious underlying pathology. Intermenstrual bleeding occurs between the menstrual periods and can be caused by local lesions of the cervix or intrauterine cavity (Fig. 1.4).

Causes of intermenstrual and postcoital bleeding

Affected region/system	Specific cause
Cervical	Ectropion
	Polyps
	Malignancy
	Cervicitis
Intra-uterine	Polyps
	Submucous fibroids
	Endometrial hyperplasia
	Endometrial malignancy
	Endometritis
Hormonal	Breakthrough bleeding

Fig. 1.4 Causes of intermenstrual and postcoital bleeding.

Postcoital bleeding is precipitated by intercourse and is caused by similar conditions. Investigation should aim to exclude local causes for menorrhagia.

Painful periods

Pain associated with menstruation is called dysmenorrhea and can be either primary or secondary. There are two definitions of primary and secondary dysmenorrhea:
- Primary dysmenorrhea occurs from menarche, whereas secondary dysmenorrhea occurs in women who previously had normal periods.
- Primary dysmenorrhea occurs from menarche, but secondary dysmenorrhea describes painful periods that are caused by, or are "secondary" to, pathology.

Severe primary dysmenorrhea occurs in up to 10% of women. The cause is not well understood, but prostaglandins, which can cause uterine contractions and vasoconstriction, have been implicated. Rarely, primary dysmenorrhea can be caused by a particular müllerian abnormality, whereby a rudimentary, functioning uterine horn does not connect with the vagina (Fig. 1.5).

Secondary dysmenorrhea can be caused by conditions occurring in the uterus, cervix and the pelvis (Fig. 1.6).

History

Dysmenorrhea is usually described as cramping pain that often radiates into the back or the upper

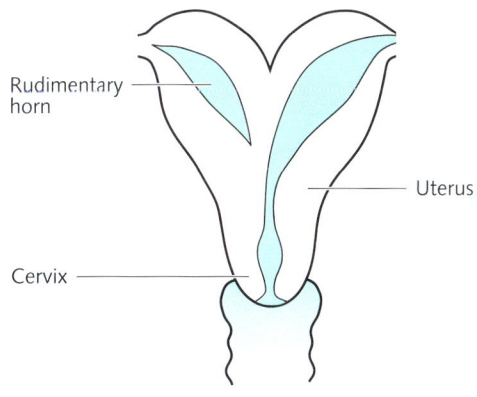

Fig. 1.5 A rudimentary uterine horn.

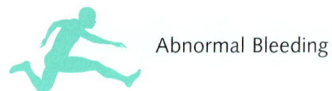

Abnormal Bleeding

Causes of secondary dysmenorrhea	
Affected region/structure	Cause of secondary dysmenorrhea
Uterine	Fibroids
	Endometrial polyps
	Asherman's syndrome
	Infection
	Endometriosis
Cervical	Stenosis
Pelvic	Pelvic inflammatory disease
	Endometriosis

Fig. 1.6 Causes of secondary dysmenorrhea.

thighs. Primary dysmenorrhea presents in young women in their early teens and usually starts within the first year of menarche as ovulation is established. There is often a family history.

Women with secondary dysmenorrhea will previously have had normal periods; pain develops or worsens at a later date. Menstrual irregularity can suggest intrauterine pathology, such as endometrial polyps or submucous fibroids. Lower abdominal or pelvic pain and dyspareunia suggests pelvic pathology, such as endometriosis, and, if associated with fever and vaginal discharge, PID. A history of cervical surgery or pregnancy associated uterine curettage usually precedes the development of Asherman's syndrome.

Examination
Examination will be normal in women with primary dysmenorrhea. A pinpoint external cervical os may indicate cervical stenosis. Pelvic tenderness and cervical motion tenderness are usually present in the presence of pelvic pathology.

Work-up
A young woman presenting with primary dysmenorrhea who has a normal pelvic examination does not usually require any further investigation. Suitable investigations for secondary dysmenorrhea include:
- Hysteroscopy, to exclude intrauterine pathology including adhesions.
- Laparoscopy, to exclude pelvic pathology.
- Pelvic ultrasound scan, which can identify uterine fibroids; an increased endometrial thickness is suggestive of intrauterine pathology.
- Microbiological swabs to identify infection, especially gonorrhea and chlamydia.

Treatment
Primary dysmenorrhea is nearly always associated with ovulatory cycles, and inhibition of ovulation using OCPs often improves dysmenorrhea. Nonhormonal medical treatment includes simple analgesia and nonsteroidal anti-inflammatory drugs (NSAIDs; prostaglandin synthetase inhibitors). A rudimentary horn might require surgical excision.

Submucous fibroids, endometrial polyps, and uterine adhesions can be treated using operative hysteroscopy techniques. Open myomectomy might be required for larger fibroids, especially in women who wish to conserve their uterus. The treatments of PID and endometriosis are discussed in Chapters 25 and 21 respectively.

Causes of PMB	
Affected structure	Cause of PMB
Ovary	Carcinoma of the ovary
	Estrogen-secreting tumor
Uterine body	Myometrium submucous fibroid

	Endometrium
	   atrophic changes
	   polyp
	   hyperplasia: simple or atypical
	   carcinoma

Cervix	Atrophic changes

	Malignancy
	   squamous carcinoma
	   adenocarcinoma

Vagina	Atrophic changes
Urethra	Urethral caruncle
	Hematuria
Vulva	Vulvitis
	Dystrophies
	Malignancy

Fig. 1.7 Causes of PMB.

Postmenopausal bleeding

Vaginal bleeding more than 6 months after menopause is called postmenopausal bleeding (PMB). This is a common condition and should be investigated promptly because it could indicate the presence of malignancy.

Figure 1.7 shows the causes of PMB using the anatomy of the female genital tract as a guide. There are many causes of PMB, and using this method will help to remember them all. Atrophic changes to the genital tract are the most common cause, but they must not be assumed to be the cause until other pathology, especially malignancy, has been excluded.

Figure 1.8 provides an algorithm for the diagnosis and investigation of abnormal uterine bleeding.

History

Atrophic changes to the genital tract—the most common cause of PMB—usually present with small amounts of bleeding. Local symptoms of estrogen deficiency include vaginal dryness, soreness, and superficial dyspareunia. Pruritus of the vulva can indicate the presence of nonneoplastic disorders of the vulva (traditionally known as vulvar dystrophies), and the presence of a lump, whether painful or painless, can suggest a vulvar neoplasm.

Profuse or continuous vaginal bleeding or the presence of a blood-stained, offensive discharge is an ominous sign and can indicate cervical or endometrial malignancy. PMB is usually the only presenting symptom of other endometrial cavity pathology, such as endometrial polyps or submucous fibroids.

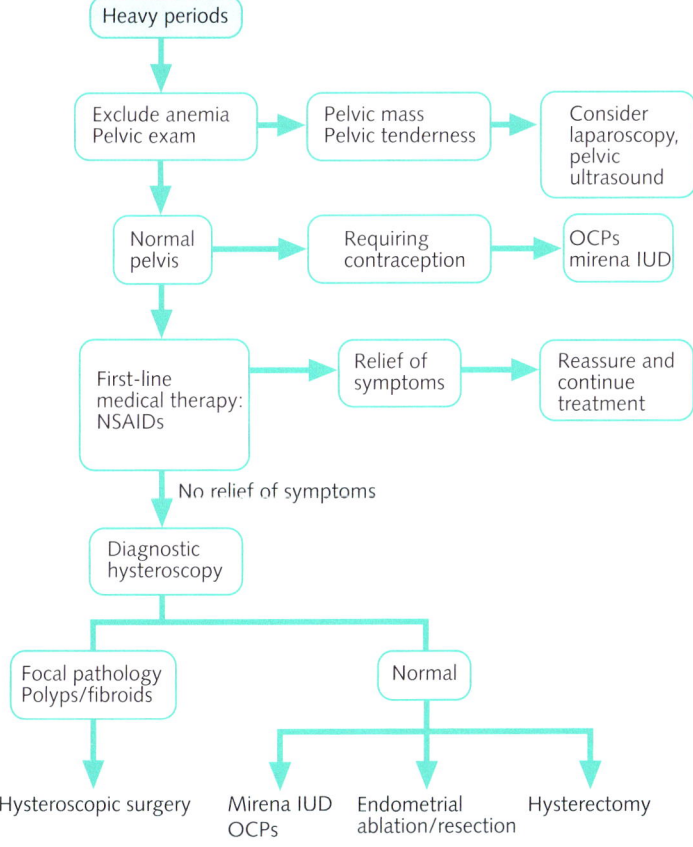

Fig. 1.8 Algorithm for abnormal uterine bleeding.

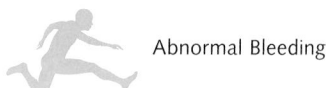

Early ovarian malignancy can be asymptomatic or present with nonspecific upper abdominal symptoms, such as epigastric discomfort or indigestion. Advanced ovarian malignancy can produce pelvic or abdominal pain and abdominal distention due to ascites.

Examination

A full gynecologic examination should be performed. Abdominal examination might reveal ascites or a mass arising from the pelvis. Vulvar lesions should be evident on examination. The vagina and cervix should be inspected using a speculum and a bimanual examination performed. Postmenopausal ovaries should not be palpable on bimanual examination.

Work-up

The following studies should be performed on all women with PMB:
- Ultrasound examination of the pelvis.
- Hysteroscopic examination of the uterine cavity.
- Endometrial biopsy.

Hysteroscopy will identify the presence of intrauterine pathology and can be performed without general anesthesia in the outpatient setting. An alternative to hysteroscopy is ultrasound scanning to assess the endometrial thickness combined with endometrial sampling (discussed further in Chapter 19). Ultrasound is also used to assess the ovaries.

When indicated, the following studies should also be performed:
- Vulvar biopsies.
- Cervical cytology or colposcopy.
- Cystoscopy.
- Sigmoidoscopy.
- Estradiol levels.

Occasionally, it is not obvious whether the bleeding is vaginal, rectal, or from the bladder, and in these cases cystoscopy and sigmoidoscopy, as well as hysteroscopy, should be performed. In the very elderly, bimanual examination might not be possible, in which case examination under anesthesia is indicated. However, elderly frail women are not always ideal candidates for general anesthesia, and less invasive investigations, such as ultrasound, might have to be relied upon.

2 Pelvic Pain and Dyspareunia

Differential diagnosis

Pelvic pain, as for any type of pain, can be either:
- Acute or
- Chronic.

Chronic pelvic pain is often associated with "dyspareunia," the term used to describe painful sexual intercourse. This is classified as superficial or deep, depending on whether it is experienced superficially at the area of the vulva and introitus or deep within the pelvis.

Figures 2.1 and 2.2 show the differential diagnoses that should be considered when the patient presents with these symptoms.

Relevant history

Because the differential diagnosis is so diverse, a thorough history is important.

Chief complaint

A detailed history of the pain is essential to distinguish between pain of acute onset and chronic pain. The following characteristics should be elicited:
- Whether the pain is continuous or intermittent.
- The duration of the pain.
- The nature of the pain: whether it is sharp or dull.

Differential diagnosis of pelvic pain

Acute	Chronic
PID (see Chapter 25) sexually transmitted infection	Adenomyosis (see Chapter 21)
	Endometriosis

Tubo-ovarian abscess
    post-termination of pregnancy
    post-insertion of IUD
    post-hysteroscopy
	Fibroids

	Adhesions secondary to:
	    gynecologic surgery
	    PID
	    appendicitis

Early pregnancy complications
(see Chapter 29)
    miscarriage
    ectopic pregnancy	

Gynecologic malignancy (see Chapter 23)	

Ovarian cyst (see Chapter 22)
    rupture
    hemorrhage
    torsion
	Gastrointestinal (GI) pathology
	    diverticulitis
	    irritable bowel syndrome

Fibroid degeneration (see Chapter 20)	
Ovulation pain (mittelschmerz)	

Labial pathology
    abscesses
    Bartholin's cyst or abscess	

Urinary tract infection (UTI)	
Renal calculi	
Appendicitis	

Fig. 2.1 Differential diagnosis of pelvic pain.

Differential diagnosis of dyspareunia

Superficial	Deep

Congenital
    vaginal atresia
    vaginal septum
	Congenital
	    incomplete vaginal
	      atresia
	    vaginal septum

Infection
    vulvovaginitis (see
    Chapter 3)
	Infection
	    PID (see Chapter 25)

Postsurgery
    childbirth injury/laceration
    pelvic floor repair
	Postsurgery
	    childbirth injury/
	      laceration
	    pelvic floor repair

Vulvar disease
    Bartholin's cyst
    vulvar dystrophies
    carcinoma of vulva
	Pelvic disease
	    endometriosis
	    fibroids
	    ovarian cyst/tumors

Psychosexual
    vaginismus
	Psychosexual
	    vaginismus

Atrophic changes postmenopausal	

Fig. 2.2 Differential diagnosis of dyspareunia.

- The position of the pain: is it unilateral or bilateral?
- The relation of the pain to the menstrual cycle.
- Its relation to bowel habits.
- Radiation of the pain to the back or the legs.
- Associated symptoms, such as nausea and vomiting, vaginal discharge, vulvar irritation.

For example, the pain related to torsion of an ovarian cyst is typically of acute onset, worse on one side of the pelvis than the other, associated with nausea and vomiting, and radiating to the upper thighs. It is important to make this diagnosis promptly, because surgery to relieve the torsion might save the ovary from irreversible ischemia.

Mittelschmerz is an acute pain associated with ovulation. To make this diagnosis, therefore, it is essential to know the timing of the pain in relation to the patient's menstrual cycle. Endometriosis is also related to menses, typically starting up to 2 weeks before the onset of menses and usually being relieved when the bleeding starts (also known as secondary dysmenorrhea). Deep dyspareunia is also commonly associated with this condition.

PID may or may not be associated with vaginal discharge. The pain is typically felt across the entire lower abdomen and there might be a history of fever.

In relation to bowel habits, appendicitis can be associated with nausea and vomiting, whereas diverticulitis is more likely to be associated with constipation and affect the older population.

Past gynecologic history

The date of the patient's last menstrual period (LMP) is important to exclude current pregnancy and the possibility of a miscarriage or ectopic pregnancy. The date and result of the last cervical Pap smear should also be checked, as well as a history of irregular or postcoital bleeding, which might be associated with malignancy.

The LMP could also be relevant if the patient has symptoms suggesting perimenopausal changes.

Recent gynecologic procedures that involve instrumentation of the uterus could put the patient at risk of developing PID (e.g. insertion of an IUD, termination of pregnancy, or hysteroscopy).

Previous PID or surgery could have resulted in adhesion formation. This is more likely to result in a picture of chronic pain and can be difficult to treat. Pelvic floor repair can alter the vagina in such a way as to cause deep dyspareunia. Recent childbirth is a common cause of superficial dyspareunia, particularly if suturing of vaginal lacerations or episiotomy was necessary.

Congenital malformations of the genital tract are rare and are likely to present before the patient is sexually active and experiencing dyspareunia. There might be a history of previous operations to restore normal anatomy.

Past medical/surgical history

A history of appendectomy excludes one of the common differential diagnoses of pelvic pain.

Drug history

A postmenopausal patient who has not been using hormone replacement therapy (HRT) might have superficial dyspareunia secondary to atrophic changes.

Sexual history

Current use of contraception must be checked, both to exclude pregnancy and to determine the

Physical exam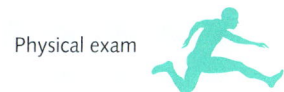

risk of PID. A recent change of partner, particularly if no barrier contraception has been used, increases the risk.

With regard to dyspareunia, there might be a history of difficulty with intercourse, suggesting vaginismus. This might be a difficult subject for the patient, and care should be taken to discuss it in a sympathetic manner.

Social history

A useful guide to the severity of symptoms in patients presenting with chronic pelvic pain is how it affects their normal life, e.g. going to school or taking time off work.

A history of sexual abuse has been shown to be relevant to presentation with chronic pain. Again, a sensitive approach is essential in questioning.

Physical exam

- General examination.
- Abdominal palpation.
- Vulvar/vaginal/cervical inspection.
- Bimanual pelvic examination.

General examination

Pyrexia and tachycardia are associated with PID. Rupture of an ovarian cyst can cause intraperitoneal bleeding and, subsequently, hypotension with tachycardia. A ruptured ectopic pregnancy would also present with these signs. It should be noted that hypotension is a late sign and its absence does not exclude these diagnoses.

Gynecologic malignancy is more likely to present with symptoms other than pelvic pain, more commonly in the older age group. However, signs such as cachexia and anemia should be excluded.

Abdominal palpation

The site of the pain should be elicited, as should the presence of guarding or rebound tenderness, which are peritoneal signs, suggesting peritonitis. An abdominal mass arising from the pelvis, such as an enlarged fibroid uterus, might be present. This could give symptoms of deep dyspareunia or of acute pelvic pain, if there is fibroid degeneration.

Vulvar/vaginal/cervical inspection

Figure 2.3 shows the diagnoses responsible for both pelvic pain and superficial dyspareunia that might affect the vulva and vagina. A speculum examination should be performed to look for discharge.

Bimanual pelvic examination
Tenderness

Generalized tenderness, including uterine, is more common with PID. Extreme pain upon moving the cervix, or cervical motion tenderness, is also called the "chandelier sign" and is highly suggestive of PID. The tenderness may be unilateral with an ovarian cyst or an ectopic pregnancy. A common site for endometriosis is the pouch of Douglas, and tender nodules can be palpated in the posterior fornix.

	Vulvar/vaginal inspection
Symptom	Cause(s)
Postmenopausal changes (see Chapter 30)	Vulvar and vaginal skin appears thin and atrophic. This can cause superficial dyspareunia
Vulvar dystrophies (see Chapter 24)	There might be patches of inflammation, leukoplakia, and ulceration, which cause superficial dyspareunia
Episiotomy/lacerations (see Chapter 41)	Injury secondary to childbirth commonly causes superficial dyspareunia
Abscesses	A Bartholin's abscess is an abscess of the gland situated towards the posterior fourchette; labial abscesses are commonly situated on the labia majora. Both types cause acute pain and need incision and drainage

Fig. 2.3 Vulvar/vaginal inspection.

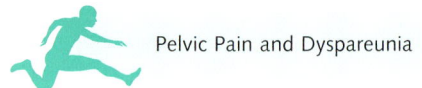

Pelvic Pain and Dyspareunia

A pregnancy test to exclude an ectopic pregnancy is mandatory in a patient of reproductive age who presents with acute abdominal pain. This is essential even if the symptoms suggest a GI cause rather than a gynecologic one, because the presentation of ectopic pregnancy can be atypical.

Mass

The following conditions may present with a pelvic mass:
- Tubo-ovarian abscess.
- Ovarian cyst.
- Endometrioma.
- Fibroid.
- Ectopic pregnancy.

The uterus is enlarged in pregnancy and the cervical os might be open if the patient is miscarrying. A fixed, tender, retroverted uterus could be a result of endometriosis or PID. The uterus typically feels tender and bulky with adenomyosis.

Appropriate work-up

A summary list of the investigations used in patients who present with pelvic pain and dyspareunia is shown in Fig. 2.4. Figure 2.5 is an algorithm for the diagnosis, investigation, and treatment of pelvic pain; Fig. 2.6 provides the same information for dyspareunia.

Blood tests

A CBC (to check hemoglobin) and T&S sample are necessary if there is an early pregnancy complication with bleeding from the vagina or intraperitoneal bleeding. A white blood cell count (WBC) will aid diagnosis of infection, along with the clinical signs.

A serum hCG or urine pregnancy test is done to exclude early pregnancy complications. This is mandatory in any patient of reproductive age who presents with acute pelvic pain, to exclude a potentially fatal ectopic pregnancy.

Work-up of patients with pelvic pain and dyspareunia	
Study	Procedure
Blood tests	CBC
	T&S
	hCG
Infection screen	Clean catch urine sample
	Vulvar/vaginal swabs
	Endocervical/urethral swabs
Radiologic studies	Pelvic ultrasound
	Abdominal X-ray
Biopsy for vulvar disease	
Laparoscopy to check for: endometriosis ovarian cyst ectopic pregnancy adhesions PID	

Fig. 2.4 Work-up of patients with pelvic pain and dyspareunia (T&S: type and screen).

Infection screen

A clean catch urine sample should be sent to exclude a UTI. Cervical swabs should be sent to check for PID, as listed in Fig. 2.4, most importantly including an endocervical swab to confirm gonorrhea and/or chlamydial infection.

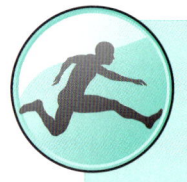

Even with a chronic pain history as opposed to an acute one, it is still appropriate to take swabs for sexually transmitted infections.

Radiologic investigations

A pelvic ultrasound is important in acute or chronic pain, as well as with deep dyspareunia, to attempt to exclude pelvic pathology. This can include ovarian cysts, uterine fibroids, ectopic pregnancy, or intrauterine pregnancy.

Appropriate work-up

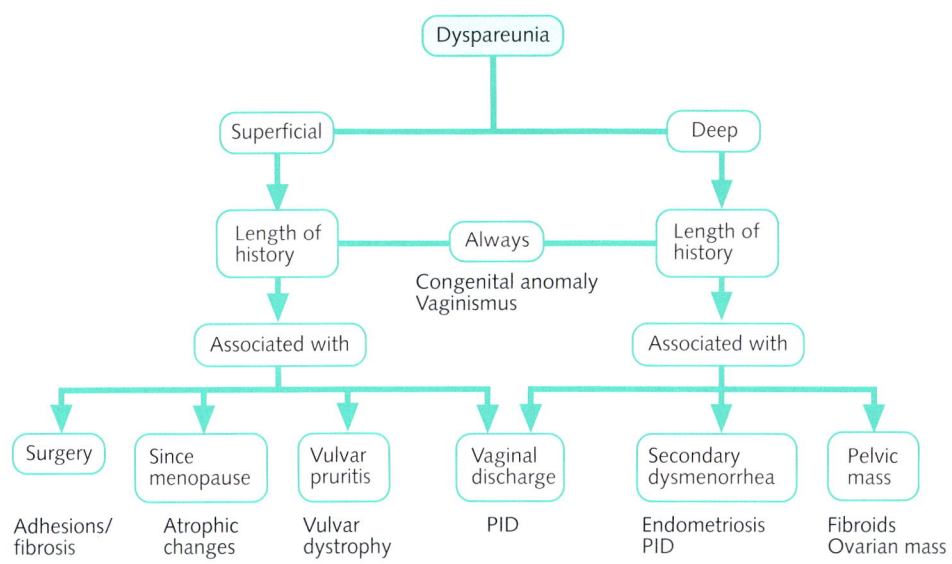

Fig. 2.5 Algorithm for dyspareunia.

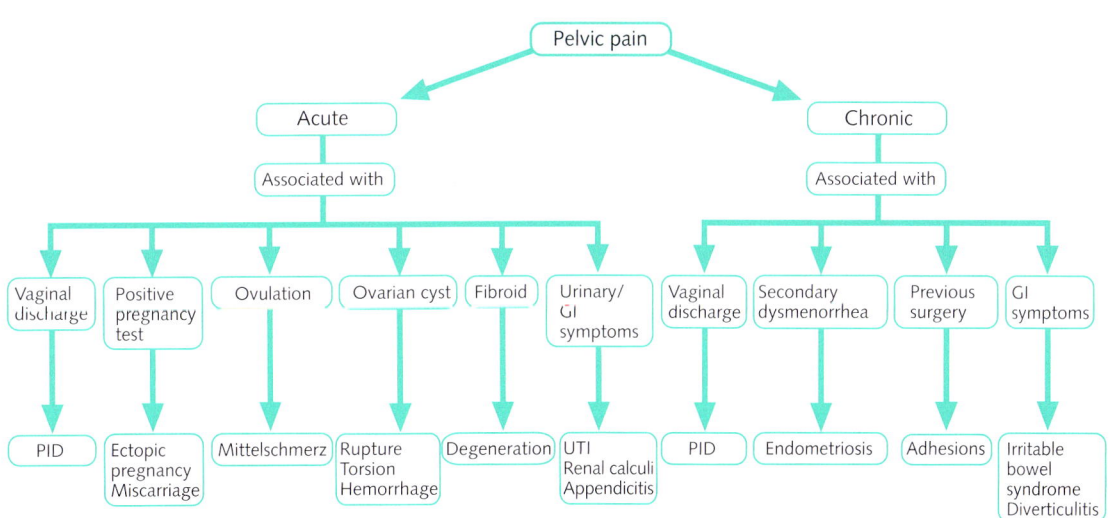

Fig. 2.6 Algorithm for pelvic pain.

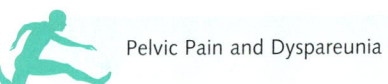
Pelvic Pain and Dyspareunia

A plain abdominal X-ray might be appropriate if the patient gives a history suggesting diverticulitis.

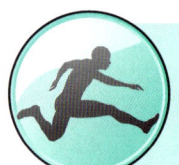 In a patient with chronic pain, assessing activities of daily living enables the physician to establish the severity of symptoms and decide on appropriate management.

Biopsy

If the appearance of the vulva is abnormal, then biopsy is indicated. This can be performed under local anesthesia, depending on the size of the lesion.

Laparoscopy

Figure 2.4 shows some of the diagnoses that can be confirmed by laparoscopy, which might be indicated by the clinical picture.

3 Vaginal Discharge

Differential diagnosis

Vaginal discharge can be either:
- Physiologic or
- Pathologic.

Physiologic discharge varies with the changing estrogen levels associated with the menstrual cycle and pregnancy. The diagnosis is usually one of exclusion, i.e. pathologic causes need to be excluded. Then the patient can be reassured that her symptoms are normal. Possible causes of physiologic vaginal discharge are:
- Vestibular gland secretions.
- Vaginal transudate.
- Cervical mucus.
- Residual menstrual fluid.

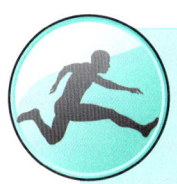

Don't forget that vaginal discharge might simply be physiologic, related to the menstrual cycle or to pregnancy.

The differential diagnoses of pathological vaginal discharge are shown in Fig. 3.1. The most common group is the infections.

Relevant history

The patient should be asked about the nature of the discharge. This includes:
- Timing of onset.
- Color.
- Odor.
- Presence of any blood.
- Irritation.
- Exacerbating factors.

For example, candidal infection is associated with a thick, itchy, white discharge, whereas with bacterial vaginosis there is typically a grey,

Differential diagnosis of pathologic vaginal discharge

Diagnosis	Cause of discharge
Infections	Sexually transmitted infection
	Chlamydia trachomatis
	Trichomonas vaginalis
	Neisseria gonorrhoeae
	Infection not sexually transmitted
	Candida albicans
	Bacterial vaginosis
Inflammatory	Allergy to soap/contraceptives etc
	Atrophic changes
	Postoperative granulation tissue
Malignancy	Vulvar carcinoma
	Cervical carcinoma
	Uterine carcinoma
Foreign body	Retained tampon/condom
	Ring pessaries
Fistula	From bowel, bladder, and ureter to vagina

Fig. 3.1 Differential diagnosis of pathologic vaginal discharge.

fishy-smelling discharge. An allergic reaction is usually associated with itching. Urinary symptoms, such as dysuria and frequency, might be present with a sexually transmitted infection.

Lower abdominal pain, backache, and dyspareunia are suggestive of PID (see Chapter 25), more commonly in a younger woman. In relation to malignancy, the patient age group is usually older than the infective group (see Chapter 23). General symptoms, such as weight loss and anorexia, should be excluded.

Past gynecologic history

The date of menopause and the last cervical Pap smear are relevant, particularly if malignancy is suspected.

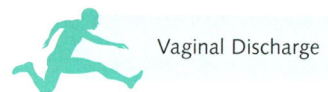

Vaginal Discharge

A ring pessary might previously have been placed to relieve genital prolapse (see Chapter 27). This should be changed every 6 months. Previous history of hysterectomy could be linked with development of a uretero- or vesicovaginal fistula. This results in constant vaginal loss that is actually urine. A history of obstructed labor, more common in developing countries, also puts the patient at risk of a vesicovaginal fistula.

Past medical history

Immunocompromised states, such as a history of human immunodeficiency virus (HIV) or diabetes mellitus, predispose the patient to candidal infection.

> Generalized symptoms can be indicative of different pathologies, depending on the age of the patient. Lower abdominal pain, backache and dyspareunia suggest infection in a younger woman but malignancy in older age groups.

Sexual history

The patient's current method of contraception is important with regard to the risk of a sexually transmitted infection, as is a recent new partner.

Drug history

Recent antibiotic therapy can precipitate candidal infection.

Physical exam

- General examination.
- Abdominal palpation.
- Speculum examination.
- Bimanual palpation.

General examination should be aimed at identifying signs of systemic infection (tachycardia, fever, local lymphadenopathy) or malignancy (cachexia, generalized lymphadenopathy).

> Always remember to perform a general examination and abdominal palpation, and not simply vulvar/vaginal examination.

Abdominal palpation should exclude any localized tenderness, which may be present if the patient is developing PID, or an abdominal mass if malignancy is suspected.

The vulva and vagina should be inspected carefully and a speculum examination should be performed to check the cervix and to confirm or exclude:

- Vaginal discharge.
- Inflammation.
- Ulceration.
- Foreign bodies.
- Local tumors.

Bimanual pelvic examination will reveal pelvic tumors. It might also elicit cervical motion tenderness, suggesting PID.

Work-up of vaginal discharge	
Investigation	Cause of discharge
Microbiologic swabs	Wet mount
	Candida albicans
	Trichomonas vaginalis
	Bacterial vaginosis
	Endocervical/urethral swab
	Chlamydia trachomatis
	Neisseria gonorrhoeae
Clean catch urine specimen	Infection
Cervical cytology	Cervical disease
Endometrial sampling/hysteroscopy	Uterine disease
Pelvic ultrasound	Pelvic mass
Laparoscopy	PID
	Pelvic malignancy

Fig. 3.2 Work-up of vaginal discharge.

Appropriate work-up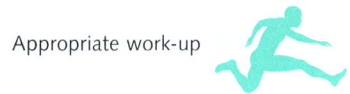

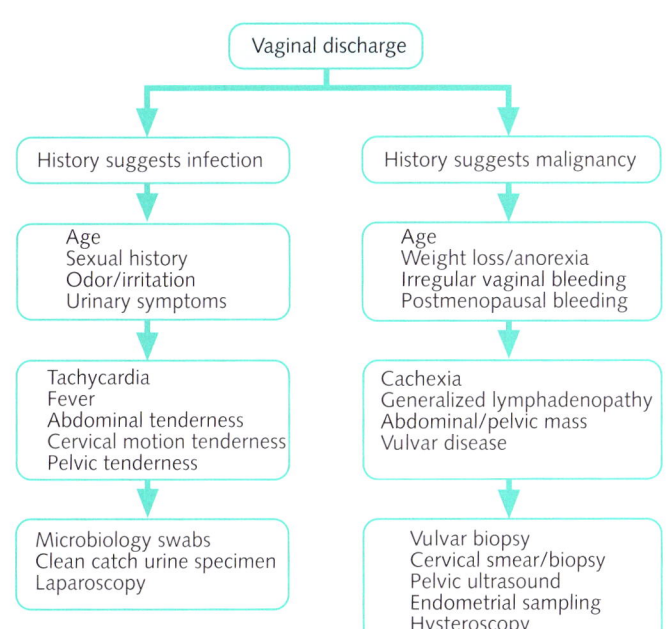

Fig. 3.3 Algorithm for vaginal discharge.

Appropriate work-up

- Wet mount/endocervical/urethral cultures.
- Clean catch urine specimen.
- Cervical cytology/biopsy.
- Endometrial sampling/hysteroscopy.
- Pelvic ultrasound.
- Laparoscopy.

Figure 3.2 shows the work-up for vaginal discharge. Figure 3.3 is an algorithm for the diagnosis and cause of vaginal discharge.

4. Vulvar Symptoms

Vulvar pruritus refers to itching or irritation of the vulvar region. This debilitating and socially embarrassing symptom is common and can be caused by a whole host of conditions. These are grouped into four broad categories (Fig. 4.1):
- Infection.
- Vulvar dystrophy.
- Neoplastic.
- Dermatologic.

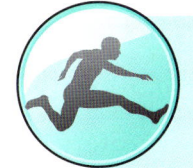

Vulvar symptoms of itching and irritation might be due to a generalized skin problem or to systemic illness.

History

The age of the patient is important, because younger women are generally more likely to have an infectious etiology, and vulvar dystrophies (more correctly termed nonneoplastic epithelial disorders of the vulva) and neoplasms are more likely in older women. Acute onset of symptoms occurs frequently with infection, whereas other causes of pruritus can have a more chronic and insidious onset. Embarrassment often delays presentation. A history of PMB is important.

Exacerbating and relieving factors can give clues as to the etiology. Symptoms of yeast and herpetic infection might worsen premenstrually. A recent change in soap or washing powder, or overzealous hygiene, can suggest a contact dermatitis. Self-treatment with emollients and antifungals is common and should be noted, as should the response.

Cervical intraepithelial neoplasia (CIN) and VIN are thought to share a common etiology, so a history of CIN should be noted. Abnormal vaginal discharge can suggest infection and, if suspected, a detailed sexual history should be taken. The discharge of infection with *Trichomonas vaginalis* and bacterial vaginosis has a typically "fishy" odor.

Dermatological conditions, such as psoriasis and eczema, can affect the vulva, and a history of these conditions elsewhere on the body might be relevant. Symptoms suggestive of diabetes mellitus, renal failure, and liver failure should be noted.

Differential diagnosis of vulvar pruritus

Type of cause	Description
Infection	Fungal
	Candida
	Tinea
	Parasitic
	Trichomonas vaginalis
	Enterobius (pinworm)
	Pediculosis pubis
	Bacterial
	Bacterial vaginosis/vaginitis
	Viral
	Herpes simplex virus
	Human papilloma virus
Vulval dystrophy	Lichen sclerosis
	Hypertrophic vulvar dystrophy
Neoplastic	Vulvar intraepithelial neoplasia (VIN)
	Squamous carcinoma
	Paget's disease of the vulva
Dermatological	Psoriasis
	Eczema
	Contact dermatitis

Fig. 4.1 Differential diagnosis of vulvar pruritus.

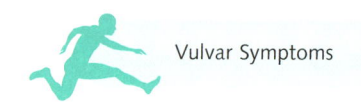

Examination

General examination of the patient includes assessment of skin surfaces prone to dermatologic conditions: face, hands, wrists, elbows, trunk, and knees. Signs of chronic renal failure and liver disease should be assessed.

Examination of the vulva, urethral meatus, and perianal region in good lighting is essential. The vagina and cervix should be inspected carefully with the aid of a speculum. Colposcopic examination of the vulva might be useful if no apparent lesion can be seen with the naked eye and to perform directed biopsies. Inguinal lymphadenopathy can occur secondary to infection or malignancy.

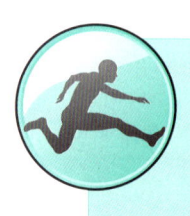

> Even if no lesion is seen, it might still be prudent to perform colposcopic examination of the area and take biopsies.

Infection

Generalized vulvitis, vaginal discharge, and ulcers suggest an infective cause, although ulceration should alert the examiner to the possibility of malignancy. Genital warts might be seen on the vulva, perianally, in the vagina, or on the cervix.

Vulvar dystrophies

Labial fusion, adhesions, stenosis of the introitus, leukoplakia (literally meaning "white plaque"), and atrophic changes are frequent signs of lichen sclerosis, the most common of the vulvar dystrophies. The lesions of hyperplastic dystrophy can be localized or extensive, and typically show thickening of the affected skin with variable color change. Thickened plaques of leukoplakia might be present.

Neoplasia

VIN lesions are variable and can be papular (similar to genital warts) or macular with irregular borders. Pigmentation (brown or black) is common, and leukoplakia and ulceration can occur. Invasive squamous carcinoma of the vulva usually appears as an exophytic tumor, often with surface ulceration. Paget's disease of the vulva can be unifocal or multifocal and the lesions are typically clearly defined, scaly, erythematous plaques with varying degrees of ulceration and leukoplakia.

> If no physical cause is found for vulvar symptoms, there might be a psychosomatic problem.

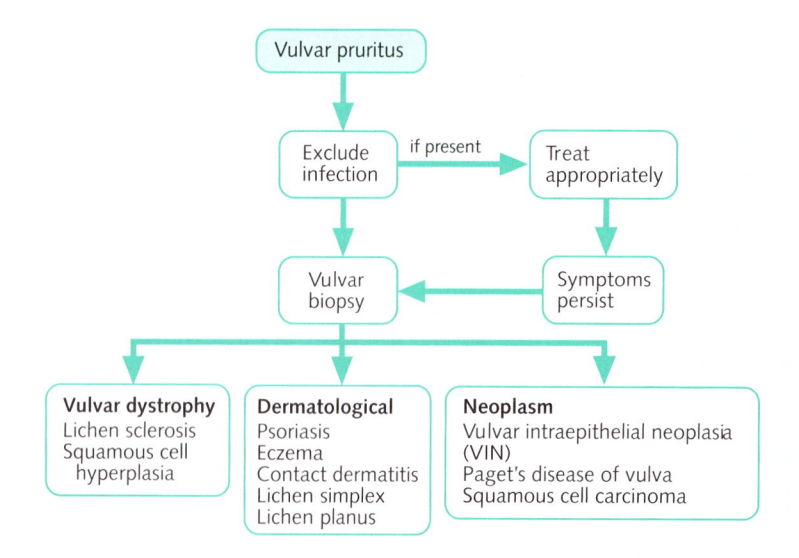

Fig. 4.2 Algorithm for vulvar pruritus.

Dermatologic

Psoriasis might appear as the typical scaly plaques, but it can also be smooth, erythematous, and fissured.

Appropriate work-up

Where systemic disease is suspected, relevant testing should include liver function, renal function, and glucose tolerance. Urinalysis might reveal the presence of hematuria, proteinuria, and glycosuria.

A saline wet prep should be performed to exclude yeast infection (Fig. 4.2), and sexually active women should be screened for sexually transmitted diseases. Pinworms might be identified by naked-eye visualization of the adult female worms in the perianal region or by microscopic identification of the ova.

Although certain conditions of the vulva have a typical appearance, many are difficult to distinguish with the naked eye. The mainstay of diagnosis of vulvar dystrophies, dermatoses, and neoplasms is histologic. Punch biopsies of the vulva can be performed under local anesthetic in the outpatient setting, with or without the aid of a colposcope. Discrete lesions can be excised in their entirety, as excisional biopsies under general anesthesia. Hysteroscopy or dilatation and curettage (D&C) is indicated to exclude endometrial pathology when PMB has occurred.

5 Urinary Incontinence

Urinary incontinence is an objectively demonstrable involuntary loss of urine that is a social or hygienic problem. The two most common causes of urinary incontinence are genuine stress incontinence (GSI) and detrusor overactivity (DO), which account for approximately 90% of incontinent women. These, and other causes, are shown in Fig. 5.1 in order of frequency of occurrence.

Female urinary incontinence

1. GSI
2. DO
3. Mixed GSI and DO
4. Sensory urgency
5. Chronic voiding problems (chronic retention)
6. Fistula

Fig. 5.1 The causes of female urinary incontinence in order of frequency of occurrence.

History

A detailed history is mandatory because of the presence of multiple symptoms that are not always apparent on initial questioning. The two symptoms of stress incontinence and urge incontinence are commonly used synonymously with the conditions GSI and DO respectively (see Fig. 5.2 for definitions of common urogynecologic terms). This is inaccurate and can lead to inappropriate treatment, because many incontinent women will admit to both symptoms, although in only 5% of women do GSI and DO coexist.

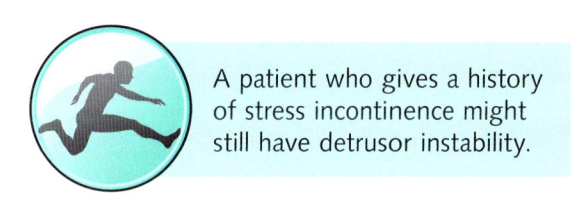

A patient who gives a history of stress incontinence might still have detrusor instability.

Commonly used urogynecologic terms

Term	Definition
Cystometry	The measurement of bladder pressure and volume
Detrusor overactivity	An overactive bladder is one that is shown objectively to contract spontaneously or on provocation during the filling phase while the patient is attempting to inhibit micturition
Frequency of micturition	Voiding more than seven times per day
GSI	The involuntary loss of urine when the intravesical pressure exceeds the maximum urethral pressure in the absence of detrusor activity
Nocturia	Voiding more than twice per night
Nocturnal enuresis	The involuntary passage of urine at night
Stress incontinence	Involuntary loss of urine associated with raised intra-abdominal pressure
Urge incontinence	Urinary leakage associated with a strong and sudden desire to void
Urgency of micturition	A strong and sudden desire to void
Urinary incontinence	Involuntary loss of urine that is a social or hygienic problem and is objectively demonstrable
Uroflowmetry	The measurement of urine flow rate
Videocystourethrography (VCU)	Combines radiologic with pressure and flow studies

Fig. 5.2 Definitions of commonly used urogynecologic terms.

Genuine stress incontinence

The most common symptom of stress incontinence is leakage of small amounts of urine. This usually occurs after an increase in intra-abdominal pressure, as with coughing, laughing, or sneezing. One-third of women with GSI will also admit to urge incontinence, and up to a half will experience urgency of micturition. Frequency of micturition and nocturia are also common symptoms.

GSI is associated with the following factors, and these must be highlighted in the history:
- Increasing age.
- Increasing parity.
- Genital prolapse.
- Postmenopausal status.
- Previous pelvic floor surgery.

Detrusor overactivity

The vast majority of women with DO will complain of urgency, urge incontinence, frequency, and nocturia. However, up to one-quarter might complain of stress incontinence because raised intra-abdominal pressure can stimulate an unstable bladder to contract and produce the symptom of stress incontinence.

The following factors should be highlighted in the history:
- Age.
- History of nocturnal enuresis.
- Neurologic history.
- Previous incontinence surgery.
- Drug history.

Sensory urgency

Sensory urgency differs from DO (motor urgency) in that the urgency occurs in the absence of detrusor activity. The presenting symptoms are the same as for DO, although incontinence is not such a common feature.

Voiding disorders

Voiding disorders can result in chronic retention, leading to overflow incontinence. As well as urgency and frequency, the following classic symptoms might be present: hesitancy, straining to void, poor flow, and incomplete emptying. Large residual volumes of urine due to incomplete emptying predispose to UTI, which aggravates the symptoms of incontinence, urgency, and frequency. Stress incontinence might be a presenting symptom.

Fistulas

Fistulas are very rare in the US, but should always be suspected when incontinence is continuous during the day and night. A fistula may occur between the urinary bladder and vagina (vesicovaginal fistula) or the ureter and vagina (ureterovaginal fistula). In developed countries, the most common cause of vesicovaginal fistula is gynecologic surgery (e.g. hysterectomy). Obstetric trauma resulting in fistula is most common in underdeveloped countries. A recent history of difficult hysterectomy followed by continuous leakage of urine from the vagina should prompt the clinician to consider vesicovaginal or ureterovaginal fistula.

Physical exam

Chronic dampness can cause excoriation of the vulva. The best way to demonstrate stress incontinence is to ask the patient to cough while standing with a moderately full bladder. Stress incontinence is not always demonstrable, especially with the patient in the supine position. Examination of the vaginal walls, using a bivalve speculum, will identify scarring from previous surgery and the presence of uterovaginal prolapse; especially important is a cystourethrocele. Bimanual examination should identify a pelvic mass.

As neurologic disease can present with urinary symptoms, including incontinence, a neurological examination should be performed.

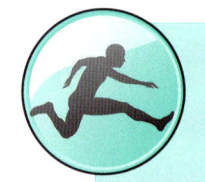

> A neurologic examination should always be carried out to exclude this cause for the incontinence problems.

Laboratory studies

As suggested above, the bladder is an "unreliable witness," and judicious investigation is important if inappropriate treatment is to be avoided. It is essential to exclude a UTI, a common cause of sensory urgency, because the UTI might be the cause of the presenting symptoms and infection

Fig. 5.3 Algorithm for urinary incontinence.

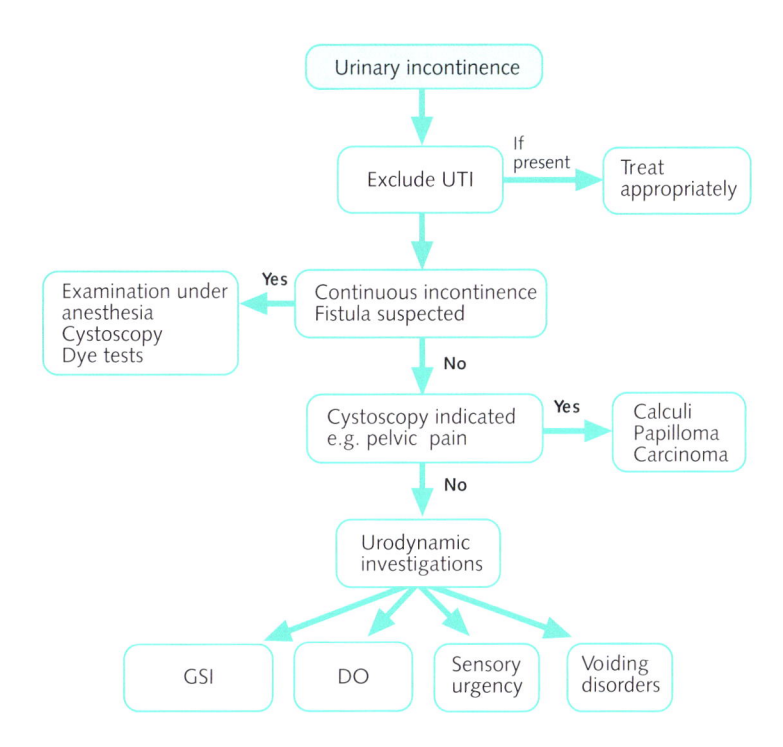

could be exacerbated by further invasive investigations (Fig. 5.3).

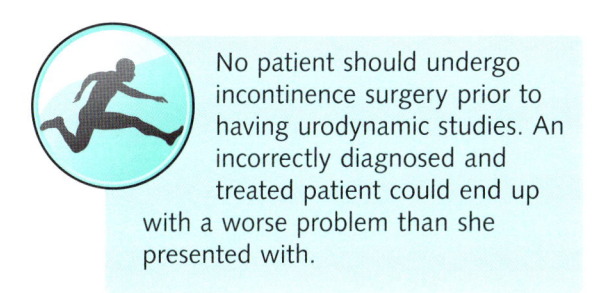

> No patient should undergo incontinence surgery prior to having urodynamic studies. An incorrectly diagnosed and treated patient could end up with a worse problem than she presented with.

Urodynamics

It could be argued that all incontinent women should have urodynamics performed (see Chapter 26). This is especially so in women about to undergo incontinence surgery.

Uroflowmetry will identify low peak urine flow rates, which suggests a voiding disorder. Cystometry is probably the single most useful urodynamic investigation and will confirm or exclude DO. Cystometry will not diagnose GSI but will suggest this diagnosis by exclusion of other disorders such as DO.

VCU combines radiologic with pressure and flow studies and gives the most information about bladder function. VCU can positively identify GSI and DO, as well as other disorders. It is a very useful test to perform prior to incontinence surgery, although not all facilities provide this service.

Cystoscopy

Although cystoscopy allows inspection of the anatomy of the bladder and bladder neck, it does not give information regarding their function. Anatomical assessment of the bladder neck is important in the presence of voiding disorders; polyps, calculi, and malignancies will be obvious, as will trabeculation. True bladder capacity can be measured under general anesthesia.

6. Prolapse

Differential diagnosis

A prolapse is the protrusion of an organ or a structure beyond its normal anatomical site. In the female genital tract, the type of prolapse depends on the organ involved and its position in relation to the anterior or posterior vaginal wall (Fig. 6.1; see also Fig. 27.1).

Cystocele/cystourethrocele
A cystocele is a prolapse of the upper anterior wall of the vagina, which is attached to the bladder by fascia. This type of prolapse can extend to include the lower anterior vaginal wall as the urethra is displaced down; this is known as a cystourethrocele.

Rectocele
A rectocele is a weakness in the levator ani muscles that causes a bulge in the mid-posterior vaginal wall, which includes the rectum.

Enterocele
An enterocele is a true hernia of the pouch of Douglas. It is a prolapse of the upper third of the posterior vaginal wall and contains loops of small bowel.

Uterine descent
The uterus cannot prolapse without carrying the upper vagina with it. This may be associated with a cystocele and/or a rectocele. Degrees of prolapse are graded based on the relationship between the location of the uterus relative to the vaginal introitus. First-degree prolapse occurs when the cervix remains within the vagina. A second-degree prolapse occurs when the cervix protrudes through the introitus. When the uterus lies entirely outside the introitus, this is called procidentia, or third-degree prolpase (see Fig. 6.3).

Relevant history

Most commonly, the patient presents with a history of local discomfort or a feeling of "something coming out," as the prolapsed organ pushes into the vagina and bulges toward the introitus. It might interfere with sexual function or be exacerbated by increasing intra-abdominal pressure, such as with coughing or straining to pass stools. Other symptoms depend on the organ/organs involved.

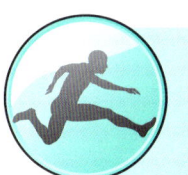

> The two most common presenting symptoms are feeling "something coming out" and backache. Don't forget that there might be other causes of backache, especially in elderly patients.

Urinary symptoms
These occur with a cystocele or a cystourethrocele. There might be urinary frequency or incomplete emptying of the bladder, which predisposes to urinary infection; there might even be overflow incontinence. Stress incontinence might be present if there is descent of the urethrovesical junction (bladder neck).

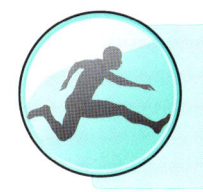

> The urinary system and the bowel are involved. Related symptoms must, therefore, be included in the history.

Differential diagnosis of prolapse	
• Cystocele	• Enterocele
• Cystourethrocele	• Uterine descent
• Rectocele	

Fig. 6.1 Differential diagnosis of prolapse.

Bowel symptoms
A rectocele may cause incomplete bowel emptying. This can be relieved if the patient pushes back the prolapse digitally.

Uterine descent
Uterine descent often gives symptoms of backache, although other causes of backache must be excluded, especially in older patients. A procidentia causes discomfort as it rubs on the patient's clothing, and this might cause a bloody, sometimes purulent, discharge.

Figure 6.2 shows factors that should be elicited in the history that may predispose the patient to prolapse in general.

vaginal wall retracted, any anterior wall prolapse will be demonstrated if the patient is asked to bear down. Conversely, if the anterior vaginal wall is retracted, then an enterocele or rectocele will be seen.

> Examination for prolapse is with the patient in the left lateral position and using a Sims' speculum. Abdominal palpation and bimanual examination must always be performed.

Physical exam

- Abdominal palpation.
- Sims' speculum examination.
- Bimanual pelvic examination.

Following abdominal palpation to exclude a mass, the patient should be examined in the left lateral position using a Sims' speculum. With the posterior

Prolapse	
Type of factor	Specific factor
Congenital	Spina bifida
	Connective tissue disorder
Acquired	Obstetric factors:
	prolonged labor
	precipitous labor
	instrumental delivery
	fetal macrosomia
	increasing parity
Chronically raised intra-abdominal pressure	Chronic cough
	Constipation
Iatrogenic	Hysterectomy
	Colposuspension
Postmenopausal atrophy	

Fig. 6.2 Factors that might predispose the patient to prolapse.

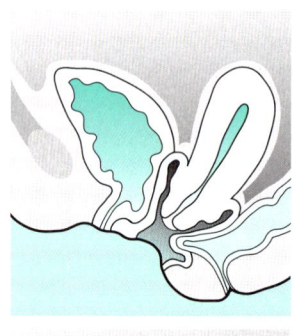

1st degree

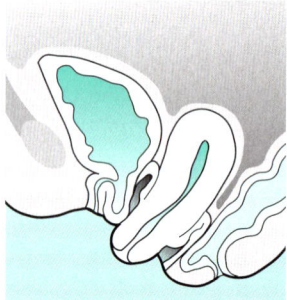

2nd degree

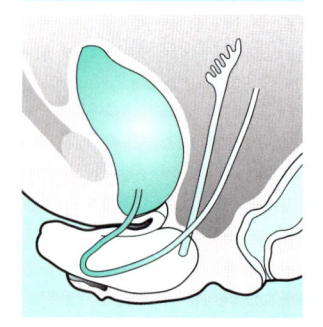

3rd degree (complete procidentia)

Fig. 6.3 Classification of uterine descent.

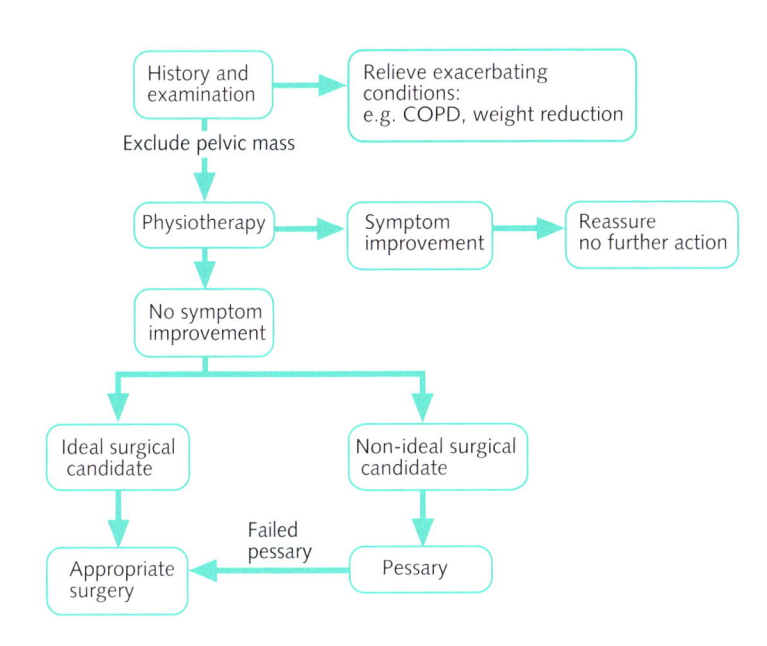

Fig. 6.4 Algorithm for prolapse (COPD: chronic obstructive pulmonary disease).

Uterine descent is assessed by examining the position of the cervix in the vagina, again with the Sims' speculum (Fig. 6.3):
- First degree: any descent of the cervix within the vagina.
- Second degree: descent of the cervix through the introitus.
- Third degree: descent of the cervix and uterus completely outside the introitus (procidentia).

If the patient has a full bladder, stress incontinence can be demonstrated by asking the patient to cough. A bimanual pelvic examination is mandatory to exclude a pelvic mass as the cause of the prolapse.

Appropriate work-up

There are few relevant investigations for prolapse because it is basically a clinical diagnosis dependent on examination findings (Fig. 6.4). In relation to patients with urinary symptoms, the following tests might be appropriate:
- Mid-stream urine specimen.
- Urodynamics.

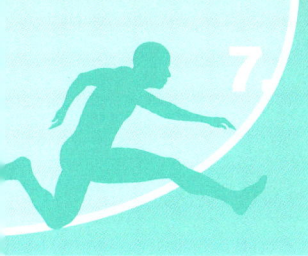

7. Bleeding and/or Pain in Early Pregnancy

The history, examination, and laboratory work must be aimed at distinguishing an ectopic pregnancy from a miscarriage (Fig. 7.1), while remembering that any woman who has pain or bleeding in pregnancy will be anxious. Any uncertainty about the diagnosis, and the reasons for it, should be explained to the patient carefully. Explain the plan for investigating the cause further. Note that the definitions in Fig. 7.2 refer to miscarriage.

Relevant history

Last menstrual period

The first day of the LMP will allow you to calculate the gestation, which is important when scanning—the absence of a fetal pole in the uterus can be explained by the fact that the pregnancy is still very early, although if the woman was further along in the pregnancy this would raise the suspicion of an ectopic pregnancy. It is important to establish whether the woman is sure of the date and whether her cycle is regular; if not, the estimate may be wrong. If she conceived while taking the pill, then the last period cannot be relied upon to predict the gestation because it was a hormonally induced withdrawal bleed.

Presenting complaint

Bleeding

Some women might not realize that there is a problem with their pregnancy until they have a scan (see Fig. 7.2). Miscarriage does not always start with heavy bleeding, and the blood loss seen with ectopic pregnancy is variable, so the amount of bleeding cannot be used to predict the problem unless the woman has seen products of conception mixed with the bleeding, in which case she is having an inevitable miscarriage. Products may be described as "pieces of tissue." You can often quantify the blood flow by asking how many pads the woman has needed to change in a day.

Differential diagnosis for bleeding in early pregnancy

- Threatened miscarriage, ongoing pregnancy (see Chapter 29)
- Nonviable pregnancy (complete, incomplete or missed abortion; see Chapter 29)
- Molar pregnancy (see Chapter 29)
- Ectopic pregnancy (see Chapter 29)
- Local cause, e.g. cervical ectropion or carcinoma (see Chapter 23)

Fig. 7.1 Differential diagnosis for bleeding in early pregnancy.

Types of miscarriage

Type of miscarriage	Description
Threatened	Bleeding occurring before 20 weeks, where the cervix is closed on examination
Inevitable	Bleeding occurring before 20 weeks, where the cervix is open on examination
Missed	Scan shows a nonviable fetus or an empty intrauterine gestation sac
	The cervix is closed on examination
	Patient might not have had any bleeding
Complete	Scan shows that there are no products of conception left in the uterus in a case where the patient has had bleeding. The cervix will be closed on examination
Incomplete	Scan shows that there are products of conception left inside the uterus in a case where the patient has bleeding. The cervix will be open on examination

Fig. 7.2 Types of miscarriage.

The woman might connect the onset of bleeding to an event such as intercourse or exercise. It is possible for the cervix, which is more friable in pregnancy, to bleed postcoitally, but actual miscarriage is not provoked by intercourse. The woman might feel guilty and blame herself, and it is important to reassure her.

Pain

Miscarriage typically causes cramping, central, low abdominal pain. The patient might describe it as "like period pains" or "like contractions." It might have started suddenly or could have been preceded by days or weeks of spotting.

The pain of a tubal ectopic pregnancy will be typically worse on one side than the other, and centered around the iliac fossa. There might have been dyspareunia on that side over the previous few days and, as a result of blood irritating the bowel, the woman might have had some diarrhea. If an ectopic pregnancy ruptures, it causes pain all over the abdomen and referred shoulder pain because of blood irritating the inferior surface of the diaphragm.

Past obstetric history

A history of miscarriage or ectopic pregnancy increases the risk of these problems happening again (see Chapter 29).

Past medical history

This should focus on any conditions that predispose to ectopic pregnancy (see Fig. 7.3 and Chapter 29). Also remember that a woman who has a nonviable or an ectopic pregnancy might need surgical intervention, so attention should be paid to conditions that may affect tolerance to anesthesia.

Physical exam

Observations

The woman might be experiencing significant pain if the uterus is expelling clots or products, or if an ectopic pregnancy has ruptured. Check her pulse and blood pressure.

Miscarriage is unlikely to cause shock due to hypovolemia, but, rarely, cervical shock is seen, in which there is a vagal response to the dilatation caused by products of conception distending the cervical canal. In this case, pulse and blood pressure would both be low.

Hemorrhage from a ruptured ectopic pregnancy can be massive; the pulse will be weak and tachycardic and blood pressure will be low. The patient will look pale, sweaty, and unwell and might collapse.

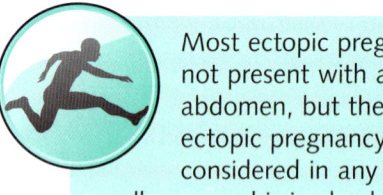

Conditions predisposing to ectopic pregnancy

Factor	Reason
PID	Tubal damage and pelvic scarring
Tubal surgery, e.g. previous ectopic or sterilization	Tubal damage
Peritonitis or pelvic surgery in past, e.g. appendicitis	Pelvic scarring
Endometriosis	Tubal damage and pelvic scarring
IUD in situ	Abnormal implantation
IVF pregnancy	Abnormal implantation

Fig. 7.3 Conditions predisposing to ectopic pregnancy.

Most ectopic pregnancies do not present with an acute abdomen, but the diagnosis of ectopic pregnancy should be considered in any woman who collapses and is in shock.

Abdominal examination

With miscarriage, the abdomen will be soft. If more than 12 weeks, or if the uterus is fibroid, it might be palpable above the symphysis pubis. With ectopic pregnancy the uterus will not be palpable abdominally. Before it ruptures there will be tenderness on the affected side, and there might be some guarding and rebound. Once ruptured, the entire abdomen will be tense and tender with guarding and rebound.

Cusco's speculum examination

The cervix should be visualized and swabs taken from the endocervix and vagina. An ectropion or, rarely, a cervical carcinoma might be visible. It might be possible to see if the os is open or closed, but this is best determined by palpation.

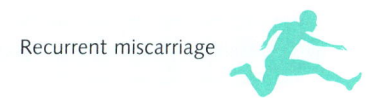

> An ectropion is not pathologic, it is simply an extension of endocervical columnar epithelium, which bleeds easily, onto the ectocervix and is common in pregnancy due to the influence of estrogen. Bleeding from an ectropion is usually light, but it can be heavier if provoked by intercourse or in the presence of infection, so cervical swabs should be taken. No treatment is necessary unless infection is proven.

Vaginal examination

Is the os open or closed? This finding is vital to help the diagnosis until a scan is available. In early pregnancy, if the woman has had a labor in the past, the external os will be open ("multiparous os"), but the internal os should be closed, so this question refers to the internal os. If it is open then there will be no resistance, and the cervix will admit a finger. An open os indicates an inevitable miscarriage; a closed os might be seen with miscarriage (see Fig. 7.2) or with ectopic pregnancy. The uterine size in weeks should be estimated. The adnexa should be examined—an ectopic pregnancy will cause fullness and tenderness on the affected side. Cervical motion tenderness may be present with an ectopic pregnancy.

> Cervical motion tenderness is sudden severe pain that occurs when the cervix is moved at the time of vaginal examination. This is different from the discomfort that many women feel at the time of examination.

Appropriate work-up

Figure 7.4 provides an algorithm for the diagnosis and findings of bleeding and/or pain in early pregnancy.

Blood tests

- CBC: the woman is unlikely to be anemic due to the bleeding of miscarriage, but there might be pre-existing anemia, which will be important from an anesthetic point of view. An ectopic, if ruptured, may result in severe anemia.
- Blood type: women who are rhesus negative will require anti-D after an operation for ectopic pregnancy, after a D&E of the retained products of conception at any gestation or after an episode of bleeding in the first trimester.
- The serum β-hCG level cannot always be used to diagnose an ectopic pregnancy, but two samples taken 48 h apart will not show the doubling in level expected in a normal intrauterine pregnancy.

Ultrasound scan

Transvaginal scans give the best view in early pregnancy (Fig. 7.5). The uterus is examined, looking for a gestation sac and fetal pole, and then for a fetal heartbeat. If the uterus is empty, raising the possibility of ectopic pregnancy, then the adnexa are scanned, looking for a mass. Sometimes a live ectopic is seen, where the ectopic gestation sac contains a fetus with a heartbeat. Free fluid, due to bleeding from the ectopic pregnancy, might be seen in the pouch of Douglas. In miscarriage, retained products of conception may be seen.

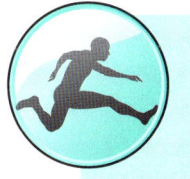

> Once a fetal heartbeat is seen on ultrasound scan there is a 90% chance of the pregnancy continuing. Fetal heart activity can be seen from around 7 weeks' gestation.

Recurrent miscarriage

A woman who has had three or more consecutive first-trimester miscarriages should have the same

Bleeding and/or Pain in Early Pregnancy

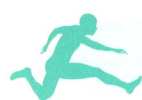

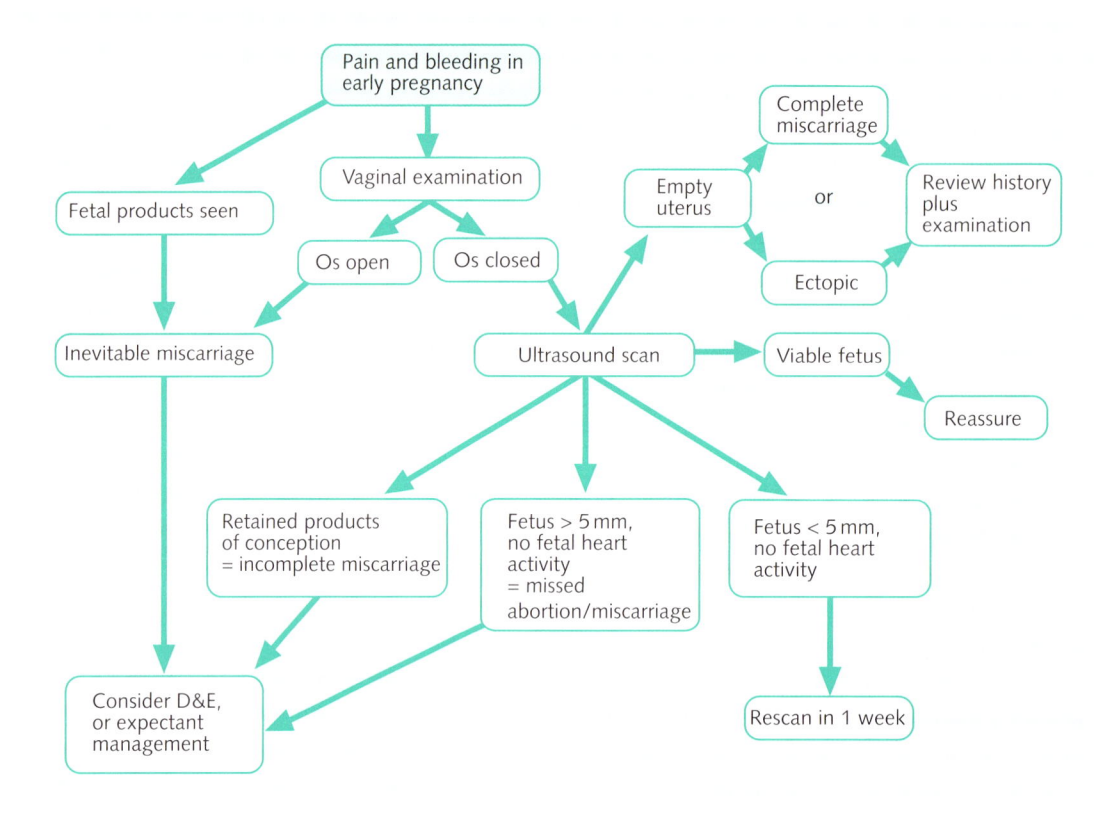

Fig. 7.4 Algorithm for bleeding and/or pain in early pregnancy (D&E: dilatation and evacuation).

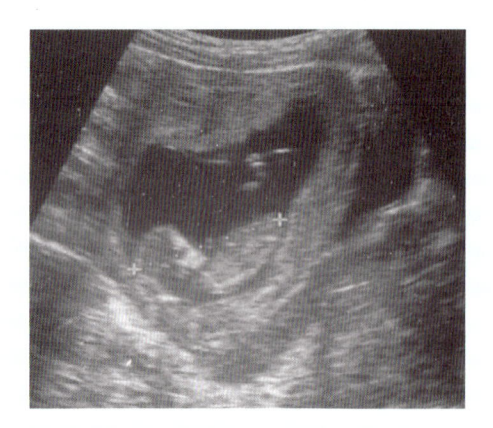

Fig. 7.5 Transvaginal scan showing intrauterine pregnancy, 7-week-sized fetus. Reproduced with kind permission from *Obstetric Ultrasound* (2nd edn), published by Churchill Livingstone.

history and examination as above, remembering to consider the causes listed in Chapter 29. Extra investigations should also be ordered:
- Karyotyping of both partners and of products of conception.
- A hysterosalpingogram (HSG) to assess the uterine cavity.
- A wet mount to screen for bacterial vaginosis.
- Antiphospholipid antibodies assay on two occasions at least 6 weeks apart. The test is performed twice to avoid the false negatives that occur due to fluctuations in antibody levels, and the false positives caused by a temporary rise in levels at times of viral illness. If the two results are different, then take the test again. The diagnosis is made after two positive tests.
- Cervical insufficiency is best diagnosed by careful history taking, where there will be a story of painless cervical dilatation or spontaneous rupture of membranes in the

second trimester. Transvaginal scan of the cervical canal can aid diagnosis, showing an open internal os and short canal.

Trophoblastic disease

Presentation can occur in several ways:
- Bleeding in early pregnancy, investigated by ultrasound, which reveals a molar pregnancy with a characteristic "bunches of grapes" appearance (Fig. 7.6). A partial mole pregnancy might not appear abnormal on scan.
- Ultrasound for dating in early pregnancy, which might have been routine or was perhaps ordered because the uterus was larger than expected by dates of LMP.
- Exaggerated symptoms of pregnancy due to the high levels of β-hCG (e.g. hyperemesis gravidarum).
- Products of conception following miscarriage and D&E are reported by the histopathologist as showing partial or complete mole.
- Persistently raised hCG following ectopic pregnancy, miscarriage, or term delivery.

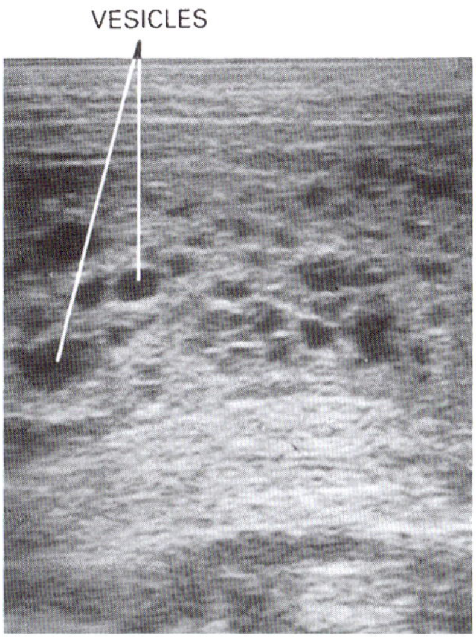

Fig. 7.6 Molar pregnancy. Reproduced with kind permission from *Obstetric Ultrasound* (2nd edn), published by Churchill Livingstone.

8. Infertility

Eighty-five percent of couples will conceive within 1 year; those that don't should be seen and investigated as a couple. The couple's infertility may be due to female factors, male factors, or both (Fig. 8.1).

Infertility affects 1 in 7 couples in the US:
- 20% = male factor alone
- 20–40% = female and male factors
- 40–60% = female factor alone

First, consider what is necessary for conception. An XX woman and an XY male must have penetrative intercourse resulting in male ejaculation. Conception occurs in the 4 days around ovulation—sperm can survive for 3 days and an egg can be fertilized for 1 day after it is released. The sperm must pass through the cervical mucus, the uterine cavity, and into the fallopian tube. The egg must have been picked up at the fimbrial end of the tube and transported down to meet the sperm so that fertilization can take place, and the fertilized embryo must be able to implant in the uterus.

Taking the history

It is helpful to bear the above sequence in mind when taking the history and examining the infertile couple to diagnose the cause of the problem (Fig. 8.2).

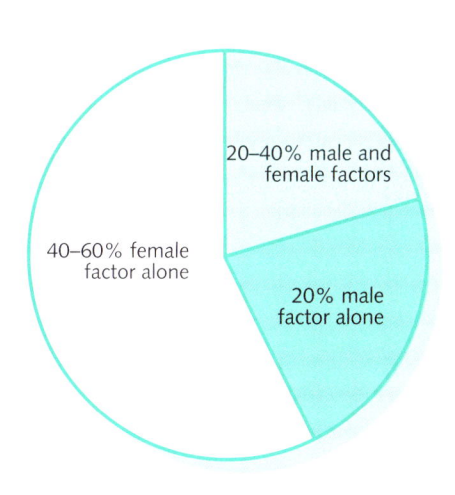

Fig. 8.1 Pie chart for infertility.

Causes of female infertility	
Type of problem	Cause of infertility
Ovulatory problem	Chronic systemic illness
	Eating disorders
	Abnormal pituitary/hypothalamic/endocrine profile • PCOS • Hyperprolactinemia • Hypo- or hyperthyroidism
	Cannabis use
	NSAIDs
Tubal problem	Previous tubal surgery
	Previous ectopic pregnancy
	Endometriosis
Uterine problem	Submucosal fibroid
	Uterine septum
	Asherman syndrome
	Uterine anomalies
Coital problem	Intercourse not occurring often enough
	Impotence
	Vaginismus

Fig. 8.2 Causes of female infertility.

History of the couple
This should include the length of time that they have been trying to conceive and whether they are having regular intercourse. Night shifts or a partner who works away or abroad could be reducing their chances of conception. The issue of sexual dysfunction should be discussed, as female vaginismus or male impotence might be the problem.

History from the woman
Past obstetric history
It should be established whether this is primary or secondary infertility, i.e. whether the woman has had a pregnancy before and, if so, whether this was with a different partner. Details of previous pregnancies must be recorded, paying particular attention to a history of ectopic pregnancy, which could point to a tubal reason for infertility.

Past gynecologic history
A menstrual history will identify heavy periods, which might be due to fibroids, and painful periods, which might suggest endometriosis. Endometriosis can cause tubal problems, either by scarring the tubes or by interfering with the ciliary action of the tubal lining. Asherman's syndrome—the presence of intrauterine adhesions that form after curettage or termination of pregnancy—causes severe dysmenorrhea. If the cycle length is between 21 and 35 days and is regular, then ovulation is more likely.

A history of chlamydial infection, IUD use, tubal surgery, or ectopic pregnancy can all raise the suspicion of PID, which can cause tubal damage. Dyspareunia is an important symptom, suggesting PID or endometriosis.

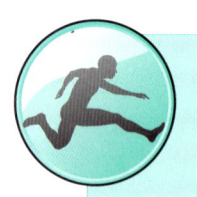

> One episode of PID gives a 10% chance of tubal blockage; three episodes of PID give a 50% chance of tubal blockage.

Women who have had treatment at colposcopy following an abnormal Pap smear have a small risk of cervical stenosis.

Past medical history
Chronic medical conditions (e.g. renal disease, hypothyroidism and hyperthyroidism) and eating disorders (especially anorexia nervosa) decrease the number of ovulatory cycles, reducing the chance of conception.

Drug history
All drugs being taken, prescription or otherwise, must be detailed. Any drugs that are not recommended for use in pregnancy can be reviewed at this visit and alternatives suggested if appropriate. All women trying to conceive should be taking prenatal vitamins, particularly with folic acid.

The regular use of NSAIDs, or of cannabis, is known to decrease the number of ovulatory cycles.

Social history
Smoking is known to decrease fertility, although the mechanism is unclear.

History from the man
Past surgical history
Ask about surgery, including that which was performed as a baby or small child. Repair of inguinal hernia might have led to obstruction of the vas deferens in its inguinal portion; undescended testes are known to predispose to poorer semen quality (regardless of timing of orchidopexy), and testicular torsion is associated with reduced fertility. Bladder neck surgery, including transurethral resection of the prostate, can result in retrograde ejaculation.

Past medical history
Epididymo-orchitis, most commonly caused by sexually transmitted infections such as chlamydia (sometimes put under the category of nonspecific urethritis) can result in epididymal obstruction. This is also common in cystic fibrosis sufferers. Postpubertal mumps orchitis can cause significant testicular atrophy, resulting in very poor quality sperm, and chronic medical conditions (e.g. renal disease) impair spermatogenesis. Diabetes can lead to retrograde ejaculation.

Drug history
Anabolic steroids, cannabis, cocaine, sulfasalazine (taken for inflammatory bowel disease), colchicine (used to treat gout), nitrofurantoin, and

tetracyclines (antibiotics) have all been shown to decrease sperm numbers and/or function. α-Blockers (used for treatment of benign prostatic hypertrophy) and some antidepressants are known to interfere with ejaculation; β-blockers can cause impotence.

Social history
Smoking can impair the quality of the sperm, but alcohol (if the intake is moderate) does not affect fertility.

Regarding occupation, it is possible that the sperm count might be lower if the testes are kept at a high temperature (e.g. the man's job entails driving all day). Heavy metals, solvents, and agricultural chemicals are all associated with oligospermia.

Physical exam

Examination of the woman
General
The BMI is calculated from height and weight (kg divided by m²). Those at the extremes, i.e. women who are obese (BMI > 30) or underweight (BMI < 19), are less likely to be ovulating. Hirsutism and acanthosis nigricans can indicate PCOS. Other syndromes linked to infertility have other typical facies (e.g. hyper/hypothyroidism, Cushing syndrome, Turner syndrome). The presence or absence of secondary sexual characteristics should be noted.

Abdominal examination
Scars from previous surgery might be seen on inspection (e.g. laparoscopy for endometriosis/PID). On palpation, the presence of a mass could point to a large fibroid uterus or ovarian cyst, and tenderness could be due to pelvic adhesions from endometriosis or PID.

Vaginal examination
The practice of female genital mutilation is widespread in some parts of the world and can make penetrative sex impossible. Occasionally, an intact hymen is discovered. Vaginal discharge can be physiologic or due to PID; if there is doubt, send cultures. The uterus is palpated; a nonmobile uterus could be due to adhesions from endometriosis or PID; an enlarged uterus is likely to be due to fibroids. The ovaries are often difficult to palpate, but might be bulky if polycystic.

Examination of the man
Obesity is known to decrease testosterone, so BMI should be calculated. The presence of secondary sexual characteristics is noted—inadequate virilization could be due to abnormal karyotype. Scars from inguinal hernia repair might point to an obstructive problem. Finally, underwear! Tight underwear raises the scrotal temperature and can impair sperm function.

Testicular presence and size are measured against an orchidometer, and the presence of the vas deferens on both sides is checked by palpation.

Work-up of infertility

Basic investigations for all couples
Blood tests
Check the following in the woman:
- Progesterone: the level rises after ovulation. The test should be performed a week before the next period is due, e.g. day 21 of a 28-day cycle, or day 28 of a 35-day cycle. If >32 nmol/L, ovulation has occurred.
- Rubella immunity: this is not an investigation of infertility, but it must be checked in any woman who is intending to conceive, so that she can be vaccinated if not immune to prevent infection in pregnancy.

Ultrasound
This can be transvaginal or transabdominal and is performed to look for:
- Presence of uterus and ovaries.
- Congenital abnormalities of the uterus.
- Bulky ovaries with multiple peripheral follicles, as in PCOS.
- Hydrosalpinx if PID appears in the history.

Microbiology
Chlamydia screening for the woman and the man in the form of urethral swabs, serum, or urine (or endocervical swab for the woman) is performed. Infection is asymptomatic in up to 70% of women, so there might be no clues in the history, but diagnosis is important. Although treatment will not improve fertility, failure to treat prior to HSG or laparoscopy and dye (see below) can lead to an

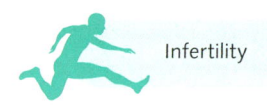

exacerbation of infection when these investigations are carried out, which may worsen infertility.

Test of tubal patency

These tests are performed in the first half of the cycle to ensure that the patient is not already pregnant.

An HSG is performed without systemic anesthesia (Fig. 8.3). The cervix is cannulated, radiopaque dye is introduced into the uterus, and an X-ray is taken to look for passage of the dye. Blockage inside or outside the tubes can prevent the dye flowing; however, tubal spasm in response to the dye can also prevent flow.

Laparoscopy and dye are performed under general anesthesia. It enables visualization of the pelvis, looking for endometriosis or scar tissue secondary to PID, the ovaries, and the tubes. Blue dye is introduced through the cervix by a second operator, and its progress through and out of the tubes can be seen with the laparoscope. Lack of 'fill and spill' of dye indicates tubal occlusion.

The choice of investigation should be dictated by the history and examination. If there is no suspicion of tubal blockage or other intra-abdominal pathology, then a HSG is preferable because it avoids the anesthetic risk; in all other cases laparoscopy should be performed.

A sonohysterogram is an ultrasound study in which the cervix is cannulated and the passage of fluid through the uterus and tubes is monitored using Doppler. This is a recently developed alternative to an HSG; the results are comparable, and it is said to be less uncomfortable for the patient. At present it is not widely used in the US.

Semen analysis

The man is asked to provide a specimen after 3 days abstinence from ejaculation and after a period of good health—a systemic illness within the previous 72 days could have affected the quality of sperm produced. The sample should be processed within 1 h of production. The sperm are counted and evaluated for motility, progression, and morphology, and the volume of the specimen is recorded (Fig. 8.4 gives the normal parameters). The presence of more than 106 white blood cells suggests epididymo-orchitis. Ideally, at least two samples should be processed. These must be produced at least 12 weeks apart to sample different populations of sperm.

Further investigations

These might be prompted by specific points in the history or examination, and include:
- Thyroid function, prolactin, LH/FSH if the woman has an irregular cycle.
- Prolactin: if either partner has galactorrhea.
- Karyotyping: if secondary sexual characteristics are absent.
- Testosterone: if the man appears hypoandrogenic (nonhirsute, small soft testes) or if the woman is overly hirsute.
- Postcoital test: if unsure whether proper sexual intercourse is taking place, or if the man refuses to provide a semen specimen for analysis (e.g.

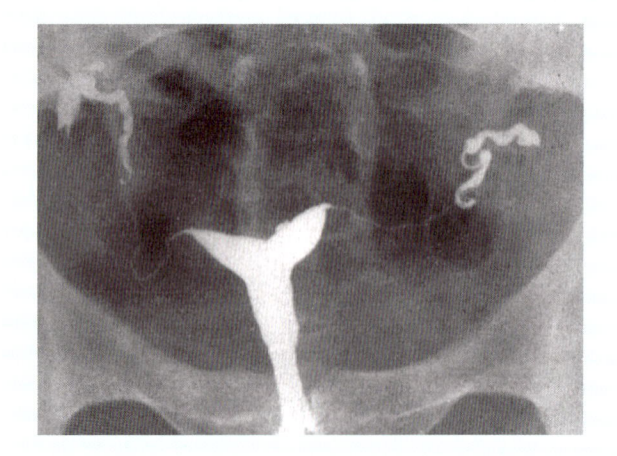

Fig. 8.3 Hysterosalpingogram. Reproduced with kind permission from *Self Assessment Picture Test Obstetrics and Gynaecology* (1st edn), published by Mosby Wolfe.

Normal parameters of semen analysis	
Volume	1.5–5 ml
Count	>20 million/ml
Progression	>50%
Normal forms	>30%

Fig. 8.4 Normal parameters of semen analysis.

on religious grounds), then a sample can be taken from the vagina, suspended in saline, and examined for the presence of sperm. This test was once more widely done to look for evidence of cervical hostility, but has now been shown to be a poor predictor.

- Antisperm antibodies: should be performed only in tertiary centers. Both women and men might have antibodies to sperm. In men they occur on the sperm surface, in the seminal plasma, and in the blood serum, whereas in women they are found in blood and in cervical mucus. They affect sperm motility and function, but their presence is not a significant predictor of infertility. They are found in 5–10% of infertile men, but also in 2% of fertile men.
- Hysteroscopy: should be performed only if the ultrasound suggests abnormality (e.g. intrauterine adhesions, endometrial polyps, or fibroids). Polyps and submucosal fibroids are associated with infertility, but the exact causal relationship is unclear.

9. Menopause

Presentation and differential diagnosis

The strict definition of menopause is cessation of menstruation for 1 year, but this is not always helpful as a basis for management because menopause is often preceded by many years of estrogen-dependent symptoms. From a biological viewpoint it is unlikely that the ovaries are suddenly switched off; their function is more likely to decline gradually, with the cessation of periods as an endpoint that is reflected by the occurrence of irregular periods, decreased fertility, increasing premenstrual syndrome, and climacteric depression before cessation of menstrual periods. This can result in difficulties in differential diagnosis, depending on which of the following menopausal symptoms predominate.

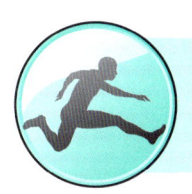

> Menstruation is a poor sign of menopausal status.

Bleeding disturbances

For example, oligomenorrhea and secondary amenorrhea. See Chapters 1 and 19 for the differential diagnosis.

Vasomotor symptoms

Vasomotor symptoms may include hot flashes, night sweats, palpitations, headaches, and dizziness. The differential diagnosis is outlined in Fig. 9.1.

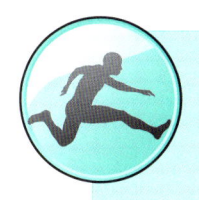

> If a woman has symptoms and is suspected of being menopausal but still has a regular cycle, then she may be treated empirically with HRT.

Differential diagnosis of vasomotor symptoms during menopause

- Cardiovascular problems (e.g. arrhythmias, coronary artery disease, valvular lesions, cardiomyopathies)
- CNS disease (e.g. transient ischemic attacks, small cerebrovascular accidents, tumors)
- Other endocrinopathies (e.g. hypo- or hyperthyroidism, hyperprolactinemia, Cushing's syndrome)
- Hematologic problems (e.g. myeloma)
- Infectious causes (e.g. tuberculosis)
- Other (e.g. malignancy)

Fig. 9.1 Differential diagnosis of vasomotor symptoms during menopause.

These symptoms affect 75% of women during natural menopause, but they are more common and severe in women experiencing acute menopause after bilateral oophorectomy or radiotherapy.

One of the greatest difficulties in diagnosing menopause is that vasomotor symptoms can occur for up to 5 years before menstruation ceases. It is crucial that the diagnosis is considered and treatment started empirically if necessary.

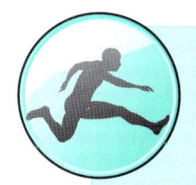

> Night sweats can be due to conditions other than the menopause, such as tuberculosis or lymphoma.

Psychologic symptoms

Psychologic symptoms may include mood swings, worsening premenstrual syndrome, decreased libido, or poor concentration. The differential diagnosis is given in Fig. 9.2.

The origin of psychologic symptoms is complex and likely to involve both biologic and psychosocial

Menopause

Differential diagnosis of psychologic symptoms during menopause
• Psychiatric disorders (e.g. major depression, anxiety, bipolar disorders) • Lesions of the CNS • Other endocrinopathies, especially hypothyroidism • Severe premenstrual syndrome • Other (e.g. malignancy)

Fig. 9.2 Differential diagnosis of psychologic symptoms during the menopause.

Differential diagnosis of systemic menopausal symptoms
• Dermatologic conditions (e.g. eczema, psoriasis) • Connective tissue disorders (e.g. scleroderma, systemic lupus erythematosus) • Other endocrinopathies (e.g. hypothyroidism) • Natural aging process • Mechanical trauma (e.g. joint sprain) • Rheumatologic conditions (e.g. rheumatoid arthritis)

Fig. 9.3 Differential diagnosis of systemic menopause symptoms.

factors. Epidemiologic studies have confirmed an increase in psychologic symptoms in women in the perimenopausal years.

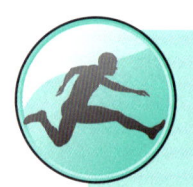

> Depression is common in the perimenopausal period because of fluctuating hormone levels, but other pathology, such as hypothyroidism, should be excluded.

There is no doubt that psychosocial issues, such as domestic stress and loss of youth and fertility, are important factors in depression. The fact that hormonal changes also play a part is suggested by the finding that the predominance of depression in women occurs between puberty and menopause and is most common at times of greatest hormonal change, such as premenstrually, post partum, and during climacteric depression. Conversely, during the last trimester of pregnancy, when hormone levels are stable, depression rarely occurs.

Again, these symptoms can occur years before menstruation ceases, and menopause must be considered as a diagnosis in women who present with depression in their 30s, 40s, and 50s (and occasionally younger) and especially after surgical oophorectomy without adequate HRT.

Systemic menopausal symptoms

- Vulvovaginal: dyspareunia, vaginal bleeding.
- Urinary: dysuria, frequency, hematuria, incontinence.
- Skin: bruising, infection, poor healing.
- Joints: pain.

The differential diagnosis is shown in Fig. 9.3 (see also Chapters 2, 4 and 5).

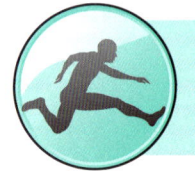

> Urinary and vaginal symptoms are often the first presenting symptoms of menopause.

Estrogen deficiency results in the rapid loss of collagen, which contributes to the generalized atrophy that occurs after menopause. In the genital tract this is manifested by dyspareunia and vaginal bleeding from fragile atrophic skin, and in the lower urinary tract by dysuria, urgency, and frequency, commonly termed the urethral syndrome. More generalized changes are seen in older women as increased bruising and thin translucent skin, which is vulnerable to trauma and infection. A similar loss of collagen from ligaments can cause many of the generalized aches and pains that are more common in postmenopausal women.

Long-term symptoms of menopause

Osteoporosis-related minimal injury fracture

Factors that might have contributed to an early presentation osteoporosis related fracture include:

Long-term symptoms of menopause

- Smoking.
- Low BMI.
- Long episodes of amenorrhea.
- Early age of menopause.
- Family history of osteoporosis.
- Systemic disease (e.g. renal disease).
- Drug usage (e.g. steroids, chemotherapy).

Osteoporosis, or osteopenia, is a disorder of the bone matrix resulting in a reduction of bone strength to the extent that there is a significant increased risk of fracture. The differential diagnosis is listed in Figure 9.4.

Osteoporosis itself is generally symptomless unless a fracture has occurred. Very rarely, the first presentation of menopause will be when a woman suffers an osteoporosis-related fracture. This could have occurred because one of the contributory factors shown above prevented that woman achieving her genetically preprogrammed peak bone mass.

There has been some enthusiasm for the implementation of a national osteoporosis screening program to measure bone density, because prediction of osteoporosis from clinical risk factors and the intensity of short-term symptoms is unreliable. However, this is premature, because no studies have yet demonstrated that bone densitometry is suitable for mass screening.

Figure 9.5 provides an algorithm for the investigation and management of menopause.

Differential diagnosis of osteoporosis-related fracture during menopause

- Fracture due to "appropriate" trauma
- Pathologic fracture (due to malignancy, e.g. multiple myeloma)
- Bone disease (e.g. Paget's osteomalacia)
- Genetic/congenital disorders

Fig. 9.4 Differential diagnosis of osteoporosis-related fracture during the menopause.

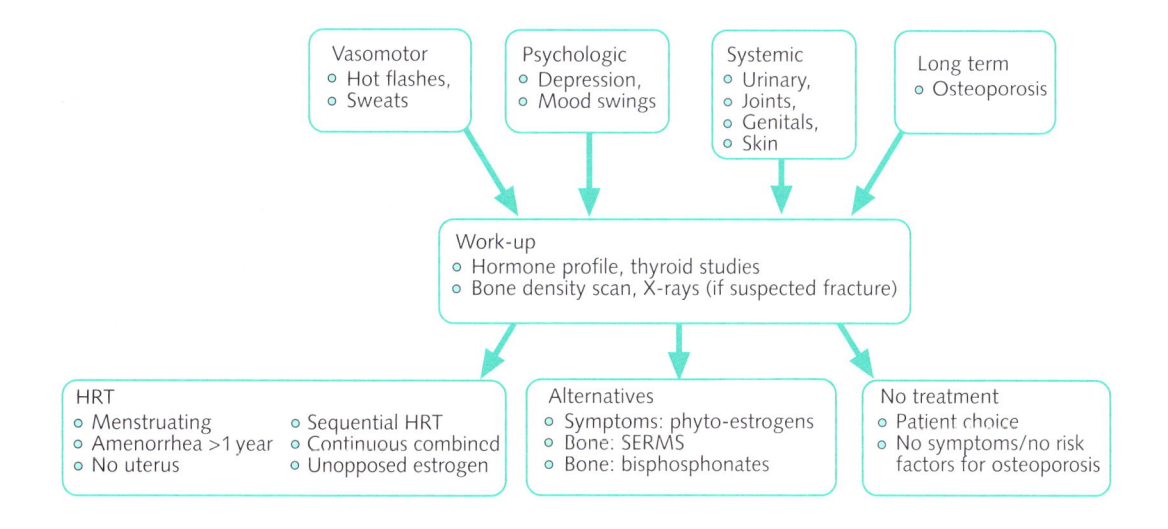

Fig. 9.5 Algorithm for the management of menopause (see Chapter 30 for details about investigation and treatment).

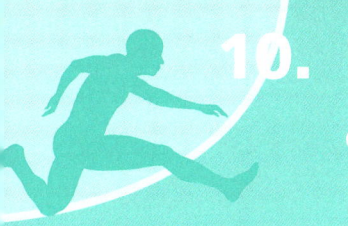

10. Bleeding in the Second and Third Trimesters of Pregnancy

Differential diagnosis of bleeding

Antepartum hemorrhage (APH) is defined as vaginal bleeding after 20 weeks' gestation, i.e. it is a separate entity from bleeding in early pregnancy associated with miscarriage (see Chapter 7). Figure 10.1 gives an overview of the differential diagnoses. Approximately 50% of cases of APH are caused by either a placenta previa or a placental abruption; the bleeding is unexplained in the remaining 50%.

> With any bleeding in pregnancy, the patient must be assessed and the amount of bleeding should be measured as accurately as possible; resuscitation of the patient must be initiated if necessary.

Differential diagnosis of APH

Source of hemorrhage	Type of hemorrhage
Uterine source (see Chapter 37)	Placenta previa
	Placental abruption
	Vasa previa
	Circumvallate placenta
Lower genital tract source (see Chapter 23)	Cervical ectropion
	Cervical polyp
	Cervical carcinoma
	Cervicitis
	Vaginitis
	Vulvar varicosities
Unknown origin	

Note: bloody mucoid vaginal loss may be the "show" associated with the onset of labor.

Fig. 10.1 Differential diagnosis of APH.

It is important to note that perinatal mortality following even minor episodes of bleeding is double that of a normal pregnancy. Also, a patient who presents with an APH has an associated risk of a PPH.

Relevant history

Figure 10.2 gives an algorithm for diagnosis of APH. Important points to elicit are:
- The amount of bleeding.
- Whether the blood is fresh or old.
- Any association with mucoid discharge.

There might be an obvious trigger event such as recent sexual intercourse (causing bleeding from a cervical lesion) or a motor vehicle accident (causing a placental abruption). The result of the patient's Pap smear is relevant to exclude a cervical cause for the bleeding. The patient should be asked about the presence of fetal movements.

The presence or absence of constant abdominal pain is particularly important, because it will help in the clinical differentiation between a placenta previa and an abruption (see Chapter 37). Remember that a placental abruption does not have to be associated with visible bleeding, as occurs with a concealed abruption (see Chapter 37).

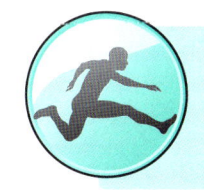

> The presence of abdominal pain typically distinguishes placental abruption from placenta previa.

The pain might be caused by uterine contractions. In the case of an abruption, the uterine myometrium becomes infiltrated by blood, which can initiate contractions or simply make the uterus irritable.

Bleeding in the Second and Third Trimesters of Pregnancy

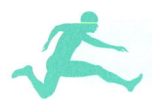

Fig. 10.2 Algorithm for APH.

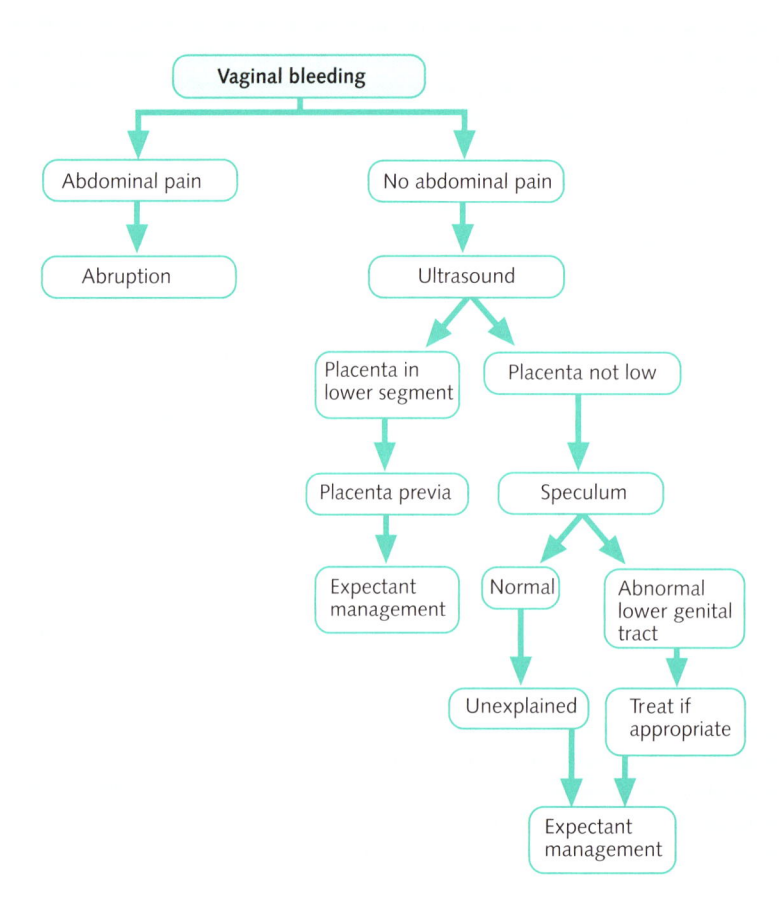

```
Vaginal bleeding
├── Abdominal pain → Abruption
└── No abdominal pain → Ultrasound
    ├── Placenta in lower segment → Placenta previa → Expectant management
    └── Placenta not low → Speculum
        ├── Normal → Unexplained → Expectant management
        └── Abnormal lower genital tract → Treat if appropriate
```

Physical exam

The aim is to assess maternal and fetal well-being.

Maternal well-being
- Pulse and blood pressure.
- Maternal pallor.
- Abdominal palpation to elicit uterine tenderness and/or uterine contractions.
- Speculum examination—*only if placenta previa has been excluded*—to exclude cervical abnormalities.
- Digital examination—*only if placenta previa has been excluded*—and/or the patient appears to be in labor, to assess cervical change.

Fetal well-being
- Abdominal palpation to assess the lie and presentation of the fetus, as well as engagement of the presenting part; it might be difficult to palpate fetal parts in the case of an abruption.
- Auscultation of the fetal heart to determine fetal viability.

Appropriate work-up

Blood tests
Initial investigations include taking blood for a hemoglobin level and T&S. Blood might need to be cross-matched if the bleeding is heavy, especially with a complete placenta previa. If a patient is rhesus negative, then she should be given anti-D immunoglobulin (Ig) to prevent hemolytic disease of the newborn in a future pregnancy.

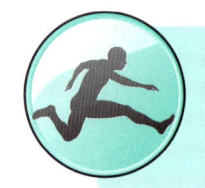

> Even with a minor degree of antepartum bleeding, the patient should be given anti-D Ig if she is rhesus negative.

50

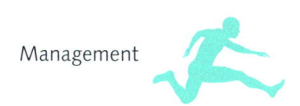

Fetal monitoring

Nonstress test (NST) should be done to confirm fetal well-being. It will also assist in monitoring uterine activity, either established contractions or an irritable uterus.

Ultrasound scan

Part of the routine 20-week anatomy scan is to check the placental site. An ultrasound scan should be arranged if it has not already been done. This can be performed by the transvaginal route to check the position of the leading placental edge in relation to the internal cervical os, particularly if the placenta is posterior. It is important to differentiate between complete and partial placenta previa (see Chapter 37).

The scan might also reveal a retroplacental hematoma, suggesting placental abruption, but this diagnosis is normally made on clinical grounds—a small hematoma might be missed, especially if the placenta is posterior.

Management

Management of the pregnancy depends on the amount of bleeding, the condition of the mother and the fetus, and the likely cause of the bleeding. If a cervical cause is suspected, then the patient might need to be referred for further investigations, such as colposcopy (see Chapter 23).

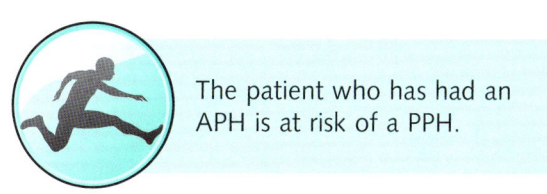

> The patient who has had an APH is at risk of a PPH.

Placenta previa

Conservative management is appropriate if the bleeding is only mild to moderate in the second trimester, especially in a preterm pregnancy. If delivery is anticipated in such a case, then intramuscular steroids should be administered to improve fetal lung maturity (see Chapter 38).

Inpatient care is advised for women with complete placenta previa in the third trimester because of the unpredictability of the timing of labor and the potential for heavy vaginal bleeding. If the placenta is within 2 cm of the internal cervical os, then cesarean section is necessary and should be performed by a senior obstetrician.

Placental abruption

Again, with mild to moderate bleeding, expectant management is appropriate. However, depending on the clinical scenario, including the amount of bleeding and the status of the fetus, immediate delivery might be necessary in the interests of the mother and the fetus.

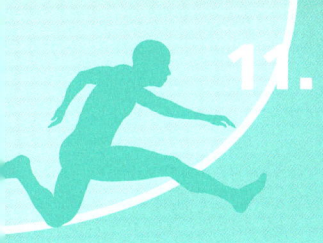

11. Large- or Small-for-Dates

Differential diagnosis

The growth of a pregnancy is estimated by measuring the fundal height (see Chapter 46). This takes into account the size of the fetus, the amniotic fluid volume, and the maternal structures, including the uterus. Before deciding whether it is abnormal or not, the dates of the LMP and the previous scan reports should be checked to confirm the gestation of the pregnancy, and also whether it is a singleton.

The differential diagnoses of size greater than dates (S>D) or size less than dates (S<D) can be considered in two categories:
1. Fetal/placental.
2. Maternal.

A fetus found to be S<D can be categorized according to its growth pattern:
- Small for gestational age (SGA): the fetus is small for the expected size at a certain gestation but continues to grow at a normal rate.
- Intrauterine growth restriction (IUGR): the fetus is small or normal-sized for the expected size at a certain gestation but the growth rate slows down as the pregnancy advances.

Relevant history

Past obstetric history
With respect to the S>D abdomen, a patient who had gestational diabetes in a previous pregnancy is at risk of developing the same condition again (see Chapter 36). This disorder puts the pregnancy at risk of fetal macrosomia and polyhydramnios (increased amniotic fluid volume).

A previous history of a baby that was SGA or IUGR, whether in relation to pre-eclampsia or not, increases the risk of a future pregnancy being affected.

Past gynecologic history
The patient might have been diagnosed with uterine fibroids or with an ovarian cyst, either prior to pregnancy or in early pregnancy. Both conditions can cause the fundal height to present as S>D.

Past medical history
Diabetes mellitus increases the chance of fetal macrosomia and polyhydramnios. The abdomen may seem S>D, as in gestational diabetes. Fetal infection with toxoplasmosis, cytomegalovirus (CMV), rubella, or herpes may produce polyhydramnios, so the mother should be asked about recent flu-like illness or rash.

Current maternal disease increases the risk of IUGR and, therefore, an S<D abdomen (see Chapter 36):
- Renal disease including renal transplantation.
- Hypertension.
- Congenital heart disease.
- Severe anemia.
- Sickle-cell disease.
- Systemic lupus erythematosus.
- Cystic fibrosis.

Family history
In relation to an S>D uterus, it is important to ask about a family history of diabetes mellitus. A positive family history will put the patient at increased risk of developing gestational diabetes in her current pregnancy.

There is also evidence that a family history of pre-eclampsia is relevant, and this disorder can be associated with IUGR (see Chapter 35).

Social history
The ethnic group of the patient can be relevant in an S<D patient. The growth charts used in most units were derived from Caucasian populations, in whom the average birth weight is greater than, for example, an Asian population. Hence, some units have developed customized growth charts for each particular patient group.

Smoking in pregnancy is a major cause of a fetus being SGA, so that the abdomen palpates as S<D. It affects growth in the third trimester. Alcohol and illegal drug use are also causes of being SGA, and so all these factors must be investigated in the antenatal history.

Large- or Small-for-Dates

Examination of the patient with an S>D or S<D uterus

Chapter 46 discusses examination of the pregnant patient and the uterus. This should include checking blood pressure, and urinalysis for proteinuria or glycosuria. The following should be noted on abdominal palpation in relation to S>D or S<D:
- Fundal height.
- Number of fetuses.
- Fetal lie.
- Amniotic fluid volume.
- Presence of uterine fibroids.
- Presence of adnexal masses.

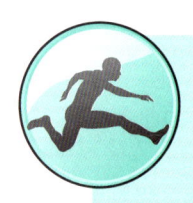

> If the fundal height is larger or smaller than expected for the gestation, then the first check is that the dates of the LMP and the first dating scan agree.

Investigation of the patient with an S>D or S<D uterus

Figures 11.1 and 11.2 provide algorithms for the investigation of the S>D and S<D uterus.

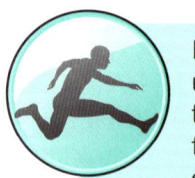

> If there is no evidence of uteroplacental insufficiency, then the other causes of the fetus being S<D should be excluded. Ultrasound scan should examine for fetal abnormalities and check for signs of in utero infection. Prior screening for chromosomal abnormalities should be reviewed.

Blood tests

In the case of an S>D patient, a glucose tolerance test should be arranged to establish whether

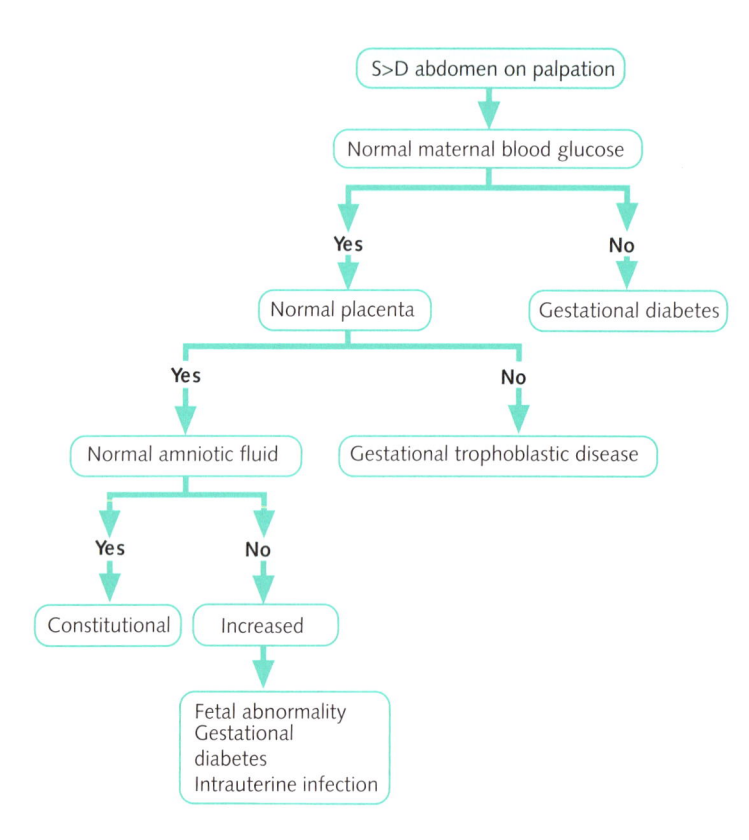

Fig. 11.1 Algorithm for an S>D abdomen.

54

Investigation of the patient with an S>D or S<D uterus

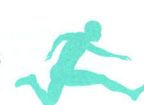

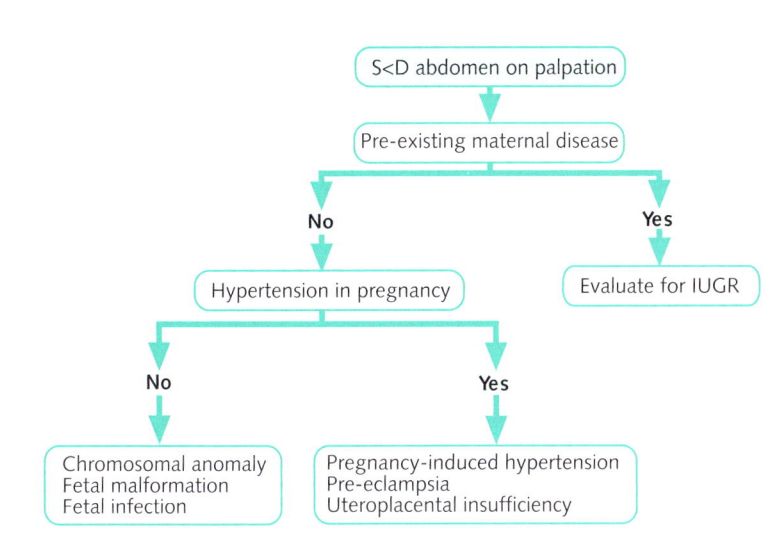

Fig. 11.2 Algorithm for an S<D abdomen.

```
S<D abdomen on palpation
        ↓
Pre-existing maternal disease
   ↓No            ↓Yes
Hypertension    Evaluate for IUGR
in pregnancy
 ↓No      ↓Yes
Chromosomal anomaly      Pregnancy-induced hypertension
Fetal malformation       Pre-eclampsia
Fetal infection          Uteroplacental insufficiency
```

gestational diabetes has developed (see Chapter 36). Fetal infection may be the cause if polyhydramnios is found in the absence of diabetes, so maternal antibodies (IgM and IgG) to *Toxoplasma* sp., rubella, CMV, and herpes should be investigated.

A patient who is S<D and is also hypertensive should be investigated for pre-eclampsia (see Chapter 35). The blood investigations include platelet count, liver function tests (LFTs), uric acid level, serum creatinine, and lactate dehydrogenase.

Ultrasound

Fetal ultrasound
Plotting ultrasound measurements of biparietal diameter (BPD), head circumference, abdominal circumference, and femur length on a growth chart is the main method of monitoring fetal growth, either S>D or S<D. In the case of S<D, then serial measurements, at least 2 weeks apart, should be taken to distinguish between SGA and IUGR.

There are two types of IUGR. Typically, asymmetric IUGR is associated with uteroplacental insufficiency, whereas symmetric IUGR is more commonly seen with other conditions. With uteroplacental insufficiency, the fetus preferentially diverts blood to the vital organs. There is less blood to the kidneys and, therefore, reduced production of amniotic fluid (oligohydramnios), as well as less storage of glycogen in the fetal liver. This results in a discrepancy between the growth of the fetal head and the abdomen.

> The fetal causes of oligohydramnios are related to its ability to produce urine, and thus amniotic fluid. The fetal causes of polyhydramnios are secondary to its inability to swallow amniotic fluid.

Placenta/amniotic fluid ultrasound
Trophoblastic disease is usually excluded at the 12-week dating scan by checking the structure of the placenta (see Chapter 29). Otherwise, this condition can present later in pregnancy with a uterus that palpates S>D.

A scan can also be used to measure the amniotic fluid volume. The amniotic fluid index (AFI) is the sum of the fluid pockets in four quadrants of the abdomen.

Maternal ultrasound
Ultrasound scan is useful to diagnose uterine fibroids or the presence of ovarian cysts.

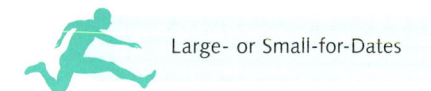

Doppler studies

In conjunction with growth scans and measurement of the amniotic fluid volume, Doppler waveforms of the blood flow in the uteroplacental and fetoplacental circulations can be used to assess the SGA or IUGR fetus. Increased placental vascular resistance, e.g. in pre-eclampsia, changes the pattern of the flow in the umbilical artery. There is normally flow towards the placenta during fetal diastole. However, as the placental resistance increases, diastolic flow becomes absent and then reversed. Other vessels can also be examined within the fetus, including the middle cerebral artery and the ductus venosus, to look for patterns of flow redistribution if the placental blood flow is insufficient.

Nonstress test

The NST can be used to assess the IUGR fetus. When not in labor, the tracing might be abnormal when the uteroplacental insufficiency is severe. The presence of the following should be excluded:
- Reduced variability.
- Bradycardia.
- Tachycardia.
- Decelerations.

The SGA fetus can only be distinguished from the IUGR fetus by serial growth scans. Further investigation includes Doppler studies and NSTs.

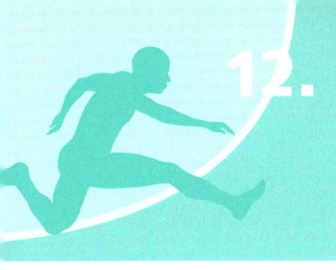

12. Abdominal Pain in the Second and Third Trimesters of Pregnancy

Differential diagnosis

The important differential diagnosis when assessing abdominal pain in pregnancy is whether the cause is obstetric or nonobstetric. Figure 12.1 shows the systems that might be involved.

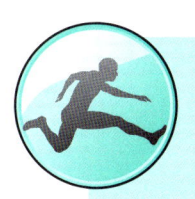

> Don't forget the nonobstetric causes of abdominal pain. Some of them are more common than the obstetric causes, such as a UTI.

Differential diagnosis of abdominal pain in 2nd and 3rd trimesters	
System involved	Pathology
Obstetric	Labor: preterm, term
	Placental abruption
	Symphysis pubis dysfunction
	Round ligament pain
	Pre-eclampsia/HELLP syndrome
	Acute fatty liver of pregnancy
Gynecologic	Ovarian cyst rupture/torsion/hemorrhage
	Uterine fibroid degeneration
Gastrointestinal	Constipation
	Appendicitis
	Gallstones/cholecystitis
	Pancreatitis
	Peptic ulcer
Genitourinary	Cystitis
	Pyelonephritis
	Renal stones/renal colic

Fig. 12.1 Differential diagnosis of abdominal pain in the second and third trimesters of pregnancy (HELLP: hemolysis, elevated liver enzymes, low platelets).

Relevant history

With diverse differential diagnoses, the history is very important to identify the cause of the pain. Figure 12.2 gives a summary of the points elicited from the history and examination that help to make the diagnosis.

Current obstetric history
This should include the current gestation and the parity. The antenatal history might be relevant. For example, if the patient has a history of pre-existing or pregnancy-induced hypertension (PIH; see Chapter 35), then she is at risk of pre-eclampsia and placental abruption (see Chapter 10). She might have already been admitted earlier in the pregnancy with suspected preterm labor (see Chapter 38). A urinary tract infection might have been treated earlier in this pregnancy.

Presenting symptoms
As with any history of pain, its characteristics are important:
- Nature: continuous or intermittent.
- Quality: stabbing, burning, tightening, etc.
- Duration.
- Site: generalized or specific.
- Radiation: to the pelvis or to the back.
- Exacerbating factors.

It is important to ask about other symptoms, particularly GI and genitourinary, such as dysuria, frequency of bowel habits, or nausea.

Past obstetric history
There might be a history of pre-eclampsia or preterm labor in a previous pregnancy, which puts the patient at increased risk in her current pregnancy.

Past gynecologic/medical/surgical history
Ultrasound scans earlier in the current pregnancy might have alerted the medical staff to the presence of an ovarian cyst or uterine fibroids. There might be a history of peptic ulcer disease or

57

Abdominal Pain in the Second and Third Trimesters of Pregnancy

Making a diagnosis from the history and examination	
Differential diagnosis	Clinical features
Labor (see Chapter 40)	Intermittent pain, usually regular in frequency, associated with tightening of the abdominal wall. The presenting part of the fetus is usually engaged. Vaginal examination shows cervical change
Placental abruption (see Chapter 37)	Mild or severe pain, more commonly associated with vaginal bleeding. The uterus is usually tender on palpation and can be irritable or tense. There might be symptoms and signs of pre-eclampsia
Symphysis pubis dysfunction	Pain is usually low and central in the abdomen just above the symphysis pubis, which is tender on palpation. Symptoms are worse with movement
Round ligament pain	Commonly described as sharp pain, which is bilateral and often associated with movement
Pre-eclampsia/HELLP syndrome (see Chapter 35)	Epigastric or right upper quadrant pain, associated with nausea and vomiting, headache and visual disturbances. On examination, there is hypertension and proteinuria
Acute fatty liver of pregnancy	Epigastric or right upper quadrant pain, associated with nausea, vomiting, anorexia and malaise
Ovarian cyst (see Chapter 22)	Unilateral pain, which is intermittent and might be associated with vomiting
Uterine fibroid (see Chapter 20)	Pain is localized and constant. Fibroid is noted on palpation and is tender
Constipation	Usually suggested by the history, can cause lower abdominal discomfort and bloating
Appendicitis	Pain associated with nausea and vomiting. Tenderness with guarding and rebound might be localized to the right lower quadrant
Gallstones/cholecystitis	Right upper quadrant or epigastric pain, which might radiate to the back or to the shoulder. Tenderness in the right upper quadrant and pyrexia with cholecystitis
Pancreatitis	Epigastric pain radiating to the back, associated with nausea and vomiting. Occurs most commonly in the third trimester
Peptic ulcer	Epigastric pain associated with food. There might be heartburn, nausea and even hematemesis
Cystitis	Usually suggested by history, with pain and tenderness in the low abdomen or suprapubically
Renal stones/renal colic/pyelonephritis	Flank pain that might radiate to the abdomen and groin, possibly associated with vomiting and rigors. Pyrexia is present with pyelonephritis

Fig. 12.2 Making a diagnosis from the history and examination.

gallstones. The patient might have had a previous appendectomy or a cholecystectomy.

Physical exam

General examination
As with any clinical examination, the general condition of the pregnant patient should be assessed, including:

- Temperature.
- Pulse.
- Blood pressure.
- Respiratory rate.
- Cardiovascular system.
- Respiratory system.

Abdominal palpation
The abdomen should be inspected for any previous operation scars. In the presence of a

gravid uterus, abdominal palpation to establish the cause of the symptoms might not be straightforward. Compared with examining a nonpregnant patient, the site of the tenderness might not be typical. Examining a nonpregnant patient who has an ovarian cyst torsion is likely to elicit tenderness and guarding in the lower quadrant. Depending on the gestation, this might not be so specific in a pregnant patient because the gravid uterus might be interfering with the usual anatomical markings. Tenderness at McBurney's point, which is typical of appendicitis (see *Crash Course, Surgery*) might also be difficult to elicit in a patient who is late in the second or in the third trimester of pregnancy.

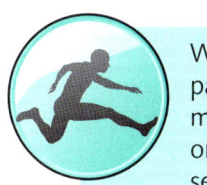

> When examining an obstetric patient, remember that she might feel faint if she lies flat on her back for too long, secondary to pressure on the large vessels reducing venous return to the heart and causing supine hypotension. She should be examined with a left lateral tilt.

The uterus should be palpated to determine:
- Lie, presentation, engagement depending on gestation (see Chapter 46).
- Presence of uterine contractions.
- Generalized or specific uterine tenderness.
- Presence of uterine fibroids.

Vaginal examination
A speculum examination is appropriate if there is vaginal bleeding, to exclude cervical causes (see Chapter 37). A vaginal examination may be indicated if the history and abdominal palpation suggest that the patient is in labor, in order to determine if there is cervical change (see Chapter 46).

Appropriate work-up

Figure 12.3 gives a summary of the investigations that should be considered and Fig. 12.4 provides an algorithm for the investigation of abdominal pain.

Summary of laboratory studies for abdominal pain
- CBC
- Clotting studies
- T&S
- Urea/electrolytes
- LFTs
- Glucose
- Urinalysis/clean catch urine/24-h urine collection for protein
- NST
- Ultrasound scan of the uterus, ovaries, kidneys, liver, and gallbladder

Fig. 12.3 Summary of laboratory studies to be considered in a patient with abdominal pain.

Blood tests
Complete blood count/clotting studies
The CBC can show a reduced hemoglobin if the patient has been bleeding, e.g. in the case of a placental abruption. The platelet count might be low in association with pre-eclampsia or HELLP syndrome, possibly associated with abnormal clotting studies. A T&S sample of serum is appropriate if there is bleeding, in case cross-matched blood is required for transfusion. With the nonobstetric causes of pain, the white blood cell count will be raised if there is infection, for example, with pyelonephritis or cholecystitis.

Urea/electrolytes/glucose/liver function tests
These tests might be abnormal in pre-eclampsia or HELLP syndrome, with raised urea and creatinine suggesting hemoconcentration, and with raised liver transaminases. Serum uric acid is high in pre-eclampsia and in acute fatty liver, whereas in the latter there is also hypoglycemia.

Urinalysis/clean catch urine sample
In pre-eclampsia, there is proteinuria on dipstick urinalysis, and a 24-h urine collection to quantify the amount of protein might be indicated to determine the severity of the disease. Proteinuria can also be present with a UTI and might be associated with microscopic hematuria, particularly in the presence of renal stones.

Nonstress test
The fetal heart should be auscultated before 24 weeks' gestation with a doptone. An NST is

59

Abdominal Pain in the Second and Third Trimesters of Pregnancy

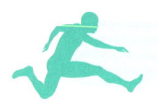

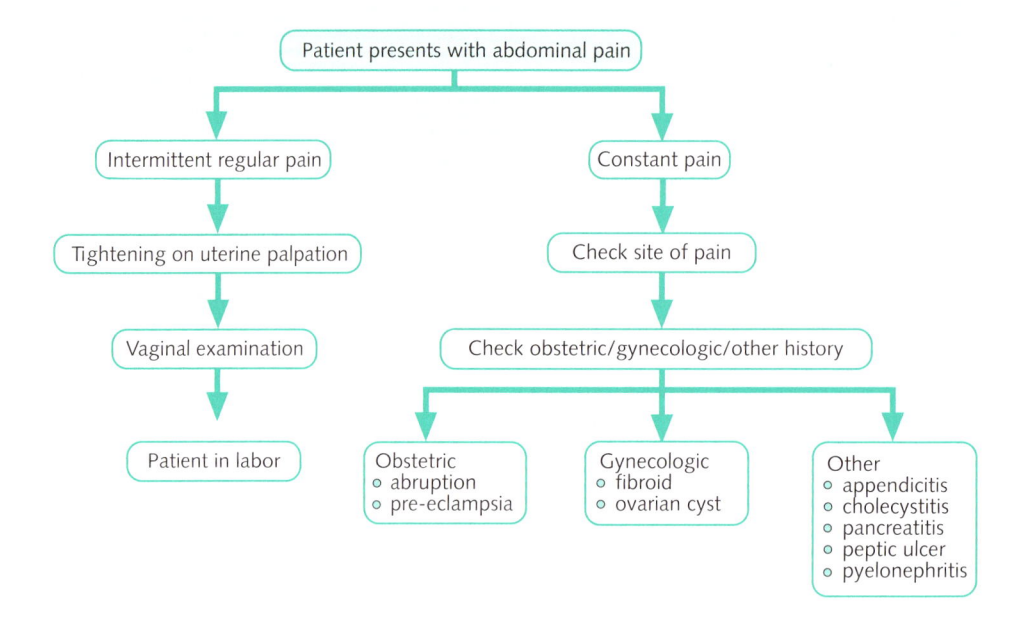

```
Patient presents with abdominal pain
   │
   ├──────────────────────────────┐
Intermittent regular pain      Constant pain
   │                               │
Tightening on uterine palpation  Check site of pain
   │                               │
Vaginal examination            Check obstetric/gynecologic/other history
   │                               │
Patient in labor      ┌────────────┼────────────┐
                   Obstetric    Gynecologic    Other
                   ○ abruption  ○ fibroid     ○ appendicitis
                   ○ pre-eclampsia ○ ovarian cyst ○ cholecystitis
                                                ○ pancreatitis
                                                ○ peptic ulcer
                                                ○ pyelonephritis
```

Fig. 12.4 Algorithm for abdominal pain.

performed after this gestation (see Chapter 16) and will help determine fetal well-being, particularly in the case of placental abruption. The recording will also detect uterine activity, including the presence and frequency of uterine contractions.

Ultrasound scan (uterus/ovaries/kidneys/liver/gallbladder)

An obstetric scan might show a retroplacental hematoma in the case of severe placental abruption. If preterm delivery is necessary, e.g. in acute fatty liver, fetal well-being and growth should be assessed, and the fetal weight estimated.

For the other systems, ultrasound examination can assist diagnosis and management. An ovarian cyst might be seen if hemorrhage, rupture, or torsion of the cyst is suspected. Renal stones or gallstones can be visualized.

Management

This depends on the cause of the pain and the gestation of the pregnancy. With regard to the obstetric causes, cesarean section or induction of labor might need to be considered. In severe pre-eclampsia, for example, the benefits of delivery to the mother's health can outweigh the risks to the fetus of preterm birth. Placental abruption might be severe enough to compromise the fetus, and then delivery should be expedited.

However, most conditions can be managed conservatively with treatment such as analgesia, e.g. with renal stones, or antibiotics for pyelonephritis. Multidisciplinary management with other specialties might be appropriate, e.g. with gastroenterology in a patient suspected of having gallstones or a peptic ulcer. Occasionally, an operation is necessary for an acute appendicitis or for ovarian torsion.

Remember to coordinate with other specialists in the management of conditions such as renal stones or cholecystitis. In the case of preterm labor, discuss management with the pediatricians.

13. Hypertension in Pregnancy

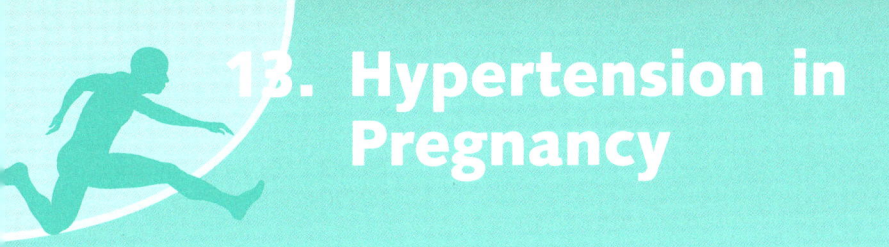

Differential diagnosis

Blood pressure problems in pregnancy can be divided into two groups:
1. Pre-existing hypertension, where the blood pressure was high prior to pregnancy and, therefore, presents either as a woman who is known to have hypertension or because a reading taken in the first trimester is high.
2. Pre-eclampsia, a multisystem disorder, one of whose manifestations is high blood pressure, but where renal, liver, and clotting functions are also affected.

History and examination are aimed at differentiating these problems, remembering that the two may coexist, as essential hypertension predisposes to pre-eclampsia.

History

Chief complaint

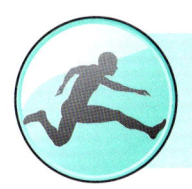

> The absence of symptoms does not exclude the diagnosis of pre-eclampsia.

The woman is often asymptomatic of her high blood pressure, which is picked up as part of the routine antenatal check, but she might be experiencing symptoms of pre-eclampsia (Fig. 13.1). You must ask specifically about:
- Headache.
- Visual disturbance (in the form of flashing lights, not the "black dots" associated with postural hypotension).
- Right upper quadrant or epigastric pain (due to edema of the liver capsule).
- Facial swelling.

Past gynecologic history
A history of high blood pressure when taking the OCP indicates a susceptibility to high blood pressure in pregnancy.

Past obstetric history
If the blood pressure was high in previous pregnancies because of essential hypertension, it is very unlikely to be normal in this pregnancy. Pre-eclampsia, however, does not always recur with every pregnancy; it is most common in primigravida or in the first pregnancy with a new partner.

Past medical history
Conditions that predispose to hypertension include diabetes and renal and cardiac disease.

Family history
Pre-eclampsia does "run in families," with the strongest association being if the patient's sister was affected in her pregnancy.

Drug history
Some women with hypertension prior to pregnancy might already be on medication. This might need to be changed to avoid drugs contraindicated in pregnancy (see Chapter 40).

Physical exam

The points to note are shown in Fig. 13.1.

General examination
- Severe pre-eclampsia can cause an altered level of consciousness.
- Look for facial edema—if you are not sure if her face is swollen, ask her partner or family member if she looks different.
- Check the blood pressure.
- Check the reflexes and examine for clonus.
- Perform fundoscopy to look for papilledema in pre-eclampsia. Retinopathy might be seen in severe, chronic cases of essential hypertension.

Hypertension in Pregnancy

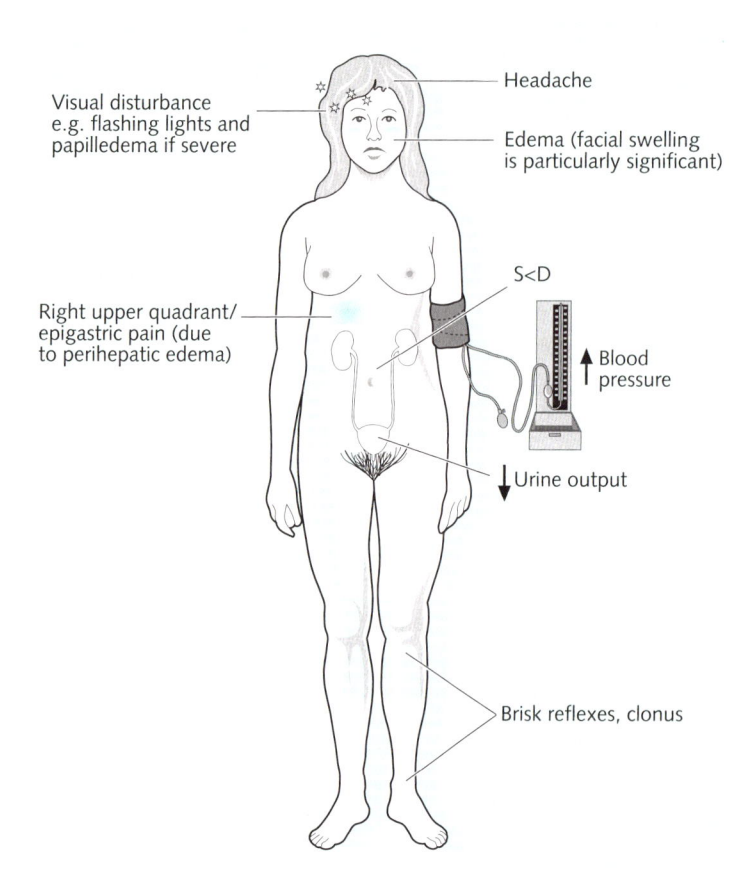

Fig. 13.1 Signs and symptoms of pre-eclampsia.

- Visual disturbance e.g. flashing lights and papilledema if severe
- Headache
- Edema (facial swelling is particularly significant)
- Right upper quadrant/epigastric pain (due to perihepatic edema)
- S<D
- ↑ Blood pressure
- ↓ Urine output
- Brisk reflexes, clonus

Blood pressure should be measured with the patient sitting or lying propped on pillows, with the arm the same level as the heart, using the disappearance rather than the muffling of sound as the cut-off for the diastolic. The correct size of cuff must be used; if a small cuff is used for a large woman, then the blood pressure will be artificially (and worryingly) high.

Abdominal palpation
- Feel for liver tenderness.
- Palpate the uterus to see whether the growth seems appropriate for the gestational age.

Work-up

Figure 13.2 provides an algorithm for the investigation of hypertension in pregnancy.

Urinalysis

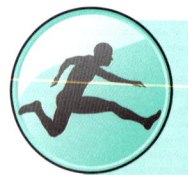

If told that you are to see a pregnant woman with raised blood pressure, one of your first questions must be "What does the urinalysis show?" The presence of proteinuria raises the suspicion of pre-eclampsia.

The urine should be dipped. The presence of protein might be due to pre-eclampsia, but it could also be the result of contamination with

Work-up

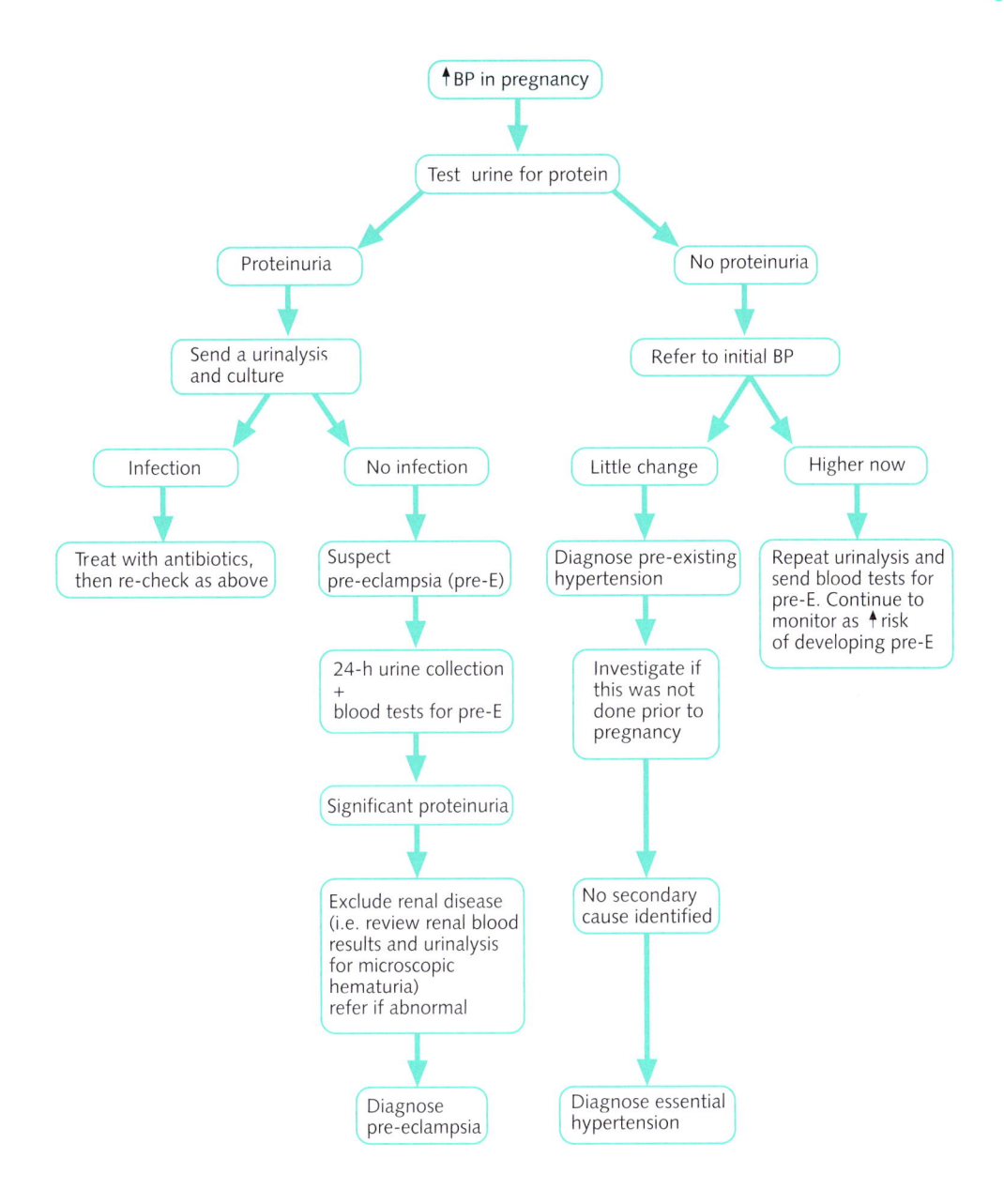

```
                    ↑BP in pregnancy
                           │
                           ▼
                  Test urine for protein
                    ╱             ╲
             Proteinuria        No proteinuria
                 │                    │
                 ▼                    ▼
          Send a urinalysis     Refer to initial BP
          and culture            ╱          ╲
           ╱         ╲      Little change   Higher now
      Infection   No infection      │            │
          │          │              ▼            ▼
          ▼          ▼        Diagnose      Repeat urinalysis and
    Treat with     Suspect    pre-existing  send blood tests for
    antibiotics,   pre-eclampsia hypertension pre-E. Continue to
    then re-check  (pre-E)        │           monitor as ↑risk
    as above         │            ▼           of developing pre-E
                     ▼       Investigate if
              24-h urine     this was not
              collection     done prior to
              + blood tests  pregnancy
              for pre-E          │
                     │           ▼
                     ▼      No secondary
              Significant   cause identified
              proteinuria        │
                     │           ▼
                     ▼      Diagnose essential
              Exclude renal hypertension
              disease (i.e. review
              renal blood results
              and urinalysis for
              microscopic hematuria)
              refer if abnormal
                     │
                     ▼
              Diagnose
              pre-eclampsia
```

Fig. 13.2 Algorithm for hypertension in pregnancy.

blood, amniotic fluid (if the membranes have ruptured), or vaginal discharge, or be caused by a UTI. It is important that the sample is a "clean catch."

Check the other findings on dipping. Lots of leukocytes and protein might indicate UTI, especially if nitrites and/or blood are also present. Even if a UTI is suspected, do not dismiss the proteinuria, because the consequences of missing pre-eclampsia could be grave. Send a urinalysis for microscopy and culture, but continue checking for pre-eclampsia.

To quantify proteinuria, a 24-h collection should be performed. The result is suggestive of pre-eclampsia if the 24-h urine protein is more than 0.3 g.

Blood tests

Uric acid, renal function tests, LFTs, a CBC, and a clotting screen are sent. The results would be expected to be normal in women with essential hypertension (unless there was an underlying cause for her hypertension, such as renal disease) but become deranged as pre-eclampsia develops (Fig. 13.3). In pre-eclampsia the following abnormalities may be found on investigation:
- Raised serum urate/uric acid.
- Raised transaminases (e.g. alanine transaminase [ALT] and aspartate transaminase [AST]).
- Raised hematocrit.
- Decreased platelets.

Ultrasound

Pre-eclampsia can cause IUGR, oligohydramnios, and abnormal Dopplers because of placental insufficiency. Essential hypertension, if poorly controlled, can also affect fetal growth.

Changed parameters in pre-eclampsia
Platelets ↓
Serum urate ↑
Liver transaminases (ALT, AST) ↑
Serum bilirubin ↑
Serum urea and creatinine ↑
Urinary protein ↑

Fig. 13.3 Changed parameters in pre-eclampsia.

Supplementary investigations

If there is any suspicion of an underlying cause for hypertension in pregnancy then it should be further investigated with a chest X-ray, electrocardiogram (ECG) and echocardiogram, and a 24-h urine collection for creatinine and (if pheochromocytoma is suspected) for catecholamines.

14. Stillbirth

The terms "stillbirth" and "intrauterine fetal demise" are used to describe the intrauterine death of a fetus after 20 weeks' gestation, which is diagnosed before or during labor or at delivery. The woman might present with symptoms of the event that caused the baby to die or simply because she has not felt fetal movements. Figure 14.1 summarizes the common causes of stillbirth.

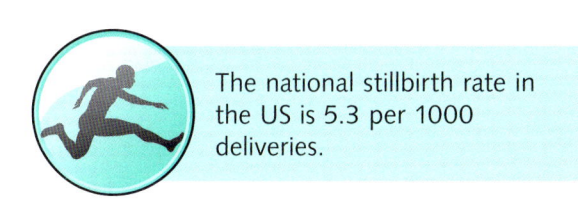

> The national stillbirth rate in the US is 5.3 per 1000 deliveries.

If fetal death is suspected antenatally, then an ultrasound scan is performed to look for absence of fetal heart activity. It is recommended that the finding of intrauterine death is confirmed by a second sonographer. The rate of stillbirth varies with maternal age (Fig. 14.2), being lowest when the mother is aged between 25 and 29.

History

Finding out when the mother last felt fetal movements can help to determine how recently fetal death occurred, but this will not help with the diagnosis of the underlying cause unless it can be linked to a particular occurrence.

History of the pregnancy
The following points might be helpful:
- Rhesus group: if the woman is rhesus negative, then isoimmunization is a possibility.
- Down syndrome screening: if the woman is high risk, a chromosomal abnormality might be present.
- Ultrasound for anomaly/growth: any structural abnormalities or a history of IUGR increase the risk of stillbirth.

Causes of stillbirth	
Type of condition	Cause of stillbirth
Maternal condition	Diabetes (pre-existing and gestational)
	Pre-eclampsia
	Sepsis
	Cholestasis of pregnancy
	Acute fatty liver
	Thrombophilias, e.g. protein C and protein S deficiency, factor V Leiden mutation, antithrombin III deficiency
Fetal condition	Infection: *Toxoplasma*, *Listeria*, *Syphilis*, parvovirus
	Chromosomal abnormality
	Structural abnormality
	Rhesus disease leading to severe anemia
	Twin-to-twin transfusion syndrome (affects monochorionic twins only)
	IUGR
	Alloimmune thrombocytopenia
Placental condition	Postmaturity
	Abruption
	Placenta previa: significant bleed
	Cord prolapse

Fig. 14.1 Causes of stillbirth.

- Recurrent APH: repeated small abruptions can compromise fetal well-being and cause IUGR.

Ask about any leaking of fluid or bleeding in the recent history. Ruptured membranes allow infection to ascend and infect the membranes and placenta (chorioamnionitis) and, therefore, the fetus. Bleeding might be due to abruption. Abruption and chorioamnionitis would both cause uterine pain. Bleeding from placenta previa is

65

Stillbirth

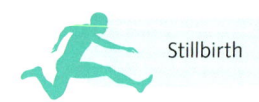

Rates of stillbirth in relation to maternal age

Maternal age	Rate of stillbirth per 1000 deliveries
<25	5
25–29	4
30–34	4.3
35–39	5
40–44	6.5
45 and over	7

Fig. 14.2 Rates of stillbirth in relation to maternal age.

painless; the mother might have had a scan earlier in pregnancy that diagnosed a low-lying placenta.

Signs of maternal illness (fever, feeling unwell, flu-like symptoms, GI upset) are also suggestive of fetal infection. *Listeria*, *Toxoplasma*, and parvovirus can cause very mild illness in the mother, but can cause death in the fetus.

Rhesus disease and twin-to-twin transfusion syndrome (TTTS) cause sudden polyhydramnios, so the mother might describe feeling suddenly larger.

> If one twin dies in a dichorionic twin pregnancy, then the chance of the other twin dying is <5%; so, the mother can be managed expectantly if the pregnancy is preterm. There is a risk that she could develop coagulopathy, so her platelets need to be monitored regularly. If one of a pair of monochorionic twins dies, compromise of the other twin is far more likely and so delivery is advisable.

Cholestasis of pregnancy causes a characteristic pattern of itching, affecting particularly the palms of the hands and the soles of the feet (see Chapter 36).

Past obstetric history

If the woman has had a previous stillbirth, then it is important to find out if an underlying cause was discovered. Rhesus disease gets more severe with successive pregnancies, so a first child might be unaffected or suffer only mild jaundice. Gestational diabetes in a previous pregnancy is likely to recur.

Past medical history

Maternal medical conditions, such as diabetes and renal disease, increase the risk of stillbirth. A personal or family history of thrombosis might point to an underlying thrombophilia.

Physical exam

General examination

The mother's pulse, blood pressure, and temperature are taken. Maternal infection can cause tachycardia and fever. A significant bleed due to abruption or bleeding placenta previa can cause hypovolemic shock. The itching of cholestasis might be evident from scratch marks on the skin—there is no rash in cholestasis of pregnancy.

Examination of the uterus

Assess the following:
- Uterine size: small-for-dates suggests IUGR or that the fetus died some time ago; large-for-dates might be due to polyhydramnios (diabetes, isoimmunization, TTTS).
- Uterine consistency: abruption causes the uterus to feel tense, tender, and hard, and it might be irritable (i.e. palpation provokes contractions). With chorioamnionitis the uterus will be soft and tender and might be irritable.
- Fetal presentation: breech presentation is associated with fetal abnormality.

Work-up

Urinalysis

The urine is dipped, looking particularly for protein as a sign of pre-eclampsia. If significant proteinuria is found, then a 24-h collection is commenced, and a urine culture is sent to exclude infection.

Blood tests

The tests below are sent to investigate the cause of fetal death. At the time of diagnosis a CBC and a sample for T&S should be sent due to the risk of disseminated intravascular coagulation (DIC) following stillbirth:
- Glycosylated hemoglobin (HbA1c): if raised, this suggests maternal diabetes.
- Coombs' test to look for evidence of rhesus disease.
- Infection screen: blood cultures and antibody levels for *Toxoplasma*, parvovirus, *Listeria*, and syphilis.
- Kleihauer–Betke (KB) test: looks for evidence of fetomaternal hemorrhage, as can occur with abruption.
- Thrombophilia screen.

Ultrasound scan

Once the diagnosis of fetal death has been made, a scan will not add much information unless the parents do not wish a postmortem of the baby, in which case the scan is an opportunity to look for evidence of internal structural anomalies.

Pathology

Parents are encouraged to allow a postmortem/autopsy examination of their baby so that all possible information is collected. They should be reassured that this will not prevent them from arranging a funeral or cremation for the baby. The placenta should be sent to pathology for evaluation. In addition, the parents should be offered genetic analysis of the fetal tissue for karyotype. If the parents do not consent to the full post-mortem, then they should be offered a more limited examination consisting of X-rays and external examination of the baby, or solely examination of the placenta.

Management of stillbirth

In most cases, labor is induced using prostaglandins and oxytocin. Occasionally, a cesarean section is performed because the mother is unwell and delivery needs to be expedited, or because induction of labor would pose a significant risk, e.g. if the mother had had several cesarean sections in the past.

Some women will opt to continue the pregnancy. More than 90% will spontaneously labor within 3 weeks. By 4 weeks after fetal death (which might have occurred some time before diagnosis) there is a 1 in 4 risk of developing coagulopathy, so these women should have their platelets monitored regularly.

> After death the fetal body releases procoagulant factors into the mother's circulation, leading to intravascular coagulation, with consumption of clotting factors and platelets, and deposition of fibrin, resulting in DIC, which can cause catastrophic hemorrhage.

After delivery, the parents should be encouraged to hold their baby. Footprints, handprints, and photographs can be taken and the parents might choose to have some form of blessing or religious ceremony at this stage.

Follow-up

Psychological and social support is extremely important. The mother should be seen approximately 1 week after delivery by the physician for a post-partum visit. Information about parent support groups should be given.

A follow-up appointment should be made with the physician, who often chooses to see the parents in the gynecology rather than the prenatal clinic. All the results will be reviewed and any questions can be answered, even if only to explain that the stillbirth was unexplained.

15. Failure to Progress in Labor

Labor and delivery require the interaction of three components: the passage, the passenger, and power—as part of a dynamic process:
- Passage: the shape and size of the hard bony pelvis and soft tissues.
- Passenger: the size and presentation of the fetus.
- Power: this is both involuntary (strength and frequency of uterine contractions) and voluntary (diaphragm and abdominal muscles).

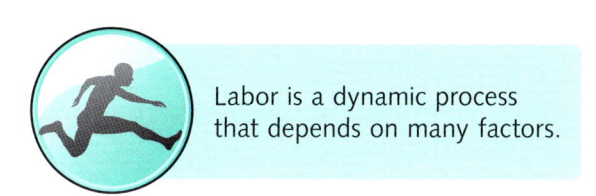

> Labor is a dynamic process that depends on many factors.

Any of these factors can be involved in the failure of labor to progress normally. Once the diagnosis of labor has been made (see Chapter 40), a primiparous patient is expected to progress at approximately 1 cm/h and a multiparous patient at approximately 2 cm/h.

A labor curve (see Fig. 40.1) gives a graphic representation of this progress; hence, failure to progress normally can easily be detected (Fig. 15.1). Examination and investigation of the causes of the resultant prolonged labor should be considered in terms of the three factors mentioned above. Figure 15.2 shows the differential diagnoses that should be excluded.

Relevant history

Passages
Bony passages
Figure 40.16 gives some of the causes of abnormalities of the bony passages that can cause failure to progress in labor.

Soft passages
The patient might have previously been diagnosed with fibroids, either prior to pregnancy or on antenatal ultrasound scans. A cervical fibroid can interfere with cervical dilatation.

A history of cervical surgery may cause scarring, which can then prevent cervical dilatation. This is particularly relevant with a cold knife cone procedure, but seems to be less common with the loop electrosurgical excision procedure (LEEP) that is more frequently performed nowadays (see Chapter 23).

Female circumcision (also known as female genital mutilation) usually makes the vaginal

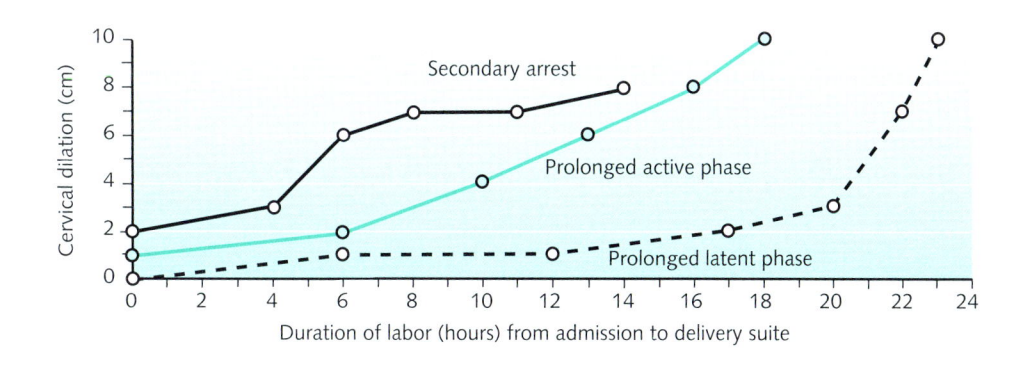

Fig. 15.1 Abnormal patterns of cervical dilatation in labor.

Failure to Progress in Labor

Causes of failure to progress in labor	
Bony passages	Abnormal shaped pelvis
	Cephalopelvic disproportion
Soft passages	Uterine/cervical fibroids
	Cervical stenosis
	Circumcision
Passenger	Fetal size
	Fetal abnormality
	Fetal malposition
	Fetal malpresentation
Power	Lack of coordinated regular strong uterine contractions

Fig. 15.2 Differential diagnosis of the causes of failure to progress in labor.

Power
There need to be three or four uterine contractions every 10 min, each lasting approximately 60 s, to maintain adequate progress in labor. This can be assessed by asking the patient or checking the tocometer.

> In the presence of efficient contractions, a malposition of the vertex usually corrects; this might require an oxytocin infusion to improve contractions, particularly in a primiparous patient.

introitus smaller and thus can affect progression to normal vaginal delivery in the second stage of labor.

Passenger
It is often useful, in a multiparous patient, to check the weights of previous deliveries as an assessment of ability to deliver the current infant.

A history of diabetes, either long standing or gestational, puts the fetus at risk of macrosomia, which means that the fetal size might be out of proportion to the size of the maternal pelvis (cephalopelvic disproportion [CPD]; see Chapter 40), resulting in failure to progress in labor.

Antenatal diagnosis of a fetal abnormality can inhibit normal progress. For example, a congenital goiter causes extension of the neck so that the normal process of flexion cannot occur. In anencephaly, a form of spina bifida in which the fetal skull fails to develop, the head is less able to engage and, therefore, labor might not progress normally.

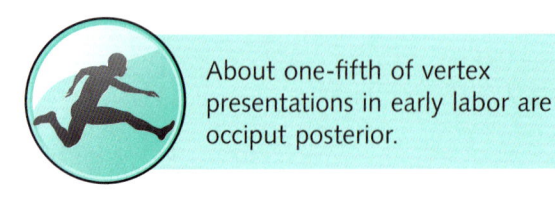

> About one-fifth of vertex presentations in early labor are occiput posterior.

Physical exam

Examination of the patient should always include checking the color of the amniotic fluid to exclude meconium. This is relevant when considering fetal well-being in a patient who is making slow progress. It should be assessed in conjunction with the fetal monitoring (see Chapter 16).

Passages and passenger
Short stature puts the patient at risk of CPD; so, traditionally, maternal height is checked at the booking visit (see Chapter 45). Chapter 46 discusses in detail the examination of the maternal abdomen and the vagina to assess the size and position of the fetus. Figure 15.3 lists the factors that should be checked.

Labor can be slow if the fetus is not in a longitudinal lie. Similarly, a malpresentation (see Chapter 39) or a malposition (see Chapter 40) causes failure to progress. The uterus should always be palpated to check engagement, i.e. how much of the fetal head is palpable above the pelvic brim.

When the cervix is fully effaced at the onset of labor, it is thin. However, if progress is slow, then it becomes thicker on palpation as it gets edematous. A cervical fibroid should be excluded.

Figure 15.4 demonstrates how the station of the presenting part is assessed. Caput and molding (see Chapter 40) increase as the progress of the labor slows. Molding is graded according to whether the overlapping of the skull bones is reducible or not.

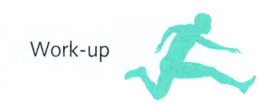

Power

Abdominal palpation assesses the following features of the contractions:
- Frequency.
- Strength.
- Length.

Work-up

Assessment of the passage and the passenger is made clinically as described above (Fig. 15.5). The tocometer can be used to assess frequency of

Examination of the patient who is making slow progress in labor	
Type of examination	Procedure
Abdominal examination	Uterine size by measuring fundal height
	Fetal lie
	Fetal presentation
	Fetal position
	Engagement
Vaginal examination	Cervical dilatation
	Cervical thickness or effacement
	Station
	Position of the presenting part
	Presence of caput or molding
	Pelvic outlet (less commonly performed nowadays)

Fig. 15.3 Examination of the patient who is making slow progress in labor.

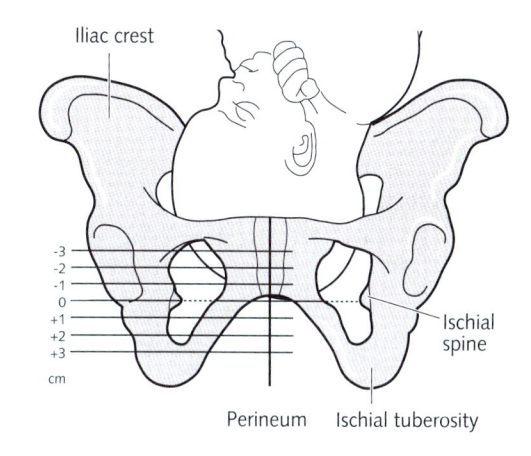

Fig. 15.4 Station of the head.

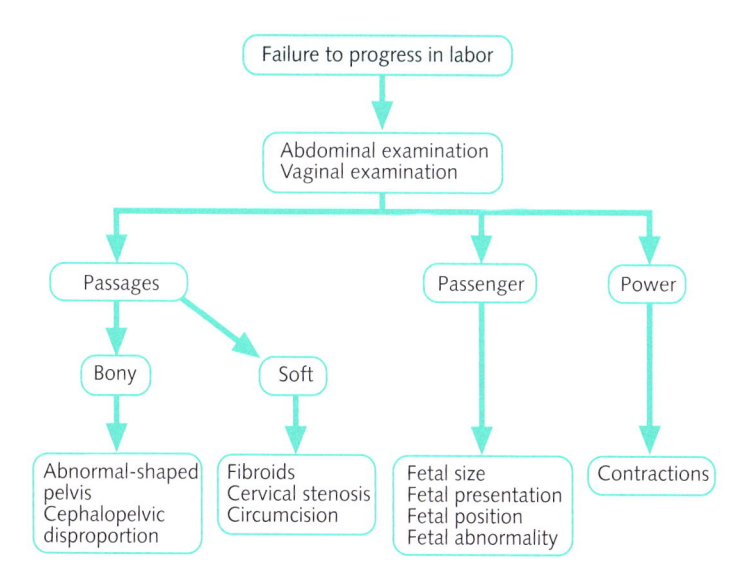

Fig. 15.5 Algorithm for failure to progress in labor.

71

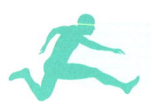

uterine contractions, in conjunction with uterine palpation. The fetal heart rate (FHR) tracing also assesses the risk of fetal hypoxia (see Chapter 16).

Management

This depends on the cause. Artificial rupture of the membranes (AROM) is thought to release local prostaglandins and can increase the rate of labor progression. The strength and frequency of the uterine contractions can also be improved.

An intrauterine pressure catheter (IUPC) may be inserted to measure the strength of contractions. If the contractions do not seem adequate, then pitocin may be started. Adequacy of contractions is assessed by montevideo units (MVU). The strength of each contraction in mmHg is multiplied by the frequency of contractions in 10 min. The contractile force must exceed 200 MVU/10 min for labor to be considered adequate. An arrest disorder is not diagnosed until adequate contractions for 2 h do not produce cervical change.

Regular, strong contractions will help to correct a fetal malposition by rotating the head against the pelvic floor muscles, as well as improving descent. However, caution must be exercised in a multiparous patient. Generally, labor proceeds more rapidly in a second pregnancy. Therefore, if progress is slow, fetal size and the risk of CPD must be considered so that excessive contractions do not put the patient at risk of uterine rupture.

Failure to progress in the second stage of labor should be assessed in the manner already described and instrumental delivery considered (see Chapter 41). If the head is almost crowning, then an episiotomy might be all that is necessary.

> Oxytocin infusions can correct prolonged labor, but particular care must be taken to exclude CPD if there is secondary arrest in a multiparous patient.

16. Abnormal Fetal Heart Rate Tracing in Labor

The FHR tracing is a form of electronic FHR monitoring used to evaluate fetal well-being before and during labor. It has been used increasingly in the US since the 1970s, with the aim of detecting fetal hypoxia before it causes perinatal mortality or cerebral palsy.

However, the expected reduction in hypoxia-induced intrapartum perinatal mortality has not occurred and the role of FHR monitoring has been questioned. Recently, the need to educate staff about FHR interpretation and audit standards has been highlighted.

> When presenting tracing, note the:
> - Patient's name.
> - Date.
> - Baseline FHR.
> - Baseline variability.
> - Presence of accelerations.
> - Absence of decelerations if the tracing is normal.

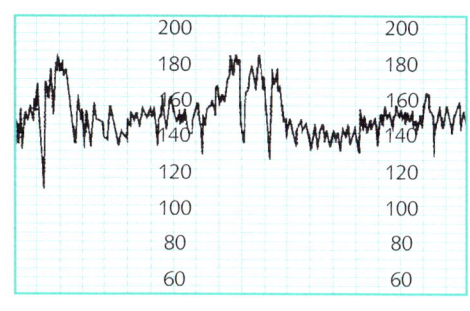

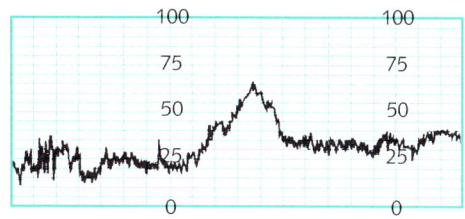

Fig. 16.1 Fetal heart acceleration during a uterine contraction with normal baseline variability.

Features of the fetal heart rate tracing

There are four features of the FHR tracing, which should all be assessed individually and then taken together with the clinical picture to determine the appropriate management of the patient. For example, the progress of the labor or the presence of meconium-stained amniotic fluid might be important considerations. Figure 16.1 shows a normal CTG tracing.

- Baseline FHR: this is the mean level of FHR over a period of 5 to 10 min. It is expressed as beats per minute (bpm) and is determined by the fetal sympathetic and the parasympathetic nervous systems. The normal range is 110–160 bpm. In the preterm fetus, the baseline tends to be at the higher end of the normal range.
- Baseline variability: minor fluctuations occur in the baseline FHR at 3 to 5 cycles per minute. It is measured by estimating the difference in beats per minute between the highest peak and the lowest trough of change in a 1-min segment of the trace. Normal baseline variability is 5–25 bpm above and below the baseline.
- Accelerations: these are increases in the FHR of 15 bpm or more, lasting 15 s or more. These are a feature of a normal strip and are very reassuring.
- Decelerations: these are falls in the FHR below the baseline of more than 15 bpm, lasting 15 s or more. Different patterns of decelerations can be seen, depending on their timing with the uterine contractions:
  ○ Early decelerations: the FHR slows at the same time as the onset of the contraction and returns to the baseline at the end of the contraction. These are an indication of fetal head compression and are reassuring in labor.
  ○ Late decelerations: the FHR begins to fall during the contraction, with its trough more than 20 s after the peak of the contraction

Abnormal Fetal Heart Rate Tracing in Labor

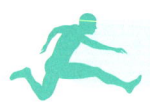

and returning to baseline after the contraction. These are indicative of uteroplacental insufficiency and are the most ominous decelerations in labor.

○ Variable decelerations: the timing of the slowing of the FHR in relation to the uterine contraction varies and can occur in isolation. There is typically rapid onset and recovery. However, other features might make this type of deceleration more suspicious, such as loss of the normal baseline variability. These reflect cord compression.

○ Sinusoidal pattern: there is regular oscillation of the baseline, with absent variability. The pattern lasts at least 10 min and has an amplitude of 5–15 bpm above and below the baseline. This pattern is indicative of severe fetal anemia.

Figure 16.2 shows an abnormal FHR tracing. The tracing can be categorized into:
- Normal: all four features are reassuring.
- Suspicious: one feature is nonreassuring, the others are reassuring.
- Pathologic: two or more features are nonreassuring, or more than one is abnormal.

Figure 16.3 shows how the features of the strip are categorized.

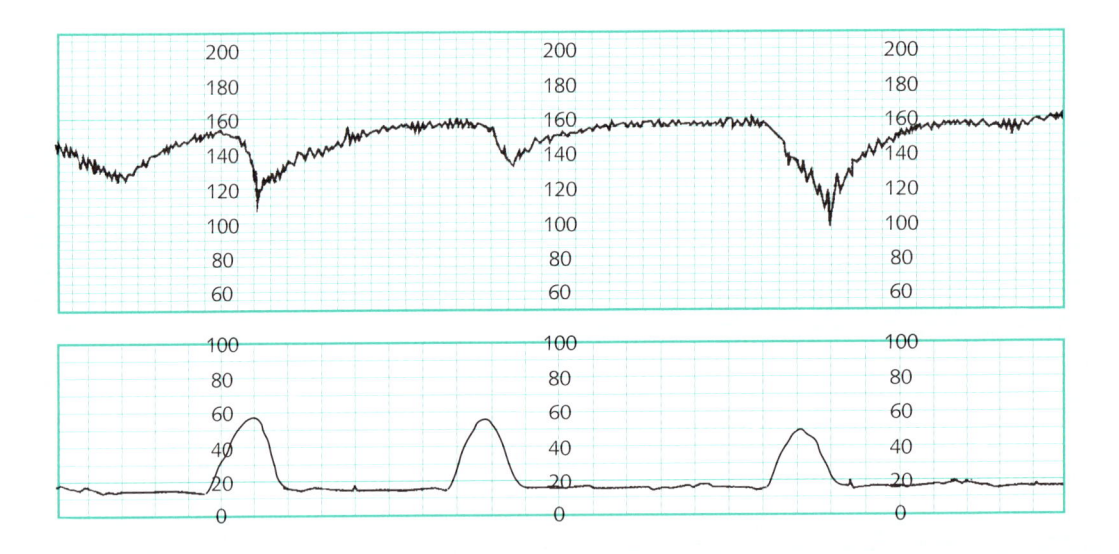

Fig. 16.2 Late decelerations occurring after uterine contractions with reduced baseline variability.

	Features of the FHR tracing			
Feature	Baseline (bpm)	Variability (bpm)	Decelerations	Accelerations
Reassuring	110–160	5–25	None present, early or mild variable decelerations	Present
Nonreassuring	100–109	<5 for ≥40 min	Severe variable decelerations Single deceleration 3 min	None present
Abnormal	<100 >180 Sinusoidal pattern	<5 for ≥90 min >10 min	Late decelerations Single deceleration >3 min	None present

Fig. 16.3 Categorization of the features of the FHR.

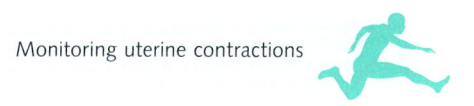

Physiology

The principle of monitoring during labor is to detect fetal hypoxia and, therefore, prevent acidemia and cell damage.

Acute fetal hypoxia
This can occur secondary to:
- Uterine hyperstimulation.
- Placental abruption.
- Umbilical cord compression.

These conditions can result in a decrease in the FHR, with decelerations or bradycardia. This is produced by chemoreceptor-mediated vagal stimulation and then by myocardial ischemia.

Chronic fetal hypoxia
If there has been chronic uteroplacental insufficiency during the pregnancy (e.g. secondary to pre-eclampsia), then the fetus might be at increased risk of hypoxia during labor. Reduced intervillous perfusion during uterine contractions or maternal hypotension can exacerbate underlying reduced placental perfusion. This might result in an increase in the fetal cardiac output with an increase in the baseline heart rate and could be followed by reduced heart rate variability due to brainstem hypoxia. Continuing hypoxia eventually produces myocardial damage and heart rate decelerations.

Monitoring uterine contractions

As well as monitoring the FHR, the tracing also monitors the frequency of the uterine contractions. This can be important, e.g. if the patient is having intravenous oxytocin to stimulate the contractions. It is essential that frequency of contractions and the return to resting tone between contractions is noted.

The actual strength and the length of each contraction should be checked by palpation of the uterus, because the size of the peaks shown on the tracing might be related to positioning of the monitor on the maternal abdomen or thickness of the maternal abdominal wall. If this proves difficult, an IUPC may be inserted.

Monitoring in an uncomplicated pregnancy
Intermittent auscultation of the FHR might be appropriate for a healthy woman in labor who has had an uncomplicated pregnancy. This involves documenting the heart rate for a minimum of 60 s at least:
- Every 15 min in the first stage of labor.
- Every 5 min in the second stage of labor, including after a contraction.

Continuous monitoring might be recommended if any abnormal features develop or any risk factors develop, such as meconium-stained amniotic fluid.

Who should have continuous fetal heart rate monitoring?
Figure 16.4 shows the maternal and fetal indications for recommending continuous monitoring.

	Indications for monitoring
Maternal	Previous cesarean section
	Pre-eclampsia
	Diabetes
	APH
	Other maternal medical disease
Fetal	Intrauterine growth restriction
	Prematurity
	Oligohydramnios
	Abnormal Doppler artery studies
	Multiple pregnancy
	Breech presentation
Intrapartum	Meconium-stained amniotic fluid
	Vaginal bleeding in labor
	Use of oxytocin for augmentation
	Epidural analgesia
	Maternal fever
	Post-dates pregnancy
	Prolonged rupture of membranes >24 h
	Induced labor

Fig. 16.4 Indications for recommending continuous FHR monitoring.

Abnormal Fetal Heart Rate Tracing in Labor

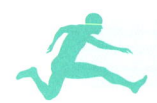

> The maternal and fetal indications for advising continuous FHR monitoring relate to the underlying physiology related to changes in the FHR during normal and abnormal labor. Don't forget that intermittent monitoring might be appropriate in some patients.

> For FBS, the following are required:
> - Appropriate equipment.
> - Cervix ≥2 cm dilated.
> - Mother in left lateral position.

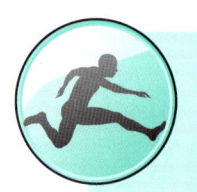

History of the patient who presents with an abnormal fetal heart rate tracing in labor

The need to act on an abnormal FHR tracing in labor can be influenced by maternal, fetal, and intrapartum factors. Figure 16.4 gives the indications for continuous FHR monitoring, but this list also shows the relevant points in the patient's antenatal history that might make the attending physician more concerned if the tracing is suspicious.

Particularly important are the intrapartum factors. In the presence of meconium-stained amniotic fluid, for example, the tracing should be acted upon promptly. If the cervix is not yet dilated, fetal blood sampling (FBS) might not be possible (see below). If progress in labor is slow (see Chapter 15), then operative delivery might be necessary.

Examination of the patient who presents with an abnormal fetal heart rate tracing in labor

Baseline maternal observations
Temperature
A raised temperature might explain fetal tachycardia.

Pulse
This might be raised in conjunction with maternal fever. In the presence of fetal bradycardia, maternal pulse should be checked to ensure that the monitoring is recording FHR and not the mother.

Blood pressure
Epidural anesthesia can be associated with maternal hypotension as it is administered. This results in reduced flow to the uterus and can cause fetal bradycardia. Therefore, blood pressure should be regularly checked when the medication is given.

Abdominal palpation
- Size.
- Engagement of presenting part.
- Scar tenderness in a patient with a previous cesarean section.
- Uterine tone.

The size of the maternal abdomen should be assessed to check whether it is large or small for dates (see Chapter 11). The engagement of the presenting part is important to assess progress in labor (see Chapters 15 and 40). In a patient who has previously had a cesarean section, the presence of scar tenderness should be elicited; scar rupture is commonly associated with an abnormal FHR tracing and vaginal bleeding. Another cause of vaginal bleeding with an abnormal FHR tracing is placental abruption (see Chapter 37). If this is suspected, then the uterus will typically feel hard and tender.

The uterine contractions should be palpated, especially if the patient's labor is being stimulated by intravenous oxytocic agents. It is important to check that the uterus is not hyperstimulated, as this can cause an abnormal tracing. There should be resting tone between contractions.

Vaginal examination
As well as assessing the dilatation of the cervix to determine the progress in labor and the ability to perform a fetal blood sample, the presence of the fetal cord must be excluded. A cord prolapse, as it is known, is associated with a fetal bradycardia, and this is an emergency situation requiring immediate delivery by cesarean section.

Investigating the abnormal fetal heart rate tracing

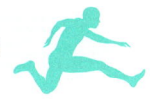

Fig. 16.5 Algorithm for FHR monitoring.

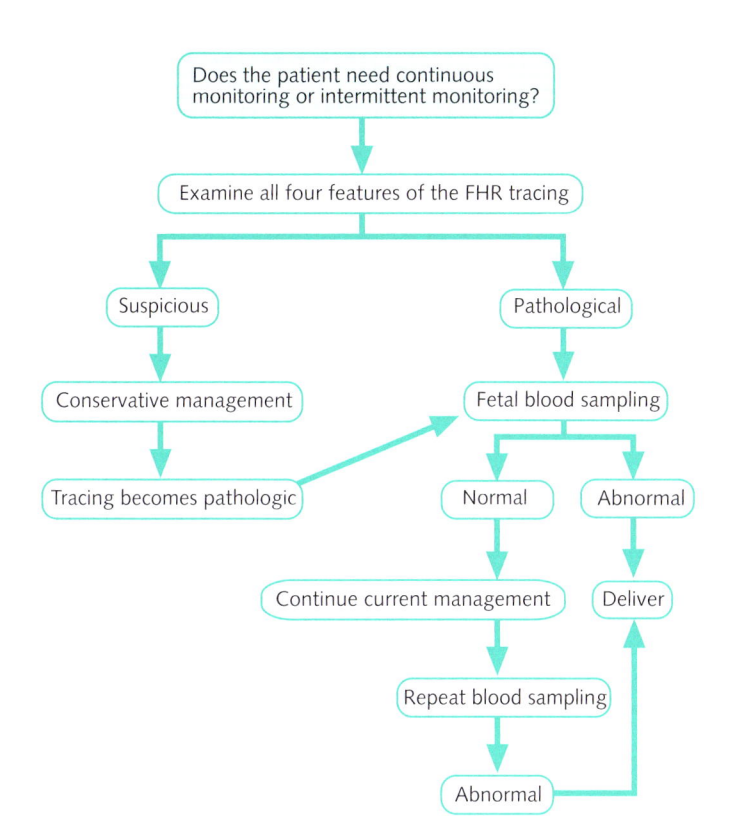

```
Does the patient need continuous
monitoring or intermittent monitoring?
              ↓
Examine all four features of the FHR tracing
         ↙              ↘
    Suspicious        Pathological
         ↓                 ↓
  Conservative      Fetal blood sampling
  management          ↙        ↘
         ↓        Normal      Abnormal
  Tracing becomes              ↓
  pathologic                 Deliver
         ↓
  Continue current management
         ↓
  Repeat blood sampling
         ↓
      Abnormal
```

Investigating the abnormal fetal heart rate tracing

Using the criteria described above, if the tracing is suspicious, then the patient can be managed conservatively (Fig. 16.5).

If the tracing is pathologic, FBS should be performed if there are the appropriate facilities. The procedure is performed with the mother in the left lateral postion and the cervix should be dilated at least 2 cm. A sample of blood from the fetal scalp gives the fetal pH (i.e. a measure of acidosis). It might indicate that delivery is necessary (pH ≤ 7.20), or that the test should be repeated within 30 min (pH 7.21–7.24).

If FBS is not possible, then delivery should be expedited. Contraindications to FBS are given in Fig. 16.6.

Contraindications to FBS

- Maternal infection (HIV, hepatitis B, herpes simplex)
- Fetal bleeding disorder (hemophilia, thrombocytopenia)
- Prematurity (<34 weeks)

Fig. 16.6 Contraindications to FBS.

17. Bleeding after Delivery

Postpartum hemorrhage

The presenting complaint in PPH is bleeding from the genital tract of more than 500 mL after a vaginal delivery or more than 1000 mL after a cesarean delivery. It is classified as either early or late:
- Early PPH: bleeding within 24 h of delivery.
- Late PPH: bleeding that starts 24 h after delivery and occurs within 6 weeks.

Figure 17.1 gives the differential diagnoses that should be considered. About 90% of cases of PPH are caused by uterine atony; about 7% are due to genital tract trauma.

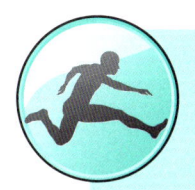

Differential diagnoses of postpartum hemorrhage	
Type of PPH	Differential diagnosis
Early	Uterine atony
	Genital tract trauma (cervix/vagina/perineum)
	Retained placenta/placenta accreta
	Coagulation disorders
	Uterine inversion
	Uterine rupture
Late	Retained products
	Endometritis
	Persistent molar pregnancy/choriocarcinoma

Fig. 17.1 Differential diagnoses of postpartum hemorrhage (see Chapter 42).

When the patient presents with early PPH, always check that the placenta and membranes are complete to exclude retained products of conception.

Don't forget to check the genital tract for signs of trauma once the placenta has been delivered.

History to focus on the differential diagnosis

Early postpartum hemorrhage
Uterine atony
Certain factors in the patient's history can increase the risk of a primary PPH secondary to uterine atony:
- Multiple pregnancy.
- Grand multiparity.
- Polyhydramnios.
- Fibroid uterus.
- Prolonged labor.
- Previous PPH.
- APH.

In a multiple pregnancy, the placental site is larger than with a singleton. There is also overdistention of the uterus (see Chapter 34). This is also seen in polyhydramnios (see Chapter 11).

Mode of delivery
The mode of delivery may increase risk of PPH. Genital tract trauma can occur with a normal vaginal delivery, either from an episiotomy (see Chapter 41) or from a vaginal or cervical tear. Bleeding is more common with an instrumental delivery, especially forceps, in particular Keilland's forceps (see Chapter 41).

Average blood loss at cesarean section is 1000 mL. This might be increased if there is a placenta previa (see Chapter 37) or if delivery of the presenting part is difficult after a prolonged labor; it becomes impacted in the pelvis and delivery causes the uterus to tear.

Rarely, PPH is secondary to uterine inversion that occurs after delivery of the placenta (see Chapter 42). As well as bleeding, the patient complains of abdominal pain, which can be severe, associated with a feeling of prolapse. Rupture of the uterus is also uncommon, except in association with labor in a patient who has previously had a cesarean section.

Other causes
Coagulation disorders can be acute or chronic. The chronic conditions such as inherited vascular disorders are usually known about antenatally. DIC can present acutely, e.g. secondary to placental abruption or severe pre-eclampsia.

Late postpartum hemorrhage
In the presence of retained products of conception, either placenta or membranes, the common presenting complaint is prolonged heavy vaginal bleeding or persistent offensive discharge. If this becomes infected then the patient might present with fever and lower abdominal pain.

A molar pregnancy also presents with persistent vaginal bleeding (see Chapter 29). The rarer choriocarcinoma might metastasize to the lungs, liver, or brain. Presenting symptoms include hemoptysis and dyspnea or neurologic symptoms.

Examination

Early postpartum hemorrhage
The blood loss must be estimated as accurately as possible to manage the patient appropriately. Examination must include the ABC (airways, breathing, circulation) of basic resuscitation (see Chapter 18), as well as pallor, pulse, and blood pressure. Abdominal palpation should assess whether the uterus is contracted or not. The fundal height should be at or below the umbilicus. If it is above, then there might be retained products of conception or the uterus could be filling with clots.

Uterine inversion should be considered if the fundus is indented or cannot be palpated. Vaginal examination will assess the degree of inversion,

Early PPH

- Amount of blood loss
- Pulse
- Blood pressure
- Urine output
- Uterine contraction
- Fundal height
- Placenta and membranes complete
- Genital tract trauma

Fig. 17.2 Examination of the patient who presents with early PPH.

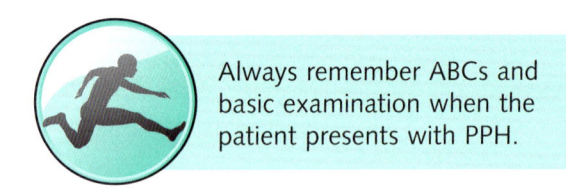

Always remember ABCs and basic examination when the patient presents with PPH.

either up to the cervical os or complete inversion of the uterus and vagina.

If the uterus is well contracted and the placenta is out, then the bleeding might be from trauma to the genital tract. The patient should be examined in sufficient light, with adequate analgesia (either regional or general), to exclude lacerations to the cervix, vagina, and perineum.

If the placenta and membranes have been delivered, then they must be carefully examined to see that the cotyledons appear complete and that there is no suggestion of a succenturiate lobe. The examination is summarized in Fig. 17.2.

Late postpartum hemorrhage
Basic observations should include pulse, blood pressure, and temperature. There might be a tachycardia and fever with endometritis. The height of the uterine fundus should be checked, because the uterus will usually remain poorly contracted if there are retained products of conception. Tenderness should be excluded to rule out endometritis.

Speculum examination assesses vaginal discharge if there is suspicion of infection. Bimanual palpation examines the size of the uterus, because it might be bulky with retained products or with a molar pregnancy. Tenderness is present with endometritis. If the cervical os is open, then there might be retained products of conception.

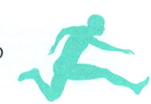

Appropriate work-up

Early postpartum hemorrhage
Having established intravenous access, blood should be sent for hemoglobin, platelets, coagulation studies (including fibrin split products), and T&S. Depending on the estimated blood loss, cross-matching blood might be necessary. Blood urea nitrogen, creatinine, and electrolytes should be tested if the urine output is poor.

Figure 17.3 provides an algorithm for the management of early PPH.

Late postpartum hemorrhage
A CBC should be ordered to estimate hemoglobin and to give an indication of infection if the WBC is raised. Again, cross-matching blood for transfusion might be necessary, depending on the clinical situation and the hemoglobin result. A cervical culture should be performed to exclude endometritis.

An ultrasound scan that is done to check that the uterus is empty will exclude retained products, including molar tissue. Care should be taken to interpret the findings in conjunction with the clinical picture, because blood clot might have a similar scan appearance.

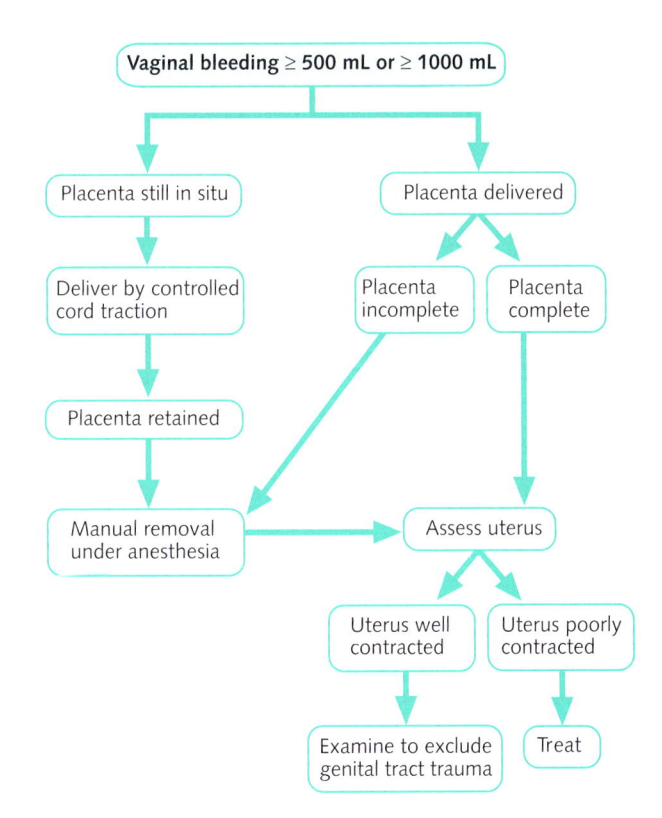

Fig. 17.3 Algorithm for the management of early PPH.

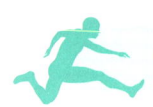

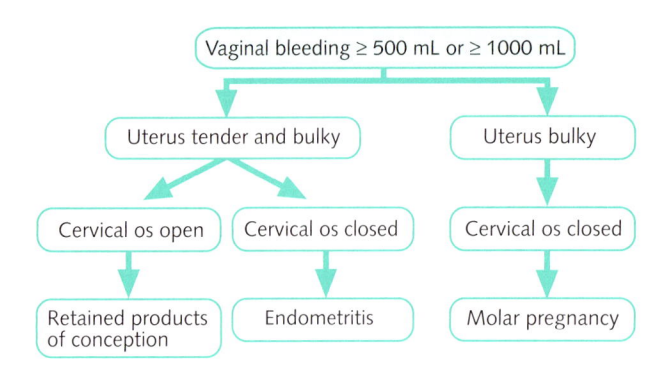

Fig. 17.4 Algorithm for the management of late PPH.

The diagnosis of a molar pregnancy is confirmed with a persistently raised serum β-hCG level. Evacuation of the uterus will yield tissue for histological analysis to confirm the diagnosis and exclude choriocarcinoma. However, if the latter is diagnosed, then LFTs and a chest X-ray should be performed to check for metastases.

Figure 17.4 provides an algorithm for the management of late PPH.

18. Maternal Collapse

Collapse of a patient on the maternity ward or delivery suite might have an obstetric or a nonobstetric cause. The danger, when faced with a collapsed pregnant woman, is to prioritize delivery because of fears for the fetus. However, it is important to remember that maternal resuscitation is the single most effective means of improving fetal health; delivery, if necessary, should be contemplated only when the mother is stable.

> The principles of first-line management are the same in all situations; check:
> - airway
> - breathing
> - circulation
>
> and call for help. If antenatal, establish fetal monitoring once the mother's initial resuscitation has commenced.

Hemorrhage

Antenatal bleeding sufficient to cause collapse will usually be due to placental bleeding, either placental abruption or placenta previa. Figure 18.1 summarizes the different presentations (see also Chapter 10). Uterine rupture can also cause collapse with bleeding. Postnatal bleeding (PPH) causes are shown in Fig. 18.2 and are covered in Chapter 17.

Placental abruption and placenta previa

Major obstetric hemorrhage can be extremely rapid and is potentially fatal, so coordinated management between midwives, doctors, anesthesiologists, and the blood bank is vital. Abruption severe enough to cause collapse or fetal distress is likely to be associated with blood loss of at least 1500 mL and a 30% incidence of coagulopathy.

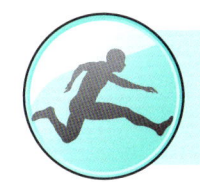

> Both abruption and bleeding placenta previa increase the risk of PPH.

It can be difficult to control bleeding from the placental site during cesarean section for placenta previa. Oxytocin infusion is used, but further measures might be required, including methergine (an ergot alkaloid), the prostaglandin analog carboprost (Hemabate), bimanual compression, internal iliac ligation, and, in extreme situations, hysterectomy. Recently, arterial embolization by radiologists has provided another alternative.

Uterine rupture

Uterine rupture is uncommon. Occasionally, trauma might be the cause (e.g. motor vehicle accident), but more commonly the woman is multiparous and in labor. Those most at risk are

Placenta previa vs. placental abruption	
Placental abruption	Placenta previa
Painful	Painless
Uterus tense, hard to palpation	Uterus soft, nontender to palpation
Amount of blood seen might not represent true loss because bleeding might be concealed	Blood loss seen reflects total loss

Fig. 18.1 Placenta previa versus placental abruption.

Maternal Collapse

Causes of PPH

- Tone: uterine atony
- Tissue: retained products of conception
- Trauma: genital tract laceration
- Thrombin: clotting abnormalities

Fig. 18.2 Causes of PPH.

women with a scar on the uterus, usually a previous cesarean section; using an oxytocin infusion in this situation increases the risk still further. Symptoms and signs include:
- Scar pain and tenderness.
- Constant pain, between contractions.
- Vaginal bleeding.
- FHR abnormalities.
- Blood-stained amniotic fluid.
- Hematuria.

Resuscitation and laparotomy are needed.

Uterine atony

When the uterus fails to contract following delivery of the placenta, the blood vessels that supplied the placenta's huge circulation are not shut off by compression, so uterine bleeding continues. Risk factors include:
- Precipitous labor.
- Induced labor.
- Augmented labor (oxytocin infusion).
- Cesarean section following prolonged/augmented labor.
- Magnesium sulfate treatment.
- Multiple pregnancy.
- Chorioamnionitis.

If medical treatment (oxytocin, methergine, Hemabate) fails, consider packing the uterus, radiological arterial embolization, or surgery—internal iliac artery ligation, B Lynch suture, or hysterectomy.

Amniotic fluid embolism

This poorly understood condition results in transient pulmonary hypertension, profound hypoxia, left ventricular failure, and secondary coagulopathy. Fetal and maternal mortality is high. The use of oxytocin and rapid labor are known to be risk factors, but amniotic fluid embolism (AFE) can also occur in nonaugmented labor.

The diagnosis might only be discovered postmortem, but could also be made on the basis of the characteristic trio of:
- Cyanosis.
- Collapse.
- Clotting derangement (DIC).

Management consists of ventilatory support and correction of the coagulopathy.

Acute myocardial infarction

Antenatal myocardial infarction (MI) carries a mortality rate of up to 45%. The resuscitation algorithm is the same as that for nonpregnant adults, but the woman must be tilted onto her left side to reduce the compression of the vena cava by the pregnant abdomen (Fig. 18.3). If it is felt that the fetus is compromising the resuscitation, then delivery should be achieved. A senior cardiologist should be involved at an early stage.

Eclampsia

Chapter 42 outlines the presentation and management of eclampsia. In summary, the management begins with controlling the seizure. A magnesium sulfate infusion is started as prophylaxis against further seizures. The blood pressure must be reduced to mean arterial pressure (MAP) levels of less than 125 mmHg. Delivery of the fetus should be considered at this point.

Diabetic emergency

Management of diabetic coma is described in *Crash Course on General Medicine*. In the acute setting it is more likely to be due to hypoglycemia, especially as the delicate balance of tight control in pregnancy and after delivery can be very difficult. Hyperosmolar nonketotic coma might be seen in a diabetic woman who has been unwell at home for some time.

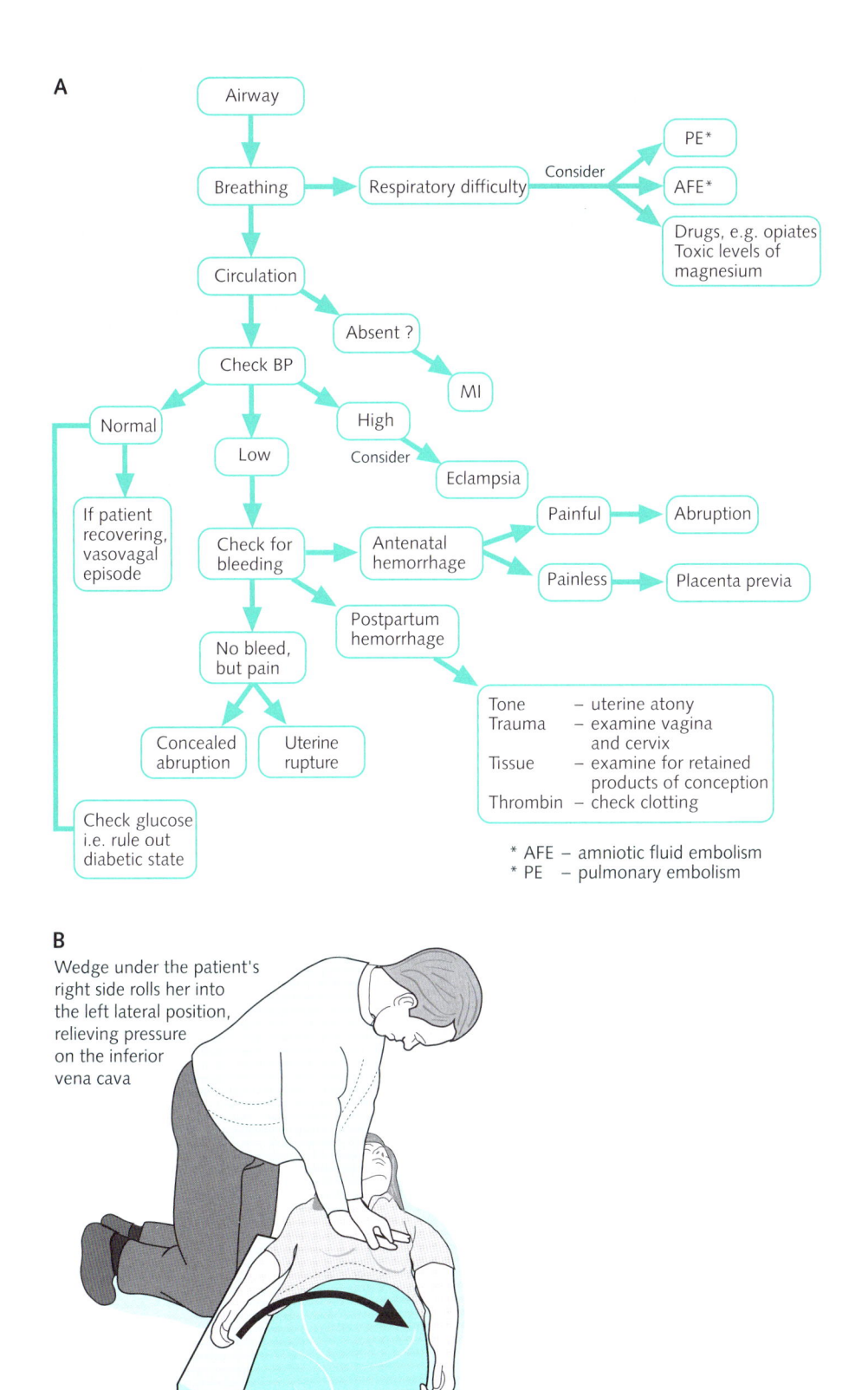

Fig. 18.3 Resuscitation. A. Algorithm. B. Position for cardiopulmonary resuscitation.

Hypoglycemia

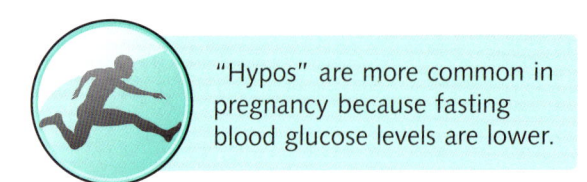

"Hypos" are more common in pregnancy because fasting blood glucose levels are lower.

Infuse 50 mL 50% dextrose intravenously over a short space of time, followed by a saline flush. Check the blood sugar again 15 min later. Once the woman is conscious, a 20 g glucose drink is given, followed by a longer-acting carbohydrate snack or meal. The blood sugar should be rechecked 1 h later.

Hyperglycemia

Rehydration, an insulin infusion to reduce serum glucose levels, and hourly assessment of serum potassium levels are the main aims of treatment of this condition. Fetal monitoring might show a nonreassuring FHR tracing, but this is likely to improve when ketosis is corrected.

Drug toxicity

Maternal collapse could be due to overdose, adverse effects or allergy to drugs administered by medical staff, or as a result of drug abuse by the patient.

Local anesthesia

High spinal anesthesia occurs when a very high dose of local anesthesia is given or due to inadvertent intravascular injection at the time of epidural anesthesia. Paralysis of the respiratory muscles requiring ventilation results. Warning signs are hypotension, nausea, dizziness, and dyspnea.

Analgesia

Opiates such as fentanyl, morphine, and demerol are used for pain relief in labor. In high doses they can cause respiratory depression. Naloxone, an opiate antagonist, will immediately reverse respiratory depression but has a short duration of action, so a further dose might be needed.

Toradol (ketorolac) is commonly used for postnatal analgesia. Any drug in this family of NSAIDs can precipitate bronchoconstriction in asthmatics. A severe asthma attack should be treated with intravenous hydrocortisone and nebulized albuterol; ventilatory support might be necessary.

Magnesium

Magnesium sulfate is used following eclampsia as prophylaxis against further seizures. Hypermagnesemia can result in coma. The signs of magnesium toxicity are shown in Fig. 18.4. Calcium gluconate injection is used to treat toxicity.

Drug abuse

Opiates, Ecstasy, and cocaine can all cause collapse and coma. Convulsions can result from Ecstasy or cocaine use and should be treated with diazepam. Opiate-induced respiratory depression is reversed with naloxone.

Loss of patellar reflex
Flushing
Slurred speech
Motor weakness
Respiratory depression
Cardiac arrest

Increasing Mg levels ↓

Fig. 18.4 Signs of magnesium toxicity.

Puerperal sepsis

Septic shock can cause collapse. There should be an attempt to establish the focus of infection, paying particular attention to the possibility of retained products of conception. Empirical antibiotic therapy should be started after consulting an infectious disease specialist and after a septic screen (blood cultures, urinalysis and culture, chest X-ray, and cervical swabs) has been performed. Renal, respiratory, and cardiac failure can ensue, and DIC often accompanies severe sepsis.

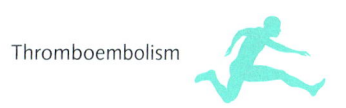

Thromboembolism

Pregnancy is a prothrombotic state, and thromboembolism is one of the most common causes of maternal mortality (see Chapters 36 and 43).

Pulmonary embolism

Smaller pulmonary emboli (PEs) will cause breathlessness and pleuritic pain, but larger emboli can present with collapse. On examination, the following may be found:
- Tachypnea.
- Tachycardia.
- Raised jugular venous pressure.
- Loud second heart sound.

The investigation of PE is detailed in Chapter 36, with first-line investigations being arterial blood gases (to look for a low P_{O_2} and P_{CO_2}), chest X-ray (to exclude infection), and ECG, followed by a ventilation perfusion (V/Q) scan or spiral CT to identify the clot. Anticoagulation with heparin is the norm, but a PE large enough to cause collapse may merit treatment with streptokinase.

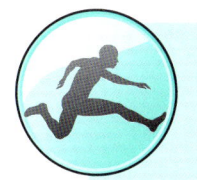

In pregnancy, arterial blood gases and ECG might be normal in the presence of a small PE, so if there is any doubt, a scan (V/Q or spiral CT) must be arranged.

Cerebral vein thrombosis

This condition is uncommon but is associated with a high mortality; it usually occurs in the puerperium. There might be focal neurological signs, but signs can be more 'general', with convulsions, headache, photophobia, and vomiting being typical. There might be a fever and raised white cell count.

The diagnosis is made on CT or MRI. Convulsions should be treated, the patient kept well hydrated, and heparin therapy considered.

DISEASES AND DISORDERS

19.	Abnormal Uterine Bleeding	91	33.	Prenatal Diagnosis	179
20.	Fibroids	103	34.	Multiple Pregnancy	183
21.	Endometriosis	107	35.	Hypertension in Pregnancy	189
22.	Benign Ovarian Tumors	113	36.	Medical Disorders in Pregnancy	195
23.	Gynecologic Malignancy	117	37.	Antepartum Hemorrhage	207
24.	Vulvar Disease	129	38.	Premature Labor	213
25.	Pelvic Inflammatory Disease	133	39.	Malpresentation and Malpositions of the Occiput	219
26.	Urinary Incontinence	137	40.	Labor	231
27.	Pelvic Organ Prolapse	143	41.	Operative Intervention in Obstetrics	245
28.	Infertility	149	42.	Complications of the Third Stage of Labor and the Puerperium	251
29.	Early Pregnancy Failure	153			
30.	Menopause	161			
31.	Contraception, Sterilization, and Unwanted Pregnancy	167	43.	Maternal Death	257
32.	Gynecologic Endocrinology	173			

19. Abnormal Uterine Bleeding

Abnormal uterine bleeding is an extremely common problem experienced by most women at some time in their life. The causes can be physiologic or pathologic and, as long as serious pathology is excluded, might not require treatment. For normal menstruation to occur, the following are necessary:
- Hypothalamic function.
- Pituitary function.
- Ovarian function.
- Endometrial function.
- Patent cervix and vagina.

Abnormal uterine bleeding can be caused by malfunction or disease at any of these levels.

Amenorrhea

This is the term used to describe absence of menstruation. Lack of menstruation after the age of 16 years is called primary amenorrhea and is relatively uncommon. Secondary amenorrhea is extremely common and implies menstruation has occurred in the past but has been absent for 6 months or more. The most common causes of secondary amenorrhea are physiologic, most frequently pregnancy and menopause.

The causes of amenorrhea can be broken down into the following five major categories:
- CNS.
- Gonadal dysfunction.
- Genital tract disorders.
- Endocrine disorders.
- Drug therapy.

Work-up of amenorrhea

Amenorrhea can be physiologic, i.e. due to the premenarche, pregnancy, lactation, or menopause. When investigating primary amenorrhea, the premenarchal state should be diagnosed only if pathology has been excluded.

Primary amenorrhea

Primary amenorrhea should be investigated from the age of 16 years or before if pubertal development has not started by the age of 14 years. Investigation should be determined by assessment of pubertal development (Fig. 19.1).

When no pubertal development has occurred by the age of 14 years, the work-up is the same as for delayed puberty (see Chapters 1 and 32).

When pubertal development is normal, genital tract anomalies, such as an absent uterus or vagina, should be excluded by examination or ultrasound

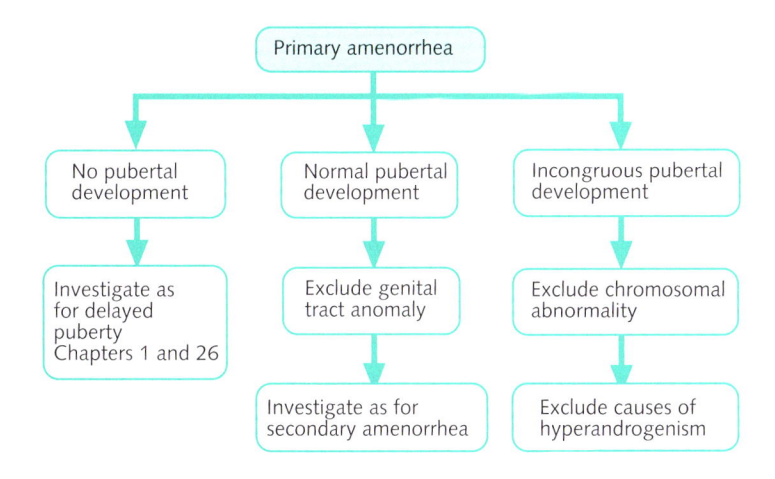

Fig. 19.1 Algorithm for primary amenorrhea.

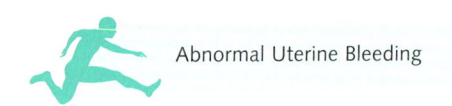

scanning. If findings are normal, then investigation should be as for secondary amenorrhea (see below).

Incongruous pubertal development can be caused by chromosomal abnormality or increased circulating androgens. For instance, women with testicular feminization often have normal or even excellent breast development in the absence of axillary and pubic hair. Poor breast development in the presence of normal or excessive axillary or pubic hair is compatible with increased circulating androgens commonly associated with PCOS, and less commonly with CAH or androgen-secreting tumors of the ovary or adrenal.

> A woman presenting with primary amenorrhea should always have her karyotype checked.

Secondary amenorrhea

The most common cause of secondary amenorrhea in women of childbearing age is pregnancy, and this should be excluded before further investigation is commenced.

Having excluded physiologic causes of secondary amenorrhea, further investigation includes measurements of serum gonadotrophins, androgens, and prolactin. Other useful investigations include a pelvic ultrasound scan, which will identify the typical appearance of polycystic ovaries and the presence of a hematometra, a lateral skull X-ray, or CT or MRI of the head to identify a pituitary tumor and exclusion of thyroid disease and diabetes mellitus (Fig. 19.2). Women under 30 years of age who have ovarian failure should have their chromosomes analyzed.

Complications of amenorrhea

Although amenorrhea itself does not cause any complications, some of the underlying conditions do carry certain risks:
- Women who carry a Y chromosome have a 25% chance of developing gonadal malignancy, usually a gonadoblastoma or dysgerminoma.
- Hypoestrogenic states characteristic of hypothalamic amenorrhea and premature ovarian failure are associated with an increased risk of osteoporosis and ischemic heart disease.
- Endometrial hyperplasia and endometrial carcinoma occur more frequently in women with PCOS because of the unopposed estrogen effect on the endometrium associated with chronic anovulation.
- Hematocolpos (accumulation of menstrual blood in the vagina, usually due to an imperforate hymen) is associated with an increased risk of endometriosis due to retrograde menstruation.
- Amenorrheic women are usually infertile.

Treatment of amenorrhea

Certain conditions can cause primary and secondary amenorrhea, depending on the age at which the condition presents. Their treatment is discussed under secondary amenorrhea.

Treatment of primary amenorrhea
Gonadal dysgenesis
Apart from the management of the psychosexual aspects of gonadal dysgenesis, these women require HRT to protect against cardiovascular disease and osteoporosis. This will also stimulate secondary sexual development in those who have not yet been exposed to estrogens (e.g. Turner's syndrome). Those women who carry a Y chromosome should have both gonads removed, because of the risk of malignancy, followed by long-term HRT.

Genital tract anomaly
Women with a congenitally absent vagina should be offered vaginal reconstruction to enable sexual activity. If the uterus is present, then this will allow drainage of a hematometria. A hematocolpos should be drained by excision of the persistent vaginal membrane.

Treatment of secondary amenorrhea
In young women who have no pathology, the condition is often self-limiting and might not require treatment.

Hypothalamic amenorrhea
Where weight loss is implicated, a return of BMI to the normal range (19–25) usually results in spontaneous menstruation, as does the removal of stressful situations or treatment of systemic illness.

Polycystic ovary syndrome
The mainstay of treatment for PCOS is weight loss. As the BMI approaches the normal range,

Amenorrhea

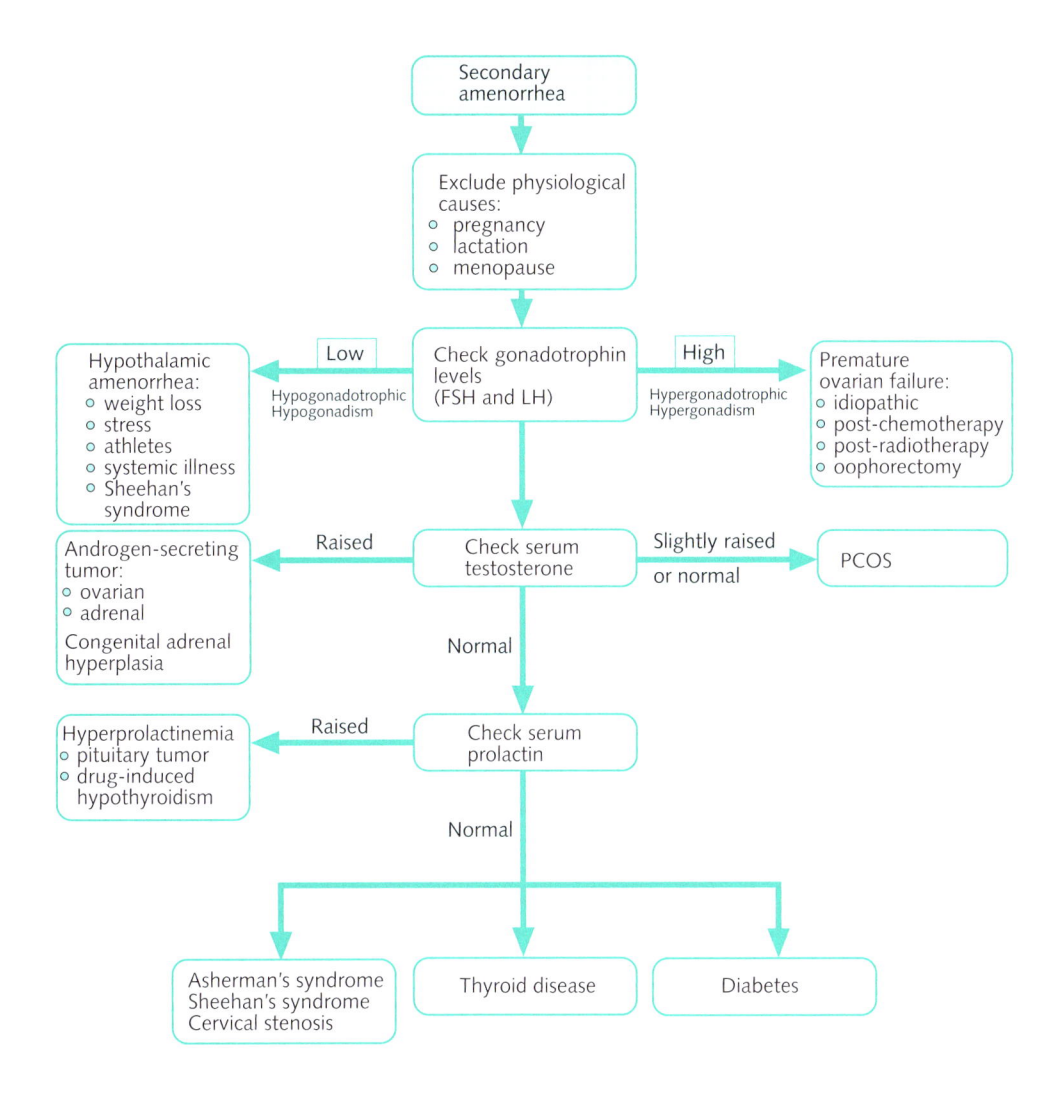

Fig. 19.2 Algorithm for secondary amenorrhea.

spontaneous ovulation and menstruation often occur. Endometrial hyperplasia should be treated with progestins. Long-term protection of the endometrium can be provided using cyclical progestins or the OCPs. A new combined pill (Yasmin®) contains a unique progestin (drospirenone) that has both a weak anti-androgenic and antimineralocorticoid activity. Therefore, it may be effective in the treatment of hirsutism.

Metformin is now being used in trials for treatment of PCOS as it is thought to be driven by insulin resistance.

Hyperprolactinemia

The treatment of hyperprolactinemia includes the following:
- Dopamine agonists for microadenoma.
- Dopamine agonists or surgery for macroadenoma.
- Cessation of drugs, where possible, in drug-induced hyperprolactinemia.
- Correction of hypothyroidism.

Treatment is advisable for pituitary microadenoma to reduce the risk of osteoporosis. Dopamine

93

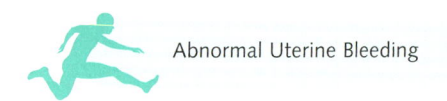

Prescribed drugs that can cause hyperprolactinemia	
Type of drug	Drug class
Antipsychotic drugs	Phenothiazines
	Haloperidol
Antidepressants	Tricyclic antidepressants
Antihypertensives	Methyldopa
	Reserpine
Estrogens	Combined OCP
H$_2$-receptor antagonists	Cimetidine
	Ranitidine
	Metoclopramide and domperidone

Don't forget chemotherapy for malignancy or immunologic disorders.

Fig. 19.3 Prescribed drugs that can cause hyperprolactinemia.

agonists, such as bromocriptine and cabergoline, should be used to reduce the serum prolactin levels. Side effects include nausea, dizziness, hypotension, drowsiness, and headaches, and are less common with cabergoline, which can be given once weekly. Cessation of therapy usually results in recurrence of hyperprolactinemia, but is recommended if pregnancy occurs.

Transphenoidal removal of pituitary macroadenoma carries a risk of diabetes insipidus, cerebrospinal fluid leakage, panhypopituitarism, and recurrence of the tumor. Shrinkage of the tumor and resolution of symptoms might occur with medical treatment, as for microadenoma.

When hyperprolactinemia is drug induced (Fig. 19.3), cessation of the drug results in a fall of serum prolactin levels to normal levels. However, this is not always advisable; depending on the condition being treated and where drug treatment is likely to be long term, estrogen replacement might be advisable to prevent osteoporosis. Hypothyroidism should be corrected with thyroxine replacement.

Asherman's syndrome
Cervical stenosis can be treated by dilatation of the cervix. Intrauterine adhesions should be divided hysteroscopically. Insertion of an IUD is advisable for at least 3 months to prevent redevelopment of adhesions. Stimulation of endometrial regrowth using exogenous estrogens (i.e. HRT) is sometimes necessary.

Hormone-secreting tumors
Ovarian and adrenal hormone-secreting tumors should be surgically removed. As much ovarian tissue as possible should be preserved, especially in younger women.

Sheehan's syndrome
Postpartum infarction of the pituitary gland due to massive obstetric hemorrhage (Sheehan's syndrome) requires estrogen replacement in the form of the combined OCP or HRT to prevent osteoporosis. In addition, replacement of other pituitary hormones might be necessary.

Menorrhagia

Menorrhagia is defined as MBL of more than 80 mL per period. This represents two standard deviations above the mean blood loss, which is about 30 mL per period. Two-thirds of women with genuine menorrhagia will have iron-deficiency anemia.

Incidence of menorrhagia
The incidence of true menorrhagia is reported to be 9–15% of population samples in the US; however, as many as one-third of women regard their menstrual loss as heavy. Early menarche, late menopause, and reduction in family size with concurrent reduction in periods of lactational amenorrhea have all contributed to an almost tenfold increase in the number of periods that women experience during their reproductive life. This, combined with the changing role of women within society, whereby many are involved in work outside the home, has meant that excessive menstrual bleeding has become one of the most common causes of concern for health in women.

Diagnosing menorrhagia
Menorrhagia can be diagnosed using the following techniques:
- Subjective assessment.
- Pictorial blood-loss assessment charts (Fig. 19.4).
- Objective assessment.

As only half of women complaining of heavy periods will have menorrhagia, reliance on

Menorrhagia

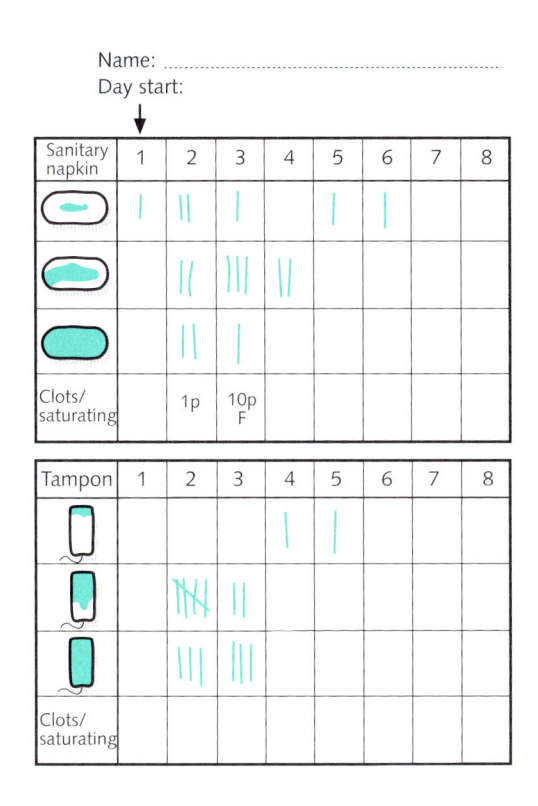

Fig. 19.4 Pictorial blood-loss assessment chart.

Etiology of menorrhagia	
Types of disorder	**Specific problem**
Systemic disorders	Thyroid disease
	Clotting disorders
Local causes	Fibroids
	Endometrial polyps
	Endometrial carcinoma
	Endometriosis/adenomyosis
	PID
	Dysfunctional uterine bleeding
Iatrogenic	IUDs
	Oral anticoagulants

Fig. 19.5 Etiology of menorrhagia.

subjective assessment alone will mean that many women are treated for a condition that they do not suffer from. A visual method of assessing MBL using pictorial charts has been shown to be more effective at diagnosing menorrhagia than subjective assessment alone. They take into account the degree to which each item of sanitary protection is soiled with blood, as well as the quantity used, but, unfortunately, are not frequently used in practice. Objective measurement of MBL is rarely performed, and usually only during clinical trials. The idea of collecting and storing soiled sanitary protection for measurement of MBL is distasteful to most and is the main reason why objective assessment is rarely performed.

Etiology of menorrhagia
There are three categories for the etiology of menorrhagia (Fig. 19.5):
- Systemic conditions.
- Local pathology.
- Iatrogenic causes.

Systemic conditions
The relationship between hypothyroidism and menorrhagia has not been confirmed because of insufficient objective data, although individual cases have been reported.

Up to 90% of women with bleeding disorders have been shown to have menorrhagia. Coagulation disorders are found in up to one-third of young women admitted to the hospital with profound menorrhagia.

Local pathology
Fibroids can increase menstrual loss in two ways. First, they can enlarge the uterine cavity, thereby increasing the surface area of the endometrium from which menstruation occurs. Second, they can produce prostaglandins, which have been implicated in the etiology of menorrhagia. In a similar way, endometrial polyps can increase the surface area of the endometrium and are also hormonally active.

Measured MBL in the presence of pelvic pathology, such as endometriosis and PID, is very variable and often in the normal range. Menorrhagia, therefore, is associated with, but not necessarily caused by, these conditions.

Dysfunctional uterine bleeding (DUB) is the most common cause of menorrhagia and is the term used when there are no local or systemic causes for menorrhagia. Therefore, it is a diagnosis made by exclusion. Altered endometrial prostaglandin metabolism would appear to have an important role in the etiology of DUB. Further evidence is given by the fact that prostaglandin inhibitors are known to decrease MBL in women with DUB.

Premalignant and malignant endometrium can present with menorrhagia and must always be excluded in women who complain of excessive MBL.

Iatrogenic causes

The presence of an IUD has been shown to increase MBL and is the most common iatrogenic cause of menorrhagia. Menorrhagia and anemia are up to five times more common in IUD users than with other forms of contraception.

Roughly one-half of women taking oral anticoagulants will be found to have objective evidence of menorrhagia.

Investigating menorrhagia

Investigation (Fig. 19.6) is aimed at excluding the systemic and local causes of menorrhagia and includes:
- CBC and, when clinically indicated, thyroid function tests and clotting tests.
- Pelvic ultrasound (vaginal ultrasound is particularly sensitive).
- Endometrial biopsy.
- Hysteroscopy.

A CBC should be performed in all cases. Thyroid function and clotting studies should be performed only where indicated by the clinical history.

A pelvic ultrasound has become almost mandatory and will identify uterine enlargement due to fibroids, as well as adnexal masses. Endometrial polyps or submucous fibroids should be suspected where the endometrial thickness is increased.

An endometrial biopsy should be performed in all women over 35 and in women under 35 if there are suspicious findings on ultrasound scan. This can be performed either in the outpatient clinic or under intravenous sedation. It might show endometrium inappropriate to the menstrual cycle secondary to anovulation, endometrial hyperplasia, or carcinoma. A cervical smear should also be performed where this is due, or sooner if there is a history of intermenstrual or postcoital bleeding.

Current methods of endometrial sampling, e.g. pipelle suctioning, appear to be at least as accurate

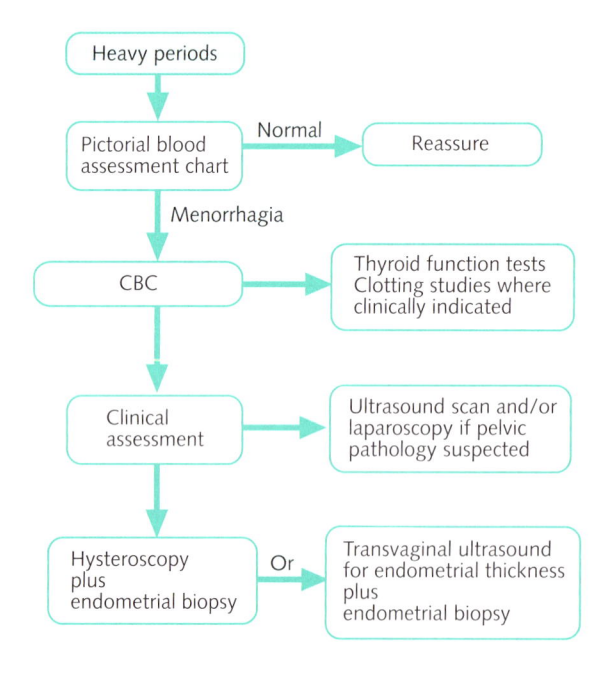

Fig. 19.6 Investigating menorrhagia.

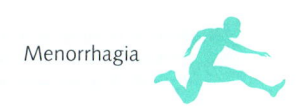

as D&C, have high levels of patient acceptability and lower complication rates, and do not require inpatient admission or anesthesia. However, they have been shown to miss benign and malignant endometrial pathology and must, therefore, be considered inadequate for the further investigation of menorrhagia that has persisted despite medical therapy. In this instance, a hysteroscopy plus sampling should be performed either as an outpatient or under intravenous sedation, depending on facilities and patient preference.

The most effective way of excluding intrauterine pathology is by diagnostic hysteroscopy. This can be performed in the outpatient setting without analgesia and will identify endometrial polyps, submucous fibroids, endometritis, and most endometrial carcinomas. Where appropriate, laparoscopy will be indicated to exclude pelvic pathology.

There would appear to be enough evidence to suggest that blind D&C, used as a diagnostic or therapeutic tool in the management of menorrhagia, is one of the most inappropriately used surgical procedures of our time.

Complications of menorrhagia

Apart from the effect on the quality of life and interference with both social life and work, which can be profound, the most common complication of menorrhagia is iron-deficiency anemia.

Treatment of menorrhagia

The treatment of menorrhagia should be tailored to the patient's needs and also to the findings of the relevant laboratory work. Practically, this usually includes the following:

- Correction of iron-deficiency anemia.
- Treatment of systemic disorders or focal pathology.
- Attempted control of menorrhagia by medical treatment.
- Surgical treatment of menorrhagia, if medical treatment fails.

Medical treatment of menorrhagia

It is generally believed, by doctors and patients alike, that most drugs used to treat menorrhagia are not only ineffective, but also produce intolerable side effects. This has led to their inappropriate use and a greater reliance on surgical techniques in the management of menorrhagia. For instance, progestogens are the most commonly prescribed drug for menorrhagia and yet are the least effective. The reduction of mean MBL for different medical therapies is shown in Fig. 19.7.

Mean percentage reduction in measured MBL in women with menorrhagia treated with medical therapy

Drug	Mean % MBL reduction
NSAIDs	
Ibuprofen	47
Hormonal therapy	
OCPs	50
Danazol	60
Levonorgestrel IUD	97
Luteal-phase progestins	15

Fig. 19.7 Mean percentage reduction in measured MBL in women with menorrhagia treated with medical therapy.

Prostaglandin inhibitors

A wide range of NSAIDs, including aspirin, indomethacin, ibuprofen, and motrin, are potent inhibitors of the cyclo-oxygenase enzyme system, which is a controlling step in the production of cyclic endoperoxides from arachidonic acid. Three-quarters of women treated with NSAIDs will find an improvement in MBL, with a mean reduction of 50%. Dysmenorrhea and menstrual headaches are also improved. As medication is taken with menstruation, side effects are usually better tolerated than with those drugs that are taken daily.

Hormonal therapy

Progestins. Oral progestogens are the most commonly used drugs for the treatment of menorrhagia and are probably the least effective. Early studies showed an improvement in subjective MBL, but objective studies have shown no statistical improvement. They are most effectively used in anovulatory menorrhagia to produce cycle control.

Intrauterine devices. IUDs impregnated with either progesterone or levonorgestrel have been shown to reduce MBL dramatically, as well as acting as a very reliable contraception. The Mirena IUD releases 20 µg of levonorgestrel every 24 h into the endometrium from a silicone barrel. As a result of minimal systemic absorption, side effects

Abnormal Uterine Bleeding

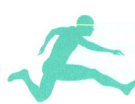

are usually limited to irregular spotting in the initial year of usage; thus, as a safe long-term medical treatment for menorrhagia, this method seems extremely encouraging. Amenorrhea is induced in up to 50% of long-term users because of endometrial atrophy. Contraceptively, it is as effective as sterilization, and yet fertility returns almost immediately on removal of the system. It is used for the treatment of menorrhagia for up to 5 years.

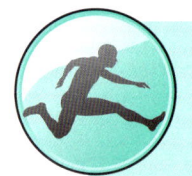

> The most effective long-term medical therapy for menorrhagia is currently the levonorgestrel IUD.

Oral contraceptive pill. When taken in a cyclical fashion, the OCP inhibits ovulation and produces regular shedding of a thin endometrium. This makes it an effective and acceptable longer term medical treatment for some women with menorrhagia. Thrombogenic side effects restrict its therapeutic use to younger women, especially in smokers.

Danazol. Danazol is a testosterone derivative producing a number of effects on the hypothalamic–pituitary–ovarian axis. The optimum dosage in the treatment of menorrhagia appears to be 200 mg daily, significantly reducing mean MBL as well as reducing dysmenorrhea. The androgenic properties of danazol produce unacceptable side effects in some women.

Gonadotrophin-releasing hormone agonists. GnRH agonists suppress pituitary–ovarian function and effectively produce a temporary, reversible menopausal state. Because of the subsequent bone density loss, their long-term use as a primary medical treatment for menorrhagia is limited unless add-back hormone therapy is given. This relegates their clinical use to that of a preoperative adjunct allowing correction of iron-deficiency anemia, reduction in the size of fibroids, and reduction in surgical blood loss (see Chapter 20).

The management of menorrhagia using medical therapies should be tailored to the patient's individual needs. Guidelines are shown in Fig. 19.8.

Surgical treatment of menorrhagia

Surgical treatment of menorrhagia depends on the diagnosis. Intrauterine pathology, such as endometrial polyps and submucous fibroids, can be removed hysteroscopically. Following hysteroscopic myomectomy, MBL has been shown to be reduced by 75%. Open myomectomy may be required in the presence of large fibroids and where the uterus is to be conserved. Endometrial ablation and hysterectomy are the most common operations performed for menorrhagia, and these will be discussed in detail.

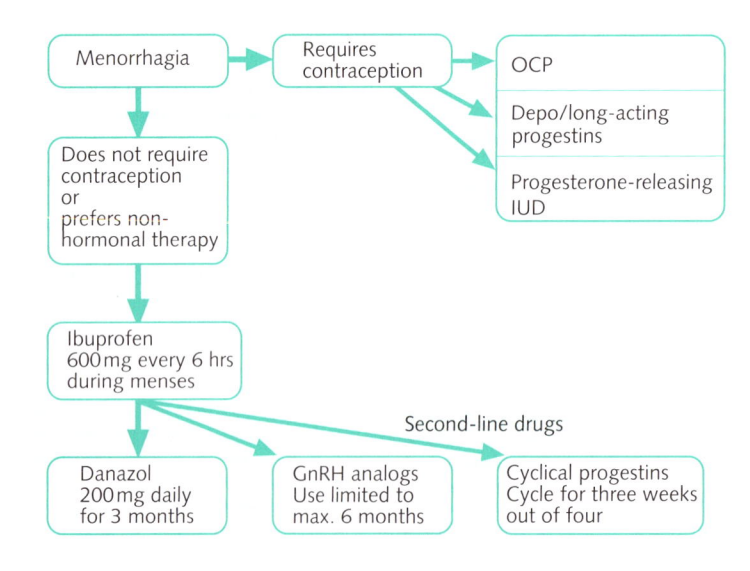

Fig. 19.8 Algorithm for menorrhagia.

> Endometrial ablative methods are becoming increasingly popular owing to rapid recovery and the possibility of outpatient treatment.

Endometrial ablation

Endometrial ablation techniques aim to reduce menstrual loss by producing an "iatrogenic" Asherman's syndrome. Endometrium is destroyed using laser, resection, or thermal ablation techniques and the ensuing intrauterine adhesions reduce endometrial regrowth from deep within crypts or glands. Although not guaranteeing amenorrhea as hysterectomy does, advantages include speed of surgery, quicker recovery, rapid return to work, and the use of local as opposed to general anesthesia. Following endometrial ablation, MBL has been shown to be reduced by up to 90%.

Deaths have occurred after endometrial ablation; these have been due to air embolism during laser ablation, toxic shock following endometrial resection, sepsis from bowel perforation, and hemorrhage following major vessel transection. The most common operative complications are:

- *Uterine perforation:* potentially one of the most serious complications of endometrial ablation, as it can be associated with fluid overload as well as trauma to the GI and genitourinary tracts and major blood vessels, resulting in peritonitis or hemorrhage. Perforation commonly occurs where the uterine wall is thinnest, such as the cornual regions and the cervical canal.
- *Fluid overload:* use of nonelectrolytic solutions, such as 1.5% glycine, for electrosurgery and the relatively high pressures needed to distend the noncompliant uterine walls predispose to the absorption of large quantities of fluid, which can result in hyponatremia due to dilutional effects of the irrigating fluid. Congestive cardiac failure, hypertension, hyponatremia, neurologic symptoms, hemolysis, coma, and even death can develop.
- *Hemorrhage:* likely to occur if the myometrium is resected too deeply and in the event of perforation of the uterus.
- *Infection:* the true incidence of pelvic infection following endometrial ablation is difficult to quantify. Infection can be overwhelming and might cause long-term pelvic pain.

Hysterectomy

Hysterectomy is one of the most commonly performed operations in the US. Each year, more than 600,000 hysterectomies are performed. The overall lifetime risk of having a hysterectomy in the US is 1/3.

The mortality rate following hysterectomy for benign disease is very low (approximately 6 per 10,000) and is usually a consequence of cardiovascular disease and sepsis.

Morbidity associated with hysterectomy is common and occurs in almost half the women undergoing abdominal hysterectomy and one-quarter of those undergoing vaginal hysterectomy. Although conditions such as thromboembolic disease should not be forgotten, the following are some of the more likely complications to be encountered:

- *Febrile morbidity.* This accounts for most of the overall morbidity following hysterectomy, with one in three women experiencing this following the abdominal approach. In one-quarter of cases the source of infection is not identifiable; the most common identifiable infection is UTI, followed by wound or vaginal cuff infection. The use of prophylactic antibiotics is associated with a lower rate of infection of the urinary tract, abdominal wound, and vaginal cuff.
- *Hemorrhage requiring transfusion.*
- *Unintended major surgery because of urinary tract damage.* Damage to the ureter occurs in approximately 1 in every 200 hysterectomies. The ureter is likely to be damaged at the infundibulopelvic ligament, beneath the uterine artery and adjacent to the cervix. Predisposing factors to ureteric damage include congenital anomaly of the renal tracts and distortion of normal anatomy from PID, endometriosis, adhesions, and malignancy. Trauma to the bladder occurs in approximately 1 in 100 hysterectomies and is much higher following vaginal hysterectomy. Predisposing factors include previous surgery and obesity.
- *Unintended major surgery because of bowel damage.* The incidence of bowel trauma is

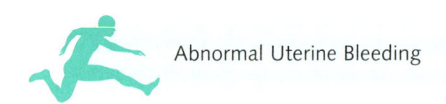

approximately 1 in 200 hysterectomies. Risk factors predisposing to bowel damage are obesity, previous laparotomy, adhesions, intrinsic bowel problems (e.g. chronic inflammatory bowel disease), and irradiation. Bowel dysfunction following hysterectomy is well documented, with constipation occurring in up to half the patients during the first 2 weeks of the abdominal approach. One in five patients will continue to complain of constipation in the first three postoperative months.

- **Long-term complications.** During the removal of the uterus, the pelvic floor and its nerve supply are disrupted. This can predispose to pelvic floor laxity with subsequent prolapse, as well as bladder and bowel dysfunction. Even when the ovaries are conserved, disruption of their blood supply is thought to interfere with their function, and might even predispose to premature ovarian failure, a risk factor for cardiovascular disease and osteoporosis.

Postmenopausal bleeding

PMB is vaginal bleeding occurring more than 6 months after menopause. In clinical practice, menopause is a retrospective diagnosis; therefore, it is important to keep in mind, and exclude, causes of secondary amenorrhea, such as pregnancy. PMB is a common disorder and requires prompt investigation to exclude malignancy.

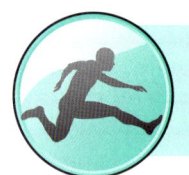

> A woman with PMB should always be investigated to exclude malignancy.

Causes of postmenopausal bleeding

There are many causes of PMB, and the simplest way of remembering them all is by anatomy (Fig. 19.9). However, although atrophic changes to the genital tract are the most common cause of PMB, malignancy of the endometrium, cervix, and ovary must always be remembered and excluded.

Disease of the ovary in postmenopausal women is uncommon, but it can present with PMB. An estrogen-secreting tumor causes PMB by stimulating the endometrium in the absence of progesterone. This is likely to cause hyperplasia

Causes of postmenopausal bleeding	
Structure affected	**Specific cause**
Ovary	Carcinoma of the ovary
	Estrogen-secreting tumour
Uterine body	Myometrium:
	• submucous fibroid
	Endometrium:
	• atrophic changes
	• polyp
	• hyperplasia—simple or atypical
	• carcinoma
	(Pregnancy)
Cervix	Atrophic changes
	Malignancy:
	• squamous carcinoma
	• adenocarcinoma
Vagina	Atrophic changes
Urethra	Urethral caruncle
	(Hematuria)
Vulva	Vulvitis
	Dystrophies
	Malignancy

Fig. 19.9 Causes of PMB.

and even carcinoma of the endometrium. Ovarian carcinoma usually causes PMB by direct invasion through the uterine wall.

Submucous fibroids can cause PMB, although these are likely to have been present from before menopause. The endometrium should be inactive in the postmenopausal years and atrophic endometritis is a common consequence. Endometrial polyps might be benign, contain areas of atypical hyperplasia, or be malignant. Endometrial hyperplasia can arise de novo, or be secondary to estrogen stimulation. Exogenous unopposed estrogens and endogenous estrogens arising from peripheral conversion of precursors in adipose tissue, or from estrogen-secreting ovarian tumors, can result in endometrial hyperplasia and adenocarcinoma. Adenocarcinoma of the endometrium is an important cause of PMB and must always be considered in the differential diagnosis.

Atrophic changes to the genital tract due to estrogen deficiency can cause bleeding and, in fact, are the most common cause of PMB. Atrophic changes can occur to the endometrium, cervix, and vagina. Urethral caruncle (prolapse of the urethral mucosa) is also associated with estrogen deficiency.

Cervical carcinoma and squamous carcinoma of the vulva can present with PMB, and although the nonneoplastic epithelial disorders of the vulva (vulvar dystrophies) do not themselves usually cause PMB, scratching because of vulvar pruritus can.

Investigating postmenopausal bleeding

Clinical examination should reveal lesions of the vulva, vagina, and cervix, as well as identifying pelvic masses. The most common cause of PMB is atrophic vaginitis; although this might be evident on clinical examination, it must not be assumed to be the cause of the PMB until other more serious causes have been excluded.

Investigation depends on the clinical findings. Vulvar and vaginal biopsies should be performed when abnormal lesions are present. Cervical pathology can be excluded by cytology or colposcopic examination (Fig. 19.10).

Intrauterine pathology is best excluded by hysteroscopic examination of the uterine cavity with endometrial biopsy, although ultrasound estimation of the endometrial thickness combined with endometrial sampling can be used. The endometrial thickness in a postmenopausal woman should be less than 4 mm. Although a negative endometrial sample is reassuring, the most common method of taking the sample in the outpatient setting is by using the "pipelle" endometrial sampler, which samples only 4% of the uterine cavity. Ultrasound with biopsy can, therefore, miss early focal pathology. Although D&C can be performed at the same time as hysteroscopy as a method of endometrial biopsy, there is no place for D&C alone in the management of PMB. The ovaries can be assessed using ultrasound, and if an estrogen-secreting tumor is suspected, then circulating estradiol levels should be measured.

Treating postmenopausal bleeding

Treatment obviously depends on the pathology. The most commonly encountered cause of PMB is atrophic change; therefore, estrogen replacement is indicated, not only to prevent a recurrence of PMB, but also to treat other symptoms associated with estrogen deficiency. Most women in this situation prefer to use topical estrogen. The newer

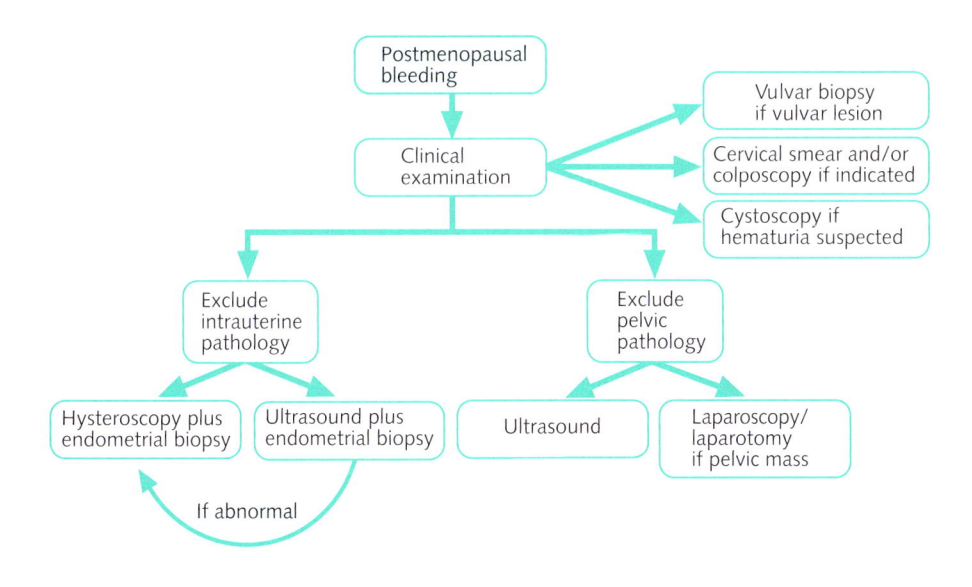

Fig. 19.10 Algorithm for PMB.

17β-estradiol-releasing creams, rings, and vaginal tablets avoid the risk of endometrial hyperplasia because of minimal systemic absorption. If systemic HRT is requested, then estrogen therapy must be combined with a progestin or progesterone in women who have a uterus.

The treatment of urethral caruncle is by surgical excision of the prolapsed urethral mucosa and is a painful and unpleasant procedure. It should, therefore, be reserved for those cases in which recurrent PMB or pain occurs. Small caruncles might recede with estrogen cream.

The treatment of vulvar, cervical, and ovarian malignancy is discussed in detail in Chapter 23.

- What are the possible diagnoses in a woman presenting with primary amenorrhea?
- What are the possible diagnoses in a woman presenting with secondary amenorrhea?
- What are the effective medical treatments for menorrhagia?
- What are the surgical options for treatment of menorrhagia?

Further reading

Rock JA, et al. (1999) *Te Linde's Operative Gynecology*, 9th ed (Lippincott Williams & Wilkins, Philadelphia).

Speroff F. (2005) *Clinical Gynecologic Endocrinology and Infertility*, 7th ed. (Lippincott Williams & Wilkins, Philadelphia).

20. Fibroids

Uterine fibroids are benign tumors of the myometrium. They are the most common benign tumors found in women, occurring in approximately 20% of women over the age of 30 years. Histologically they are composed of whorling bundles of smooth muscle cells that resemble the architecture of normal myometrium.

Although their etiology is unknown, fibroids are associated with exposure to estrogens. Factors influencing the incidence of fibroids are shown in Fig. 20.1. The hyperestrogenic state of pregnancy might stimulate the growth of fibroids already present. Fibroids can be categorized by their position within the myometrium (Fig. 20.2).

Symptoms of uterine fibroids

Symptoms associated with uterine fibroids are shown in Fig. 20.3.

No symptoms

Approximately 50% of women with fibroids are asymptomatic, diagnosis being made during incidental clinical or ultrasound assessment of the pelvis and during pregnancy.

Up to 50% of women with fibroids will be completely asymptomatic.

Menstrual abnormalities

Menstrual abnormalities occur in about one-third of women with fibroids, usually heavy periods. Submucous fibroids can also cause intermenstrual bleeding, postcoital bleeding, continuous vaginal bleeding, or dysmenorrhea. Increased MBL due to fibroids is associated with:
- Increased endometrial surface area.
- Prostaglandin production.

Abdominopelvic mass

Large fibroids growing into the abdominal cavity can cause abdominal swelling or distention.

Pain

Abdominopelvic pain can be caused by:
- Degeneration of uterine fibroids.
- The presence of associated pelvic varicosities.
- Stretching of the uterine ligaments.
- Compression of surrounding pelvic structures.

Infertility

Fibroids compressing the cornual region of the fallopian tubes can cause infertility. Submucous fibroids, especially those that are hormonally active, can affect implantation and might result in miscarriage. There is now evidence that even intramural fibroids that are not distorting the endometrial cavity can still lead to reduced embryo implantation and pregnancy rates, possibly because of interference with the endometrial blood supply.

Pressure symptoms

Urinary frequency, nocturia, and urgency can be caused by pressure on the bladder from an enlarged uterus, and incarceration of a pelvic fibroid can result in urinary retention. Pressure on the rectum might also be noticed.

Complications

Necrotic degeneration occurring in pregnancy can present with acute pain, and the subsequent massive release of prostaglandins can cause miscarriage or premature labor. Pedunculated fibroids can undergo torsion and present with an acute abdomen. Urinary retention might occur with impaction of a pelvic fibroid. Hyaline, cystic, and calcific degenerative changes can also occur. Sarcomatous (malignant) change, usually within very large or rapidly growing fibroids, is a rare (approximately 1 in 1000) but potentially fatal complication.

In pregnancy, fibroids situated low in the uterus can result in malpresentation of the fetus and obstruct delivery. They can also lead to IUGR if placental perfusion is compromised. Fibroids can also restrict postpartum involution of the uterus and predispose to PPH.

Fibroids

Fig. 20.1 Factors influencing the incidence of fibroids.

| Factors influencing the incidence of fibroids ||
Increased incidence with:	Decreased incidence with:
African-American women	Cigarette smoking
Increasing age	Use of OCP
Nulligravidity	Full term pregnancy
Obesity	

Symptoms associated with uterine fibroids

- Asymptomatic
- Menstrual abnormalities
- Abdominopelvic mass
- Infertility
- Pressure symptoms
- Pregnancy complications

Fig. 20.3 Symptoms associated with uterine fibroids.

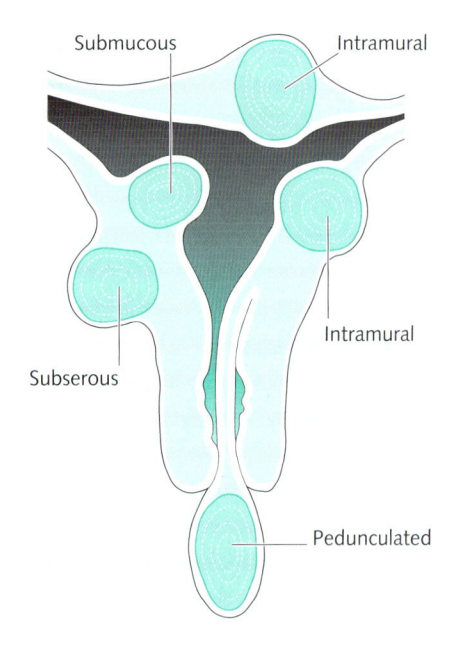

Fig. 20.2 Categorization of fibroids. (Submucous, Intramural, Subserous, Pedunculated)

Clinical evaluation

The presence of fibroids can be elicited by abdominopelvic examination; classically, the uterus feels firm and irregular. If a fibroid is moved on bimanual examination the uterus moves with it, although this can also occur with an ovarian mass adherent to the uterus. Pelvic ultrasound might show characteristic diffuse changes associated with the presence of fibroids. Individual larger fibroids can be seen and measured by ultrasound, but the best method of excluding submucous fibroids in the presence of menstrual abnormalities is by hysteroscopy. MRI has become the gold standard imaging method for differentiating fibroids from other pelvic masses. However, laparotomy might be required to be 100% certain in some cases.

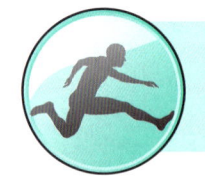

> Diagnosis is usually confirmed by ultrasound scan, which will define size and location.

Indications for treatment

Small, asymptomatic fibroids do not require intervention. Indications for treatment include:
- Symptomatic fibroids.
- Rapidly enlarging fibroids.
- Fibroids that are thought to be causing infertility.

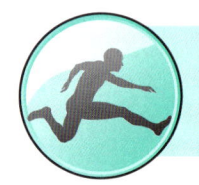

> Fibroids need treatment only if they are causing symptoms or if there is subfertility.

Medical therapy

Medical therapy is only useful as an adjunct to surgery and as an aid to correction of anemia prior to surgery. Fibroids regrow to their original size within 3 months of ceasing medical therapy without surgical intervention.

Gonadotrophin-releasing hormone analogs

GnRH analogs produce a hypogonadotrophic hypogonadal state; that is, they produce a temporary, reversible, chemical menopause that results in a reduction in fibroid volume by up to 50% with a maximum benefit within 3 months of starting therapy.

GnRH analogs have several different uses prior to surgery:
- They reduce surgical blood loss and the need for blood transfusions.
- They increase the likelihood of performing surgery through a transverse suprapubic incision rather than a midline incision.
- They reduce the risk of hysterectomy when myomectomy is planned.

The long-term use of GnRH analogs has been limited because of their side effects, which include menopausal symptoms and bone density reduction (osteoporosis). However, recent data have indicated that low-dose HRT, used concomitantly as "add back," can avoid menopausal side effects and prevent loss of bone density while maintaining the benefits of the GnRH analogs. GnRH analogs are currently licensed for 6 months use. More data are required before GnRH analogs with add back are licensed for longer-term use.

Surgical treatment

Definitive surgery includes one of:
- Myomectomy.
- Hysterectomy.

Myomectomy is the removal of fibroids with preservation of the uterus and can be performed either at laparotomy (open myomectomy), hysteroscopically, or laparoscopically.

Complications include hemorrhage, which might require blood transfusion, and (rarely) hysterectomy. Adhesion formation can impair future fertility and is most common after open myomectomy, especially for posterior wall fibroids. Fibroid regrowth is likely to occur in 40% of patients, with a reoperation rate of up to one-fifth of cases. Hysterectomy is the surgical procedure of choice in women who have completed their families.

> Surgical treatment with hysterectomy often causes less morbidity than myomectomy; the latter is performed in women who wish to preserve their fertility.

Advances in fibroid treatment

Techniques for the treatment of fibroids are currently being developed to reduce the need for laparotomy, to decrease postoperative adhesion formation, and to avoid large uterine scars. These include:
- Interstitial laser photocoagulation: laser probes are inserted into the fibroid laparoscopically to produce tissue degeneration and subsequent fibroid shrinkage.
- Laparoscopic diathermy.
- Radiologic embolization of fibroids via uterine artery catheterization using tiny silicone microbeads.
- Directed high-energy ultrasound.

- What are the different types of fibroid degeneration?
- What are the possible locations for fibroids?
- What symptoms can be caused by fibroids?
- How can fibroids be managed medically?
- How can fibroids be managed surgically?
- What are the new techniques for dealing with fibroids?

Further reading

Hillard PA, et al. (2002) *Novak's Gynaecology*, 13th ed. (Lippincott Williams & Wilkins, Philadelphia).

Rock JA, et al. (2003) *Te Linde's Operative Gynecology*, 9th ed. (Lippincott Williams & Wilkins, Philadelphia).

21. Endometriosis

Endometriosis is the presence of functional endometrium outside the uterine cavity. Endometriosis occurring in the myometrium is known as adenomyosis. The true incidence of endometriosis is difficult to ascertain, as not all women with endometriosis complain of gynecologic symptoms. Endometriosis occurs in about 10% of the female population in their reproductive years, but has been discovered incidentally in up to 25% women undergoing gynecologic laparoscopy.

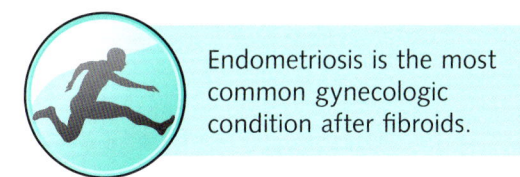

Endometriosis is the most common gynecologic condition after fibroids.

Etiology

The etiology of endometriosis is unknown, but several theories have been suggested (Fig. 21.1).

Retrograde menstruation/implantation theory
During menstruation, endometrial tissue spills into the pelvic cavity through the fallopian tubes, resulting in retrograde menstruation. This ectopic endometrium then implants and becomes functional, responding to the hormones of the ovarian cycle. This theory is supported by the association between endometriosis and increased menstruation occurring with a short menstrual cycle and prolonged periods, and by the fact that the most common sites for endometriosis are the ovaries and the uterosacral ligaments—areas in which retrograde menses spill. The implantation theory would also account for the rare cases of endometriosis found in the surgical incision following surgery on the uterus. Imperforate hymen and other outflow obstructions that exacerbate retrograde menstruation are also associated with severe endometriosis.

However, this theory does not account for the existence of endometriosis at the distant sites in the body (e.g. lungs). There is growing laparoscopic evidence to suggest that most women experience retrograde menstruation, in which case the incidence of endometriosis would be expected to be higher. This would suggest that this theory, as it stands, is too simplistic.

Lymphatic and venous embolization
This theory hypothesizes that endometrial tissue is transported through the body by the lymphatic or venous channels and would explain the rare cases of distant sites for endometriosis. However, distant endometriotic deposits would be expected to be more common if the lymphatic and venous embolization theories were the only mechanism for the development of endometriosis.

Celomic metaplasia
This theory relies on the principle that tissues of certain embryonal origin maintain their ability to undergo metaplasia and differentiate into other tissue types. This is certainly true of peritoneum of celomic origin, which can undergo metaplasia and differentiate into functional endometrium. Although this is an attractive theory, it does not explain the distribution of endometriosis within the peritoneal cavity itself (most common in the lower part of the peritoneal cavity) or the presence of endometriosis in sites of the body that are not of celomic origin.

Genetic and immunologic factors
The role of a genetic influence is supported by the strong family history seen in endometriosis sufferers. What exactly that role is has not yet been ascertained. It is possible that those women

---

Suggested theories for the etiology of endometriosis

- Implantation/retrograde menstruation
- Genetic and immunological factors
- Lymphatic and venous embolization
- Celomic metaplasia
- Composite theories

Fig. 21.1 Suggested theories for the etiology of endometriosis.

Endometriosis

with a genetic predisposition to endometriosis have an abnormal response to the presence of ectopic endometrium, which results in the development of endometriosis. There is some evidence that an altered or defective cell-mediated response is implicated.

Composite theories

None of the above theories will alone account for all cases of endometriosis; however, together, all the theories could play a role in some way. Whereas an abnormal response to the presence of ectopic endometrium might result in functioning endometrium responding to the ovarian cycle, this in turn could trigger celomic metaplasia and further development or advancement of the disease process in response to the local release of endometrial hormones and/or the inflammatory response.

Sites of endometriosis

The most common sites for the development of endometriosis are the ovaries and the uterosacral ligaments. These and other pelvic sites are shown in Fig. 21.2. Although endometriosis has been reported in nearly every organ except the spleen, extrapelvic endometriosis is rare. Assessment of the severity of pelvic endometriosis can be made using the American Fertility Society Classification (Fig. 21.3), which takes into account the site and size of endometriotic lesions, and the presence and consequences of adhesions.

Symptoms

The key to the diagnosis of endometriosis is the presence of cyclical pain associated with menstruation. Cyclical pain occurs because the deposits of endometriosis, whatever their location in the body, respond to the ovarian cycle, and bleeding from these deposits causes local irritation and inflammatory responses (Fig. 21.4). The exact location of the type of pain depends on the sites of ectopic endometrium. If the endometriosis is severe, then pain can be continuous, with exacerbations at the time of menstruation. Neural and intracranial endometriosis produce continuous pain.

Endometriosis of the lung, bladder, bowel, or umbilicus will produce bleeding from these sites associated with the menstruation.

Rupture of an ovarian endometrioma will cause severe lower abdominal pain. The release of the very irritant "chocolate" material from the cyst causes peritonitis.

Infertility

An association between infertility and endometriosis exists, with as many as one-third of infertile women being diagnosed as having endometriosis. Dense adhesions and the resultant tubal and ovarian damage and distortion caused by severe endometriosis will obviously contribute to

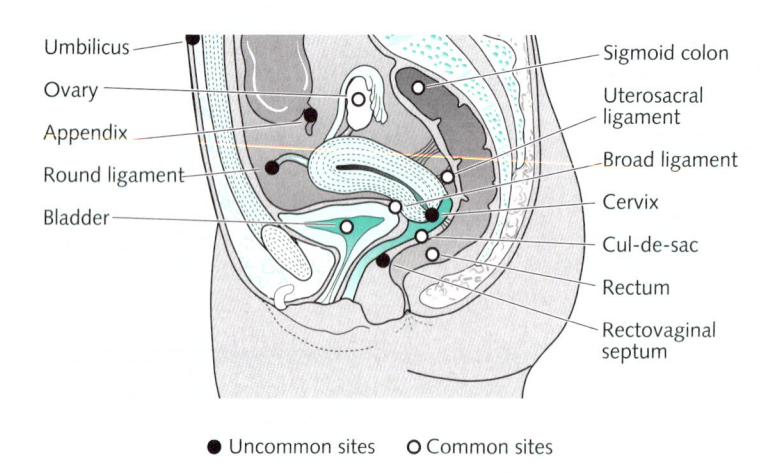

Fig. 21.2 Sites of endometriosis.

Infertility

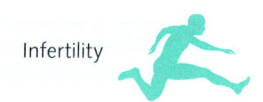

Anatomical Site	Score	1	2	3	4	6
Peritoneum	Endometriotic lesion size	<1 cm	1–3 cm	>3 cm		
	Adhesions	Flimsy	Dense with partial pouch of Douglas occlusion	Dense with complete pouch of Douglas occlusion		
Ovary [points for each side involved]	Endometriotic lesion size		<1 cm		1–3 cm	>3 cm
	Adhesions		Filmy		Dense with partial ovarian coverage	Dense completely enclosing ovary
Fallopian tubes [points for each side involved]	Endometriotic lesion size		<1 cm		>1 cm	Tubal occlusion
	Adhesions		Filmy		Dense and distorting tubes	Dense and completely enclosing tubes
			Stage I (Mild) <5 Stage II (Mod) 6–15		Stage III (Severe) 16–30 Stage IV (Extensive) >31	

American Fertility Society classification of endometriosis

Fig. 21.3 American Fertility Society classification of endometriosis.

Lungs — Cyclical hemoptysis

Urinary tract — Cyclical hematuria
ureteric obstruction

Large bowel — Cyclical tenesmus
Cyclical diarrhea
Cyclical rectal bleeding
Colonic obstruction

Surgical scars/ umbilicus — Cyclical pain
Cyclical bleeding

Pelvis — Secondary dysmenorrhea
Deep dyspareunia
Continuous pelvic/ lower abdominal pain
Menstrual abnormality
Infertility

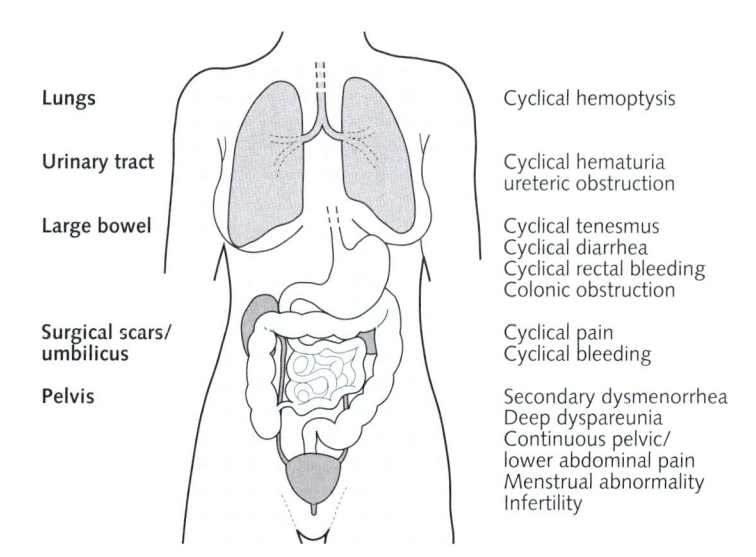

Fig. 21.4 Symptoms of endometriosis.

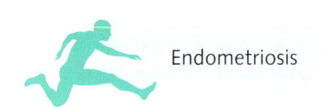

the lack of conception. The association with mild endometriosis, in which no mechanical damage has occurred, is less easy to understand. Release of substances from the ectopic endometrium, such as prostaglandins, which can affect ovulation or tubal motility, has been implicated. There is evidence that treatment of even mild disease can lead to an improvement of fertility prospects.

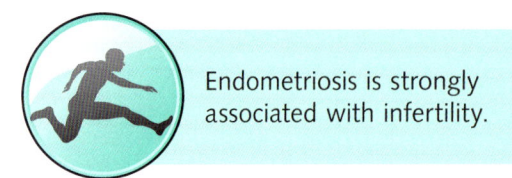

> Endometriosis is strongly associated with infertility.

Clinical evaluation

Endometriosis should be considered in any woman who presents with any of the symptoms shown in Fig. 21.4. The classic quartet of symptoms of endometriosis is:
- Secondary dysmenorrhea.
- Deep dyspareunia.
- Pelvic pain.
- Infertility.

The dysmenorrhea associated with endometriosis typically starts prior to the beginning of the period and is exacerbated by menstrual flow.

Pelvic examination can reveal a tender, retroverted, retroflexed, fixed uterus with thickening of the cardinal or uterosacral ligaments. Endometriotic nodules might be palpable in the posterior vaginal fornix, and ovarian endometriomas might be evident on bimanual palpation. The pelvic anatomy might be normal with mild disease, and a useful sign is to elicit pain on moving the cervix anteriorly. This stretches the uterosacral ligaments, which is painful in the presence of endometriosis. In the presence of adenomyosis, the uterus is typically smoothly enlarged (globular) and tender.

Diagnosis and severity of disease can only effectively be assessed through the laparoscope. The classic "powder-burn" lesions of endometriosis might be seen, but these areas of hemosiderin pigmentation might represent "burnt-out" endometriosis. Nonpigmented lesions can appear as opaque white areas of peritoneum, red lesions, or glandular lesions. If there is doubt about the macroscopic appearance, then a peritoneal biopsy should be taken. Ovarian endometriomas can be seen by ultrasound, but differentiation from other ovarian pathology can be difficult.

Differential diagnosis

Complications
Complications of endometriosis are often due to the resultant fibrosis and scarring and can affect not only the reproductive organs, but might also cause colonic and ureteric obstruction. Rupture of an endometrioma and the subsequent release of the very irritant "chocolate" material contents can cause peritonitis. Malignant change within endometriotic lesions is rare and most commonly occurs in ovarian endometriosis.

Treatment

Treatment of endometriosis is indicated to:
- Alleviate symptoms.
- Stop progression of disease and development of complications.
- Improve fertility.

Treatment depends on the severity of the disease and should be tailored to the woman's needs; it can be medical or surgical.

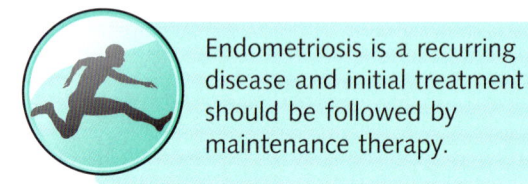

> Endometriosis is a recurring disease and initial treatment should be followed by maintenance therapy.

Medical treatment
The lesions of endometriosis regress in response to pregnancy and the menopause. Medical treatment is therefore aimed at mimicking one of these two physiological processes (Fig. 21.5).

Progestins
Continuous progestin therapy can effectively induce a state of pseudopregnancy, causing decidualization of endometriotic deposits, which then regress. Progestins can be taken orally or as depot preparations, and treatment should be for 6 months.

Treatment

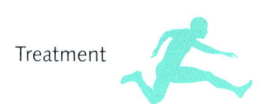

Summary of medical treatment of endometriosis

Drug	Mode of action	Side-effects
Progestins	Pseudopregnancy	Break-through bleeding, weight gain, edema, acne, abdominal bloating, increased appetite, decreased libido
Danazol	Pseudomenopause	Increased weight, break-through bleeding, muscle cramps, decreased breast size, hot flushes, emotional lability, oily skin, acne, hirsutism, headache, increased libido, hoarseness or deepening of the voice
GnRH analogs	Pseudomenopause	Hot flashes, break-through bleeding, vaginal dryness, headaches, decreased libido, bone density loss

Fig. 21.5 Summary of medical treatment of endometriosis.

Danazol
Danazol is a testosterone derivative and used to be the most common medical treatment for endometriosis. As well as its androgenic properties, danazol produces a hypoestrogenic state, and it is this pseudomenopausal state that induces endometrial regression and atrophy. The mode of action of danazol is complex: it acts at the pituitary, ovarian, and target tissue levels. It should be taken for 6–9 months and the dose should be titrated to the patient's response and presence of side effects. Patients should be warned to stop treatment if they develop deepening of the voice, as this could be irreversible.

Gonadotrophin-releasing hormone analogs
This class of synthetic drugs are GnRH superagonists. Continued administration desensitizes pituitary gondotrophs and results in a temporary, reversible state of hypogonadotrophic hypogonadism, in other words, a temporary, reversible, chemical menopause. GnRH analogs are as effective as danazol in reducing the symptoms and severity of endometriosis and are usually used for 3–6 months. Their menopausal side effects are often better tolerated than the androgenic side effects of danazol and can be reduced by using "add-back" continuous combined HRT (see Chapter 20).

Oral contraceptive pills
The OCP suppresses ovulation and the normal cyclical ovarian production of estrogen and progesterone. Mild symptoms of endometriosis can be controlled by using the OCP, but it is more often used as maintenance therapy following initial treatment. Endometriosis is a recurring disease, with up to 40% women developing recurring symptoms within 1 year of stopping treatment. Initial treatment should, therefore, be followed by maintenance therapy to reduce the chance of recurrence. Maintenance therapy aims to suppress or reduce the frequency of periods, and this can be achieved by tricycling a continuous dose combined OCP.

Surgical therapy
Surgical treatment of endometriosis can be conservative or radical. Which method is used depends on the patient's:
- Age.
- Fertility requirements.
- Response to medical treatment.

Conservative surgery
Conservative surgery can be performed through a laparoscope or at laparotomy and aims to:
- Return the anatomy of the pelvis to normal.
- Destroy visible lesions of endometriosis.
- Improve fertility.
- Conserve ovarian tissue.

Necessary procedures can include division of adhesions, destruction of endometriotic lesions using diathermy or laser, and excision of deep-seated endometriomas, which are known not to respond well to medical therapy. Complications include damage to other pelvic structures, including bowel, bladder and ureters. Recurrence of symptoms might occur not only because endometriosis is a recurring disease, but also because endometriotic deposits not visible to the naked eye will not have been destroyed. Diffuse peritoneal endometriosis might be better treated medically. Pregnancy rates following conservative surgery are directly related to the severity of the disease.

Radical surgery
Definitive radical surgery for endometriosis is reserved for women who no longer wish to maintain fertility and in whom other forms of treatment have failed. Total abdominal hysterectomy (TAH) with bilateral salpingo-oophorectomy (BSO) is the procedure of choice. It is the removal of the ovaries, the main source of estrogens, that produces a hypoestrogenic state and effectively treats the endometriosis. As many of these women are relatively young, HRT is advised. Estrogen replacement can cause a recurrence of endometriosis in a small percentage of women and should, therefore, be kept to a minimum. Continuous combined estrogen and progesterone replacement might further reduce the rate of recurrence because of the effects of progestins on endometriosis.

- What are the theories for the genesis of endometriosis?
- What are the most common sites of endometriosis?
- What are the typical symptoms of endometriosis?
- How is endometriosis thought to cause infertility?

Further reading
Hillard PA, et al. (2002) *Novak's Gynaecology*, 13th ed. (Lippincott Williams & Wilkins, Philadelphia).

Speroff F. (2005) *Clinical Gynecologic Endocrinology and Infertility*, 7th ed. (Lippincott Williams & Wilkins, Philadelphia).

22. Benign Ovarian Tumors

Incidence

Benign ovarian cysts are common and often asymptomatic, resolving spontaneously. Therefore, despite being a frequent cause for admission to hospital, their exact incidence is unknown. About 90% of ovarian tumors overall are benign, but this changes with age. Malignant tumors are most common in the postmenopausal age group.

Etiology

Ovarian tumors can be physiologic or pathologic. Classification depends on the ovarian tissue from which they arise (Fig. 22.1). Excluding the physiologic group, a germ cell tumor is the more common diagnosis in a woman less than 40 years of age, whereas an epithelial cell tumor is more likely in an older woman.

Physiologic cysts
These are often asymptomatic and occur commonly in younger women.

Follicular cysts
These are the result of either nonrupture of the dominant follicle during the normal cycle or from failure of atresia of a nondominant follicle. Smaller cysts might resolve spontaneously, but intervention could be necessary if the cyst causes symptoms or if ultrasound follow-up shows failure of resolution or an increase in size.

Luteal cysts
In contrast to follicular cysts, luteal cysts are more likely to present with intraperitoneal bleeding secondary to rupture.

Benign germ cell tumors
Such tumors arise from totipotential germ cells and thus can contain elements of all three layers of embryonic tissue: ectodermal derivatives, such as teeth and hair; endodermal tissue, such as intestine; and mesodermal structures, such as bone.

Classification of benign ovarian tumors	
Type of tumor	Name
Physiologic	Follicular cysts
	Luteal cysts
Benign germ cell tumors	Mature cystic teratoma (dermoid cyst)
	Mature solid teratoma
Benign epithelial tumors	Serous cystadenoma
	Mucinous cystadenoma
	Endometrioid cystadenoma
	Brenner tumor
Benign sex cord stromal tumors	Theca cell tumors
	Fibroma
	Sertoli–Leydig cell tumor

Fig. 22.1 Classification of benign ovarian tumors.

Mature cystic teratoma
Also known as a dermoid cyst, this type of tumor has a median age of presentation of 30 years with about 10% being bilateral. Most are asymptomatic, but they can undergo torsion or, rarely, rupture.

Mature solid teratomas
Much less common than a dermoid cyst, these tumors must be distinguished from an immature solid teratoma which is malignant.

Benign epithelial tumors
The majority of ovarian cysts arise from the ovarian epithelium. They develop from the celomic epithelium over the gonadal ridge of the embryo and might, therefore, be derived from any of the pelvic organs or the renal tract.

Serous cystadenoma
This is the most common tumor in this group. Again, they are bilateral in about 10% of cases and they contain thin serous fluid, usually within a unilocular cavity. Histologically, they appear to have a tubal origin.

Mucinous cystadenoma
In contrast to the serous cystadenomas, these tumors are usually unilateral, larger in size, and multilocular with thick mucoid fluid. The mucus-secreting cells are likely to indicate an endocervical derivation.

Endometrioid tumors
These are mostly malignant tumors arising from endometrial cells.

Brenner tumors
The majority of these tumors are benign. They arise from uroepithelial cell lines and contain transitional epithelium; 10–15% are bilateral, usually small in size, and some might secrete estrogen.

Benign sex cord stromal tumors
Such tumors account for only about 4% of benign ovarian tumors. Many secrete hormones and thus present at any age with hormonally mediated symptoms.

Theca cell tumors
These cysts are nearly always benign solid tumors presenting over the age of 50 years (in contrast, granulosa cell tumors are always malignant).

Fibroma
These tumors are rare and can be associated with ascites.

Diagnosis

History
Benign ovarian tumors can be asymptomatic, e.g. detected by routine bimanual palpation during an annual exam on routine antenatal ultrasound scan. The presenting symptoms include:
- Pain secondary to torsion/rupture/hemorrhage/infection.
- Abdominal swelling.
- Pressure effects on bowel or bladder.
- Hormonal effects secondary to secretion of estrogens or androgens.

Figure 22.2 shows the differential diagnoses that need to be considered for the history, examination, and work-up. The history must include the date of the LMP and the regularity of the menstrual cycle, as well as current contraception, if appropriate. Any history of GI symptoms might be important, e.g. a patient with an ovarian torsion might present with sudden onset of right-sided abdominal pain associated with nausea and vomiting, and appendicitis must be excluded.

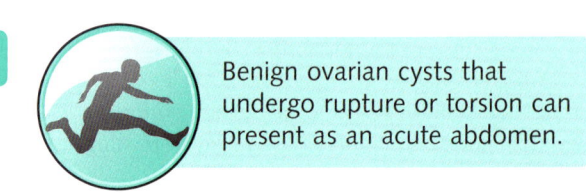

Differential diagnoses for ovarian tumors	
Symptom	Differential diagnosis
Pain	Ectopic pregnancy
	Spontaneous miscarriage
	PID
	Appendicitis
	Diverticulitis
Abdominal swelling	Pregnancy
	Fibroid uterus
	Full bladder
Pressure effects	Constipation
	Urine frequency
	Vaginal prolapse
Hormonal effects	Menstrual irregularity
	Postmenopausal bleeding
	Precocious puberty

Fig. 22.2 Differential diagnoses for ovarian tumors.

Benign ovarian cysts that undergo rupture or torsion can present as an acute abdomen.

Examination
Initial examination must include the pulse and blood pressure; rupture of an ovarian cyst can result in intraperitoneal bleeding that leads to hypovolemia. In a young patient, this might present at first with tachycardia and cold peripheries, with hypotension showing as a relatively late sign.

Distention might be seen on abdominal inspection, resulting from the cyst itself or from ascites if the cyst is malignant. If the cyst has torsed, or if there is hemorrhage into the cyst so that the capsule stretches, then abdominal palpation will elicit tenderness, typically in the lower quadrant, which might be associated with signs of peritonitis. A large ovarian tumor might rise up out of the pelvis and be palpated in the abdomen; this is done using the left hand and moving distally from the xiphoid process toward the pelvis (see Chapter 46). Ascites, associated with malignant tumors, should be excluded by testing for shifting dullness.

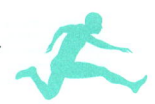

Bimanual palpation of the pelvic organs, as described in Chapter 46, is essential. If the tumor has presented acutely with abdominal pain, then adnexal tenderness or an adnexal mass will assist in excluding GI etiology. Assessing the size of the uterus will help to exclude a fibroid uterus or intrauterine pregnancy. If there seems to be an adnexal mass, then its approximate size, consistency, and the presence of any tenderness should be elicited.

Work-up

In line with the list of differential diagnoses in Fig. 22.2, investigations include:
- Hemoglobin.
- WBC.
- Urine pregnancy test and/or serum β-hCG level.
- Pelvic ultrasound scan.
- Serum CA125 level.
- Chest X-ray and intravenous pyelogram (IVP) if malignancy is suspected (see Chapter 23).

> The epithelial tumor marker (CA125) is almost always checked in the presence of an ovarian cyst to aid in the differential diagnosis.

Management of a benign ovarian tumor

The patient's management depends on the:
- Severity of presenting symptoms.
- Patient's age.
- Future fertility needs.
- Risk of malignancy.

Asymptomatic cysts

Treatment might not be warranted if an ovarian cyst is asymptomatic; this depends on the patient's age and the size of the cyst (Fig. 22.3). In a younger woman (usually taken as less than 40 years of age), the risk of the tumor being malignant is reduced and, therefore, the cyst can be monitored with pelvic ultrasound scans. A physiologic cyst is likely to resolve spontaneously, but a laparoscopy or laparotomy might be indicated if it persists or increases in size.

> Simple ovarian cysts <5 cm diameter can be managed conservatively with repeat ultrasound scans in 6–8 weeks.

In a woman who is older (e.g. at or nearing menopause), the issue of maintaining fertility is usually less important and the diagnosis of a physiologic cyst is unlikely. If the cyst is above a

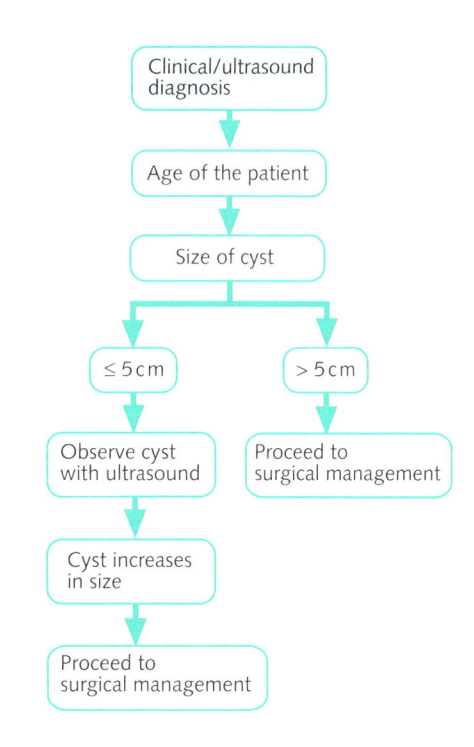

Clinical/ultrasound diagnosis
↓
Age of the patient
↓
Size of cyst
↓
≤5 cm → Observe cyst with ultrasound → Cyst increases in size → Proceed to surgical management
>5 cm → Proceed to surgical management

Fig. 22.3 Management of an asymptomatic benign ovarian tumor.

certain size (5 cm has been suggested), then malignancy must be excluded by:
- Measuring tumor markers.
- Ultrasound scan to distinguish solid elements within the cyst.
- Color Doppler studies of the blood flow around the cyst.

Laparoscopic assessment or laparotomy is then advised to obtain histological specimens.

Symptomatic cysts

If the patient presents with severe acute pain, an emergency laparoscopy and/or laparotomy is appropriate. With chronic symptoms, a procedure can be planned as above.

Thus, the appropriate treatment for an ovarian tumor depends on many factors. A woman in whom a selective cystectomy is attempted must be advised of the risk of oophorectomy if hemostasis cannot be achieved or if the cyst cannot be isolated. If the patient is young, with minimal risk of malignancy, a laparoscopic procedure might be an option. In an older woman, it might be more advisable to perform a laparotomy, possibly including bilateral oophorectomy, hysterectomy, and infracolic omentectomy (see Chapter 23).

> An ovarian cyst thought to be benign can be managed by observation, ultrasound-guided drainage, or laparoscopic or open ovarian cystectomy.

- What are the potential origins of the tissue that forms an ovarian cyst?
- List the symptoms that an ovarian cyst can cause the patient.
- What are the differential diagnoses for an ovarian cyst?
- What are the treatment options for a patient with an ovarian cyst?
- What ultrasound features would increase suspicion for malignancy within an ovarian cyst?

Further reading

Disaia PJ, et al. (2002) *Clinical Gynecologic Oncology*, 6th ed. (Mosby, St Louis).

23. Gynecologic Malignancy

Ovarian malignancy

Ovarian malignancy is the second most common gynecologic malignancy, and over 50% of ovarian cancer occurs in women aged 45–65. Ovarian tumors can be divided into different groups according to their cell of origin: epithelial, sex cord stromal or germ cell, and whether they are benign (see Chapter 22), borderline, or malignant. Most tumors are derived from epithelial cells; their particularly unpleasant characteristic is that they cause nonspecific symptoms and, therefore, women often present "late," when spread has already occurred. Their staging, treatment, and survival rates are summarized in Fig. 23.1.

> There are 25,000 new cases of ovarian cancer diagnosed each year in the US; 75% of those diagnosed will die of the disease.

Etiology

The life factors that increase and reduce the risk of developing ovarian cancer are shown in Fig. 23.2.

Women with a familial predisposition to ovarian cancer probably account for around 10% of cases, and most of these will have either the BRCA1 or BRCA2 mutations (chromosomes 17 and 13), or the Lynch II syndrome (an autosomal dominant inherited disorder that predisposes to breast, endometrial, colonic, and ovarian cancer).

Presentation

Ovarian tumors are relatively "silent," producing vague symptoms. Pain is rare, but could occur if the ovary twists (torsion) or if there is bleeding into the tumor. More common are abdominal distention, urinary frequency due to pressure on the bladder, and GI upset (e.g. vague diarrhea or constipation symptoms).

Studies
Ultrasound
Ultrasound scans will identify an ovarian mass. Features suspicious of malignancy include:
- A solid rather than a cystic mass, or a cyst containing septae.
- Mass measuring more than 5 cm.
- Presence of ascites.
- Bilateral tumors.

Staging of ovarian carcinoma

Stage	Description	Treatment	Success rate (%)
I A B C	Limited to the ovaries: One ovary, capsule intact, no ascites Both ovaries, capsules intact, no ascites Breached capsule(s) or ascites present	Surgery	80
II A B C	Presence of peritoneal deposits in pelvis: On uterus of tubes On other pelvic organs With ascites	Surgery then chemotherapy	60
III	Peritoneal deposits outside pelvis: Microscopic deposits Macroscopic <2 cm diameter Macroscopic >2 cm diameter	Surgery then chemotherapy	25
IV	Distant metastases	Surgery for palliation only	5–10

Fig. 23.1 Staging of ovarian carcinoma.

117

Gynecologic Malignancy

Risk factors for ovarian carcinoma	
Increased risk	**Reduced risk**
Few or no pregnancies	Pregnancies
Treatment with ovulation-induction drugs	Treatment with OCP
White Caucasian	Black/Asian
Blood group A	Blood group O
Higher socioeconomic status	
Late age of first conception	
Family history	

Fig. 23.2 Risk factors for ovarian carcinoma.

If cancer is suspected, then an ultrasound of the liver is performed to look for metastatic disease.

CA125
This tumor marker is often raised with epithelial tumors of the ovary, although it can also be high in the presence of fibroids, diverticular disease, and pregnancy, thus giving false-positive results. False negatives are also possible: some malignant tumors, especially mucinous tumors, will not secrete high levels of CA125.

Management
Surgery
Surgery is performed unless there are distant metastases, the aim being to remove as much tumor mass as possible. A midline incision is used. Uterus, tubes, ovaries, and omentum are removed. The pelvis is carefully explored, looking for and biopsying any deposits. Peritoneal fluid is sent for cytology.

Staging will determine further management. Unless distant metastases have been seen on scans prior to surgery, it is the operation that will define the stage, on the basis of what is found at laparotomy and the ensuing pathology report.

Stage I tumors are treated with surgery alone, but stage II and III tumors will require chemotherapy. Stage IV tumors (distant metastases present) can be operated upon, but this will not be for cure—surgery is performed for staging or to relieve bowel obstruction only.

Chemotherapy

> Another option for treatment might be to give chemotherapy prior to surgery to shrink the tumor mass. Studies are ongoing to look into this further.

Combination therapy is used; for example, cyclophosphamide + carboplatin or Taxol + carboplatin. Common side effects include:
- Myelosuppression.
- Nausea and vomiting.
- Peripheral neuropathy.
- Alopecia.

Taxol gives severe hypersensitivity reactions, so premedication with a corticosteroid and antihistamine is needed. Platins are also toxic to the kidney, ear, and eye. Cisplatin, an older platin drug, had a poor side-effect profile, so has been largely superseded by carboplatin.

> Radiotherapy is not very practical in ovarian malignancy because of the large area involved.

Screening
The rationale for screening for ovarian cancer is to reduce the late presentation that currently results in poor survival. Unfortunately, screening for this condition is very difficult. This is partly because there is no premalignant stage, but also because there is no one test to diagnose ovarian cancer. Large studies have looked at using CA125 and ultrasound (with or without Doppler), but the nonspecificity of CA125 adds to the confusion and, at present, there is no screening program.

Uterine endometrial tumors

Incidence
Endometrial carcinoma affects 34,000 women per year in the US. The median age of women affected is 61, and 80% are postmenopausal.

Risk factors
Predisposing factors are shown in Fig. 23.3 and include women who have high estrogen levels (obesity, PCOS, tamoxifen therapy) and those who have had many menses (nulliparous, early menarche, late menopause). OCPs protect against endometrial carcinoma, halving the user's risk. The protective effect is most marked where the OCP has been used for more than 10 years, and it continues for at least 20 years after the woman stops taking the pill. A family history of breast or colon cancer might point to Lynch II syndrome.

Endometrial hyperplasia is recognized as being a premalignant condition. Simple (also called cystic) hyperplasia and complex (adenomatous) hyperplasia are unlikely to progress to carcinoma, but they can be treated with progesterone to encourage regression. Atypical hyperplasia, however, is likely to progress, and in many cases might indicate that a carcinoma is already present in another part of the uterus.

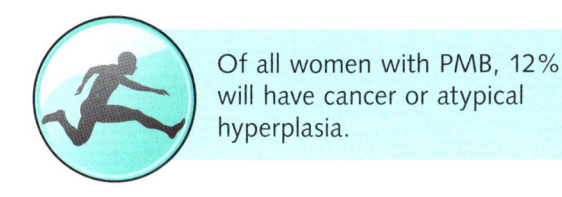

Of all women with PMB, 12% will have cancer or atypical hyperplasia.

Risk factors for endometrial carcinoma

- Obesity
- Nulliparity
- Early menarche
- Late menopause
- PCOS
- Unopposed estrogen therapy
- Tamoxifen therapy
- Diabetes
- Personal or family history of breast or colon cancer

Fig. 23.3 Risk factors for endometrial carcinoma.

Pathology and spread
Endometrial cancer is an adenocarcinoma, the most common type being endometrioid. Other subtypes are adenoacanthoma and papillary serous and clear cell adenocarcinomas. The latter two have a particularly poor prognosis.

Spread is initially local myometrial invasion and then transperitoneal. Lymphatic spread occurs to the para-aortic nodes. Staging is shown in Fig. 23.4.

Presentation
Most women present with bleeding that is either abnormal perimenopausal or postmenopausal.

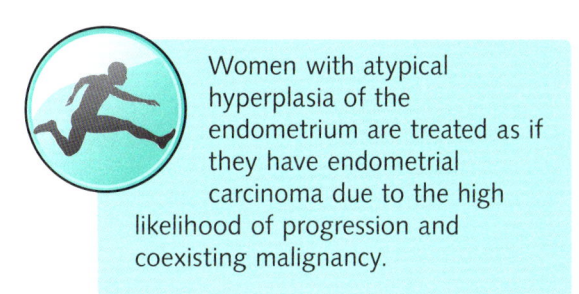

Women with atypical hyperplasia of the endometrium are treated as if they have endometrial carcinoma due to the high likelihood of progression and coexisting malignancy.

Staging of endometrial cancer

Stage	Structures involved	Survival rates
I A B C	Body of uterus: Endometrium only Extension into inner half of myometrium Extension into outer half of myometrium	85
II A B	Extension from body of uterus to cervix: Endocervical glands only Cervical stroma	60
III A B C	Spread to adnexae, or positive peritoneal cytology Metastases in vagina Pelvic or para-aortic lymphadenopathy	40
IV A B	Involvement of bladder or bowel mucosa Distant metastases	10

Fig. 23.4 Staging of endometrial cancer.

Investigation

Women with postmenopausal or suspicious perimenopausal bleeding should be investigated with ultrasound to measure the endometrial thickness and some form of endometrial sampling. Endometrial cancer causes thickening of the endometrium. Pipelle sampling involves the passage of a thin plastic tube through the cervix into the uterine cavity and uses aspiration to obtain an endometrial biopsy. It is done as an outpatient without the need for anesthetic, but it causes period-type pain during and after the procedure. The pipelle can be expected to miss a number of tumors, but in combination with ultrasound it is a useful tool. Alternatively, endometrial tissue can be sampled at the time of hysteroscopy under intravenous sedation, either under direct vision (using a resectoscope) or blind, with a curette.

Once a tissue diagnosis is obtained, ideally an MRI scan is performed to assess the extent of myometrial involvement and thus to differentiate between the different stages of endometrial cancer (see Fig. 23.4).

Treatment

Stages IA and IB are treated by TAH–BSO. The vaginal route of hysterectomy is not suitable for the treatment of cancer. The role of lymphadenectomy for treatment of these stages is unclear and is being investigated. Washings are taken from the peritoneum for cytology.

Stages IC and IIA are treated by TAH–BSO and lymph node dissection, followed by radiotherapy. This might be external beam or intravaginal (brachytherapy).

Stage IIB is treated first with radiotherapy. Stage III needs debulking surgery prior to radiotherapy. Stage IV tumors are incurable, so the woman will need palliative care and treatment as necessary.

Prognosis

The overall recurrence rate is 30%; cases with positive lymph nodes or peritoneal cytology are more likely to recur than those without (50% versus 10%). Most recurrence occurs within 2–3 years; the earlier recurrences are harder to treat and, therefore, carry a poorer prognosis. Isolated vaginal recurrences can be treated with radiotherapy. Later recurrence can be treated with progestogens in the first instance. If hormonal treatment fails, then chemotherapy is used.

Survival rates are shown in Fig. 23.4; the overall survival rate is 60%.

Uterine sarcoma

Stromal sarcoma

Tumors of stromal cells can be divided into the following categories:

- Low-grade sarcomas: look like fibroids, are slow-growing. Treatment is TAH–BSO with wide excision of the parametria.
- High-grade sarcomas: aggressive tumors with less than 50% survival rates, treated with radiotherapy.
- Mixed müllerian tumors: derived from the glandular cells within the stroma, these are aggressive tumors that commonly spread to the cervix and lymph nodes. Treatment is TAH–BSO with postoperative radiotherapy.

Myometrial sarcoma

Leiomyosarcoma could be described as a "malignant fibroid"; although only 5–10% of them arise within an existing fibroid they are macroscopically very similar, being tumors of smooth muscle cells. Often, diagnosis is not made until a TAH specimen is examined histologically, but lymph node sampling and BSO must be performed.

Atypical myometrial tumors

Leiomyoblastoma, clear cell leiomyoma, and epithelioid leiomyoma are tumors of smooth muscle that occur most often in premenopausal women and are estrogen dependent. Treatment is therefore TAH–BSO and the issue of HRT is difficult.

Cervix

Cervical intraepithelial neoplasia

CIN is a premalignant condition of the cervix. CIN is divided into three grades, although the disease itself is a continuum. CIN grading is shown in Fig. 23.5.

The national screening program was designed to detect CIN on Pap smear, thus allowing intervention before the condition progressed to

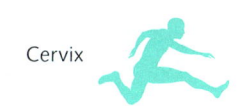

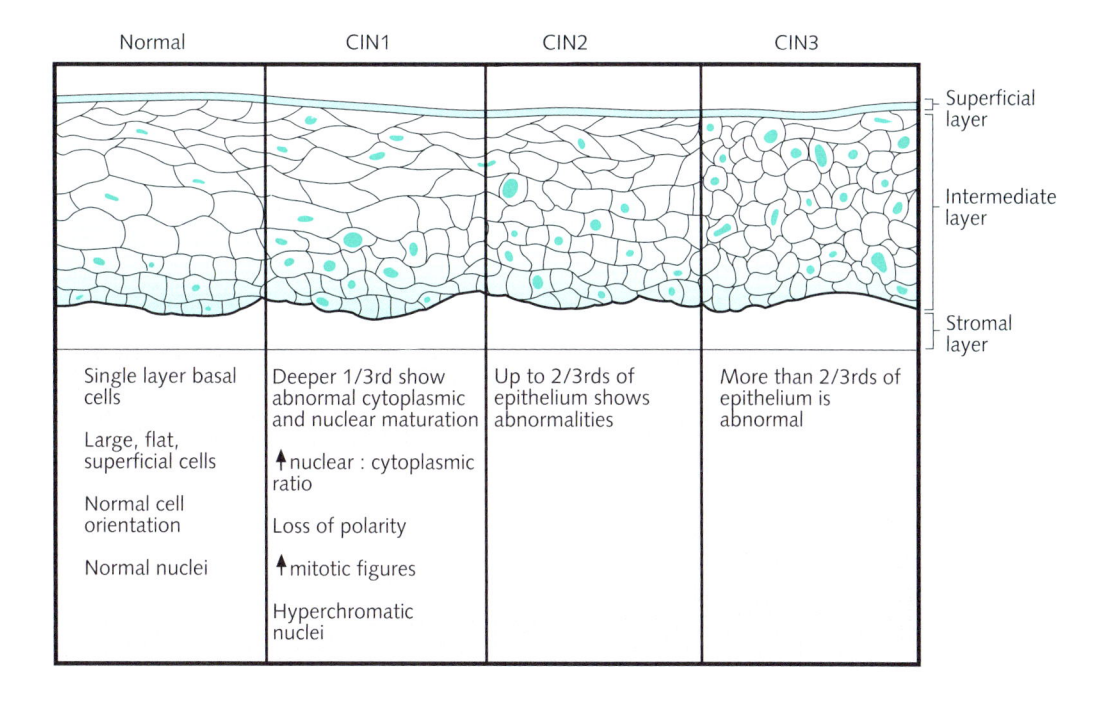

Normal	CIN1	CIN2	CIN3
Single layer basal cells Large, flat, superficial cells Normal cell orientation Normal nuclei	Deeper 1/3rd show abnormal cytoplasmic and nuclear maturation ↑nuclear : cytoplasmic ratio Loss of polarity ↑mitotic figures Hyperchromatic nuclei	Up to 2/3rds of epithelium shows abnormalities	More than 2/3rds of epithelium is abnormal

Superficial layer / Intermediate layer / Stromal layer

Fig. 23.5 Grades of CIN.

cancer. The first Pap smear is performed 3 years after first intercourse or at age 21, whichever comes first. Pap smears are then taken annually, stopping at age 64 if the previous two smears have been negative.

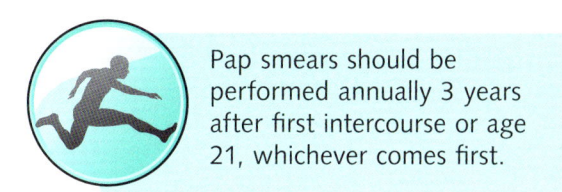

> Pap smears should be performed annually 3 years after first intercourse or age 21, whichever comes first.

The success of screening is seen in the fact that the incidence of cervical carcinoma has decreased by 25% since 1986, and mortality is decreasing. However, many women still die, and those who are missed by screening are often women who have a much higher chance of having and dying from cervical cancer because of their high-risk factor profile. Around 85% of women in the US are screened.

The Pap smear does have its limitations: the result is governed by subjective cytological assessment, the technique is subject to sampling errors, and it has false negative (2–20%) and false positive (10–13%) rates. Screening for human papilloma virus (HPV) increases sensitivity and specificity (Fig. 23.6)

Etiology of cervical intraepithelial neoplasia
The risk factors for CIN are the same as those for cervical carcinoma (see Fig. 23.9). HPV is described more fully in Fig. 23.6.

Management of cervical intraepithelial neoplasia
Figure 23.7 provides an algorithm for management of CIN based on the Pap smear result and on the patient's Pap smear history. The first smear showing mild dysplasia does not merit referral because, especially if the woman is a nonsmoker, there is a good chance that over 6 months the cells will revert to normal. The moderate and severe dysplasia cases should be referred for colposcopy.

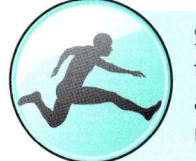

> Smoking makes it less likely that low-grade CIN will resolve and more likely that CIN will recur after treatment.

Gynecologic Malignancy

Human papilloma virus information box

- Double-stranded DNA viruses
- Over 90 different types identified, 30 of which present in the human genital tract
- Most lead to focal epithelial proliferation, some are linked to cervical cancer
- Low-risk virus types: associated with benign warts and occasionally CIN1—HPV6, HPV11, HPV42, PHV43 and HPV44
- Intermediate-risk virus types: associated with CIN2 and CIN3 but rarely seen with invasive cancer—HPV33, HPV35, HPV39, HPV45, HPV51, HPV52 and HPV56
- High-risk virus types: commonly detected in women with CIN2, CIN3 or invasive cancer—HPV16, HPV18 and HPV31
- High-risk HPV types lead to increased degradation of p53, a tumor suppressor
- Higher viral load is associated with a higher risk of developing invasive cancer
- The prevalence of HPV in sexually active women under 30 is 20–40% but most women will clear themselves of HPV within 6–8 months
- Smoking and increasing age make it less likely that the virus will be cleared

Fig. 23.6 HPV information box.

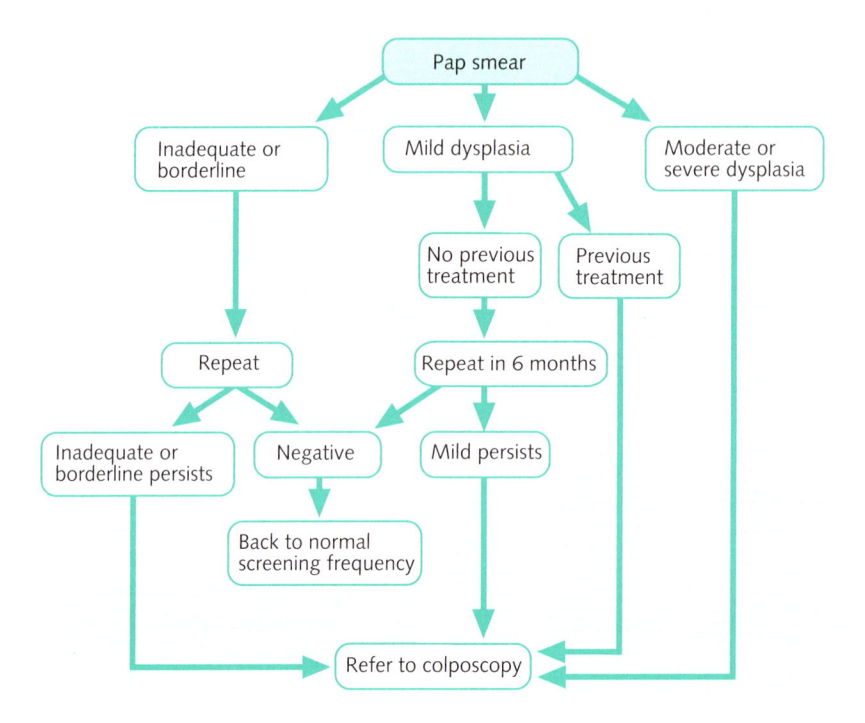

Fig. 23.7 Algorithm for abnormal Pap smears.

At colposcopy the cervix is washed with acetic acid and then with iodine. The cervix is inspected for suspicious features (Fig. 23.8). Abnormal areas can be biopsied, meaning that the patient will be invited back at a later date for treatment if appropriate, or treatment can be performed at this point.

Treatment consists of either excising or destroying the transformation zone. Excision techniques include LEEP and cone biopsy; these allow the tissue removed to be sent for histology and to be examined to confirm the diagnosis and to check the margins, ensuring complete excision.

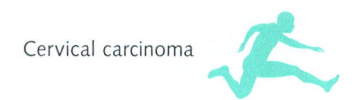

Destructive techniques include cryotherapy, cauterization, or laser.

Initial treatment has a 95% success rate. Patients are followed up with a Pap smear (see Fig. 23.7).

Cervical carcinoma

Cervical cancer affects 13,000 women per year in the US. There is a "double peak" in terms of age group affected, as it is most common in 40–44- and 70–74-year-olds. The risk factors for cervical cancer are shown in Fig. 23.9.

Pathology
Squamous cell tumors account for 90–95% of cervical cancers; the other 5–10% are adenocarcinomas derived from cervical glands. The national cervical screening program aims to detect changes in the cervix that occur before squamous cell tumors develop—it was not designed to look for adenocarcinomas.

Presentation and work-up
Women can present with symptoms of abnormal bleeding, particularly intermenstrual and postcoital, or they might be asymptomatic but have had an abnormal Pap smear result. At colposcopy, suspicious features are noted (see Fig. 23.8).

Suspicious features at colposcopy

- Intense acetowhite, pale on iodine staining
- Mosaicism and punctation due to atypical vessel formation
- Raised or ulcerated surface

Fig. 23.8 Suspicious features at colposcopy.

Risk factors for cervical cancer

- Early age of first intercourse
- Higher number of sexual partners
- HPV infection
- Lower socioeconomic group
- Smoking
- Partner with prostatic or penile cancer

Fig. 23.9 Risk factors for cervical cancer.

Staging
Staging is shown in Fig. 23.10. Staging for cervical cancer is performed by clinical examination. The procedures necessary to stage the tumor are:
- Cone biopsy, to assess depth of invasion.
- Chest X-ray.
- IVP.
- Cystoscopy and sigmoidoscopy or MRI to look for bladder/bowel involvement.

Management
Patients with cervical tumors that have progressed beyond the microinvasive stage should be referred to a gynecologic oncologist for treatment by a specialist multidisciplinary team.

Treatment is summarized in the algorithm in Fig. 23.11. Early-stage disease (stages I and IIA) can be treated equally well with surgery or radiotherapy, although surgery is preferred because it leads to fewer sexual, bowel, and bladder problems in the long term. Later-stage disease is treated with radical radiotherapy. At present, chemotherapy use is only experimental. When the disease has spread (stage IVB), palliative treatment is appropriate.

Staging of cervical cancer

Stage	Description
0	Carcinoma in situ
I A A1 A2 B B1 B2	Confined to the cervix: • Visible only under a microscope: • <3 mm in depth • >3 mm in depth • Visible without a microscope • <4 cm • >4 cm
II A B	Beyond the cervix: • No parametrial involvement • Parametrial involvement
III	Spread to the pelvic side wall, or affecting the kidney, or spread to the lower third of the vagina
IV A B	Involving the rectal or bladder mucosa Beyond the true pelvis

Fig. 23.10 Staging of cervical cancer.

Gynecologic Malignancy

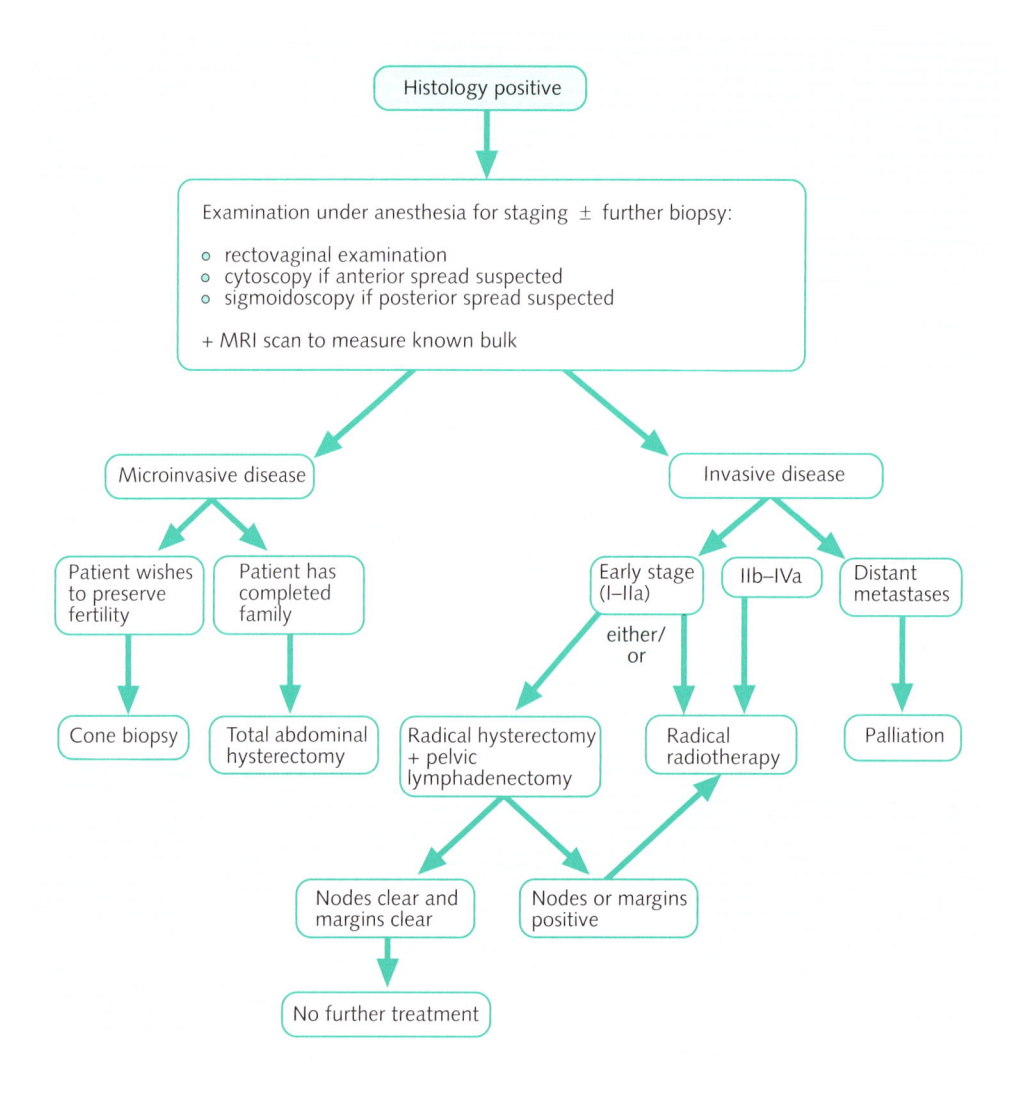

Fig. 23.11 Management of cervical cancer.

Vulvar tumors

Vulvar intraepithelial neoplasia
VIN is a premalignant condition, but the risk of progression to invasive carcinoma seems to be far less than that of CIN to cervical carcinoma. If VIN is present, then CIN is often seen too, and HPV is an underlying factor. Treatment of VIN is not clear-cut, partly due to the lack of knowledge about the danger of not treating. Presentation is usually vulvar irritation and, although vulvar colposcopy is practiced, diagnosis is based on the histopathologic study of a biopsy.

Incidence and etiology
Vulvar tumors are uncommon, affecting around 3,400 women per year in the US. The peak incidence is from the age of 63–65. Predisposing factors include:
- Smoking.
- Immunosuppression.
- Vulvar maturation disorders (e.g. lichen sclerosus; see Fig. 23.12).
- History of CIN, VIN or HPV.

Pathology
The majority of vulvar tumors are squamous cell carcinomas. Nonsquamous cell tumors include

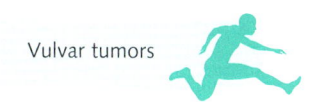

Vulvar tumors

Lichen sclerosis information box
Lichen sclerosis is a benign skin condition, with white plaques and atrophy seen in a figure-of-eight pattern around the vulva and anus. Extragenital plaques on the trunk and back might be seen. It is associated with autoimmune disorders, e.g. vitiligo. It can be classed as premalignant, as around 4% will go on to develop vulvar squamous cell carcinoma

Fig. 23.12 Lichen sclerosis information box.

melanoma, sarcoma, adenocarcinoma, and basal cell tumors. Paget's disease of the vulva is a malignant change in cells of the epidermal layer, which have a characteristic appearance. The presence of vulvar Paget's disease is associated with an adenocarcinoma elsewhere in the body in one in four cases, with the most common sites being breast, urinary tract, rectum, and genital tract.

Presentation
The most common presenting symptoms are:
- Pruritus.
- Lump/ulcer.
- Bleeding.
- Pain.

Urinary symptoms or unusual discharge can also be symptoms. The most common sites are shown in Fig. 23.13. The tumor can be multifocal.

Spread
Local spread occurs to the vagina, perineum, clitoris, urethra, and pubic bone. Lymphatic spread is to the superficial inguinal, deep inguinofemoral, and iliac nodes. Unless the tumor is central, only the nodes on the affected side are involved.

Work-up
Biopsy is performed, and at the time of biopsy the vagina and cervix are thoroughly inspected for signs of involvement. Positive nodes detected by CT or MRI scan.

Staging
Stages are shown in Fig. 23.14, but the disease can be more broadly divided into "early" and "late," with those having nodal involvement or large, multifocal lesions being in the latter group.

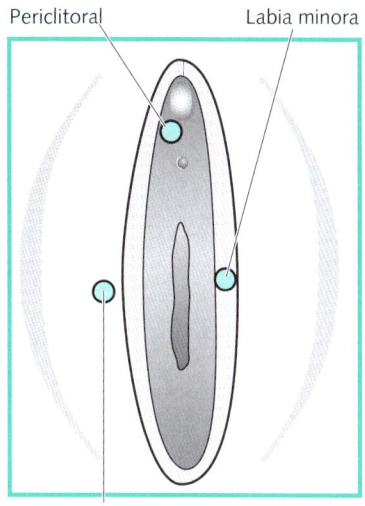

Fig. 23.13 Squamous cell carcinoma of the vulva—most common sites.

Staging of vulvar cancer	
Stage	Description
I A B	Confined to vulva: <1 mm invasion <2 cm diameter, no groin nodes
II	Confined to vulva, >2 cm diameter, no groin nodes palpable
III	Confined to vulva, suspicious nodes or beyond vulva with no suspicious nodes
IV	Obvious groin nodes or involving rectum, bladder, urethra or bone or pelvic or distant metastases

Fig. 23.14 Staging of vulvar cancer.

Management
The aim of treatment is to excise the cancer and minimize the risk of recurrence while preserving as much function as possible. Patients should be treated by a gynecologic oncologist.

The management plan depends on the stage; early tumors are treated by wide local excision. If the initial biopsy showed the depth of invasion to be more than 1 mm, then the nodes on the affected side must be dissected; if depth of

Gynecologic Malignancy

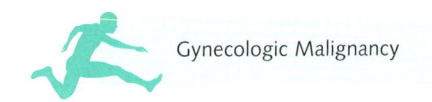

Complications of vulvectomy and radiotherapy

Type of treatment	Complication
Vulvectomy	Hemorrhage
	Thromboembolism
	Infection—wound, urinary tract
	Wound breakdown
Radiotherapy	Erythema
	Necrosis of the femoral head or pubic symphysis
	Fistula formation (urethrovaginal, vesicovaginal, or rectovaginal)

Fig. 23.15 Complications of vulvectomy and radiotherapy.

Staging of vaginal cancer

Stage	Description
0	VAIN
I	Limited to the vaginal wall
IIA	Subvaginal tissue, but not the parametrium, involved
IIB	Parametrial involvement
III	Spread to the pelvic side wall
IV	Bladder/rectum involved or distant organ spread

Fig. 23.16 Staging of vaginal cancer.

invasion is less than 1 mm, then nodal dissection is unnecessary.

Larger tumors are treated by radical vulvectomy, with ipsilateral node dissection if the tumor is less than 2 cm in diameter and bilateral if it is more than 2 cm. If groin nodes are not obviously involved, then the operation can be performed using either one incision (en bloc) or three separate incisions (the butterfly method); the latter seems to reduce the postoperative complications without increasing mortality or recurrence.

Radiotherapy is necessary if histology reveals the nodes to be positive. Chemotherapy has not been shown to be helpful.

Complications of treatment are shown in Fig. 23.15. Owing to the large area involved, wound breakdown is, sadly, relatively common. With the en bloc method it occurs in up to 80% of cases, whereas rates for the butterfly incision are between 5 and 50%. Some surgeons advocate performing skin grafts at the time of initial surgery. Radiotherapy adds extra complications.

Prognosis
The most important factor is nodal involvement, and in particular whether the pelvic nodes are positive. Overall survival rates are:
- Node negative: 70–90%.
- Node positive: 25–40%.

Patients with positive pelvic nodes, as opposed to groin nodes only, very rarely survive.

Vaginal tumors

Vaginal tumors are rare and are usually either primary squamous carcinoma or spread from vulvar or cervical squamous cancers. Even rarer tumors include endodermal sinus tumors, rhabdomyosarcoma (both are seen in children, but the latter are also seen in older women), melanoma, clear cell adenocarcinoma, and leiomyosarcoma.

Etiology
Associations are with CIN and HPV and with a history of another gynecologic malignancy in the past.

Presentation
The upper third of the vagina is the most common site, and women usually present at an early stage with abnormal bleeding.

Investigation
Staging is shown in Fig. 23.16 and requires biopsy, examination under anesthesia, and assessment of the bladder and rectum either at operation or on MRI. Chest X-ray is performed as part of the evaluation.

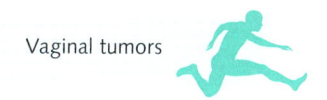

Management

Treatment is a combination of external beam and intravaginal radiotherapy, with the complications being fistulas (as with vulvar radiotherapy) and stenosis of the vagina and rectum.

Prognosis

Of the women who present, 70% have stage I or II disease, with 5-year survival rates of around 70%.

- Name three features of an ovarian cyst seen on ultrasound that raise the suspicion of malignancy.
- Give an example of a chemotherapy drug used to treat ovarian cancer and a common side effect.
- Which age group of women is most affected by endometrial carcinoma? How do they usually present?
- Who has Pap smears? How often are they performed?
- What is the treatment of a large vulvar carcinoma?

Further reading

Disaia PJ, et al. (2002) *Clinical Gynecologic Oncology*, 6th ed. (Mosby, St Louis).

Rock JA, et al. *Te Linde's Operative Gynecology*, 9th ed. (Lippincott William & Wilkins, Philadelphia).

24. Vulvar Disease

Diseases of the vulva are, to some, difficult to understand. This is likely due to a combination of the lack of information or understanding of the etiology and classification of these diseases. Although the vulvar dystrophies have recently been renamed (Fig. 24.1), the more familiar names will be used here to avoid confusion.

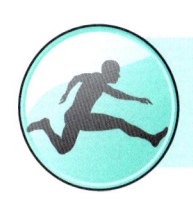

> Please take heed of the new nomenclature as this can be very confusing.

Histology of the vulva

The whole surface of the vulva up to the inner aspect of the labia minora is covered by stratified, keratinized squamous epithelium with a superficial cornified layer. The cornified layer is absent in the vagina, and there is a decreasing degree of keratinization (Fig. 24.2). The anatomy of the vulva is shown in Fig. 24.3.

Vulvar dystrophies

Histologically, the vulvar dystrophies are divided into atrophic and hypertrophic or a mixed picture of both. Atrophic vulvar dystrophy is better known as lichen sclerosis.

> Most vulvar lesions should ideally have colposcopic examination and biopsy to exclude malignancy.

Lichen sclerosis

Lichen sclerosis is the most common of the vulvar dystrophies. It usually develops in postmenopausal women, although any age group can be affected, including prepubertal girls (Fig. 24.4). The cause of lichen sclerosis is not understood.

Skin affected by lichen sclerosis is typically thin, shiny, and can be white (leukoplakia) or red due to inflammation. Anatomical changes associated with lichen sclerosis include shrinkage or loss of the labia minora and shrinkage of the introitus. Adhesions can fuse the labia together. Lichen sclerosis can affect the perineum and perianal region.

Diagnosis is made histologically from vulvar biopsies. Treatment is aimed at relieving the itching and soreness; as this is a chronic relapsing condition, treatment is usually intermittent. Simple emollient creams can relieve mild symptoms, but, if severe, short courses of potent topical steroids might be needed. Testosterone cream is sometimes used, but probably acts more as an emollient than hormonally.

Complications are unusual and include anatomical changes and the risk of malignancy. Anatomical changes can cause dyspareunia and, if fusion of the labia occurs in the midline, difficulty in micturition, which might require separation of the labia. Long-term follow-up of women with lichen sclerosis is important, as up to 5% will develop squamous carcinoma of the vulva.

Hyperplastic vulvar dystrophy

Histologically, squamous cell hyperplasia occurs which is distinguishable from vulvar intraepithelial neoplasia by the absence of atypia. Clinically, the two conditions have a similar presentation. Typical lesions are raised, thickened, and can be white, gray, or red, depending on the degree of inflammation. Treatment is with topical steroids and the condition is likely to recur.

Neoplasia

Neoplastic conditions of the vulva include what is, effectively, the carcinomas-in-situ, VIN, and Paget's disease of the vulva, and malignant squamous carcinoma.

Vulvar intraepithelial neoplasia

This is a relatively uncommon condition, although the incidence is increasing in young women. HPV (specifically HPV 16) has been implicated in the etiology. Histologically, neoplastic cells are contained within the basement membrane and the degree of dysplasia is divided into mild, moderate, and severe (VIN 1, VIN 2, and VIN 3 respectively).

Symptoms include pruritus, pain, soreness, and palpable lesions, but many are asymptomatic and found incidentally. Lesions can be papular (like genital warts) or macular with irregular borders. They can be red, brown or black (pigmented), or white (leukoplakia), and ulceration might be present. Unifocal lesions are more common postmenopausally. The diagnosis is made histologically from vulvar biopsies.

New nomenclature for the vulvar dystrophies	
Old name	New name
Vulvar dystrophy	Non-neoplastic epithelial disorders of the vulva
Lichen sclerosus et atrophicus	Lichen sclerosis
Hypertrophic vulvar dystrophy	Squamous cell hyperplasia

Fig. 24.1 New nomenclature for the vulvar dystrophies.

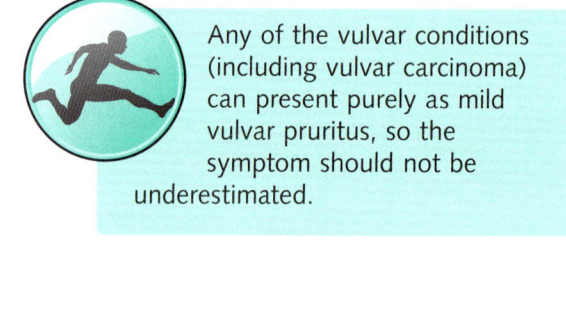

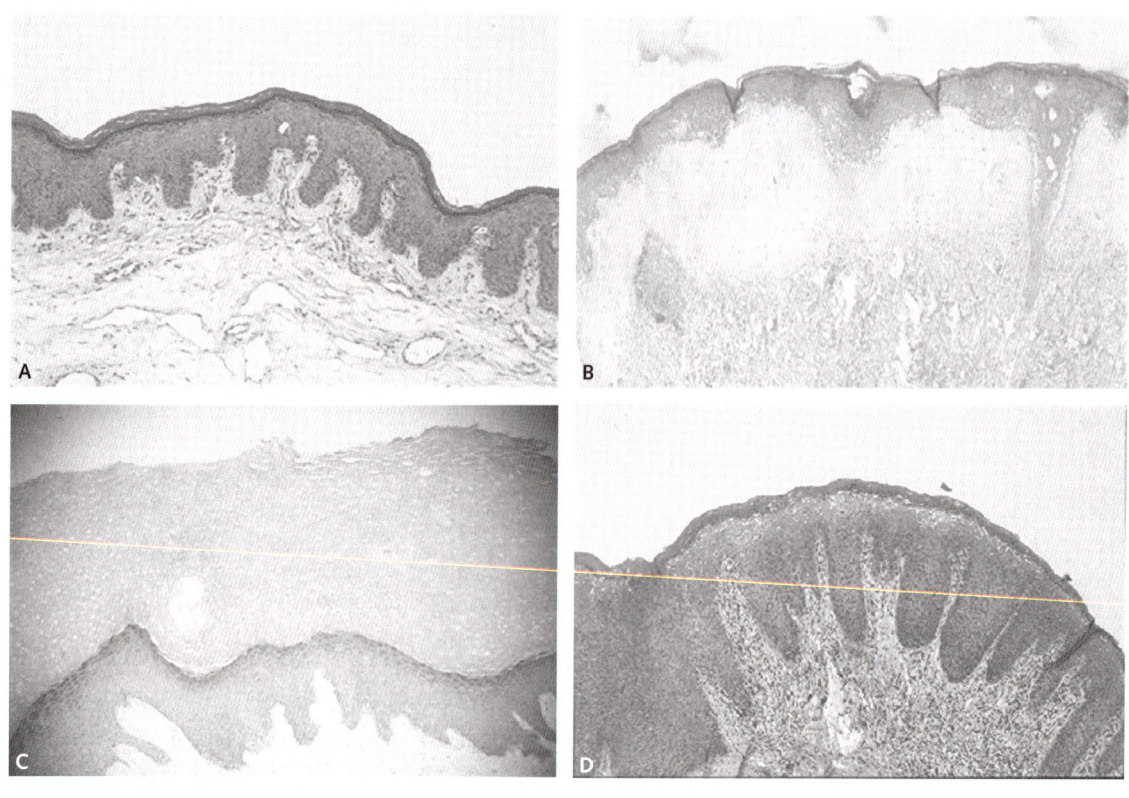

> Any of the vulvar conditions (including vulvar carcinoma) can present purely as mild vulvar pruritus, so the symptom should not be underestimated.

Fig. 24.2 Histology. (A) Normal, (B) lichen sclerosis, (C) squamous hyperplasia, and (D) dysplasia. Reproduced with kind permission from *Fundamentals of Obstetrics and Gynaecology* (7th edn), published by Mosby.

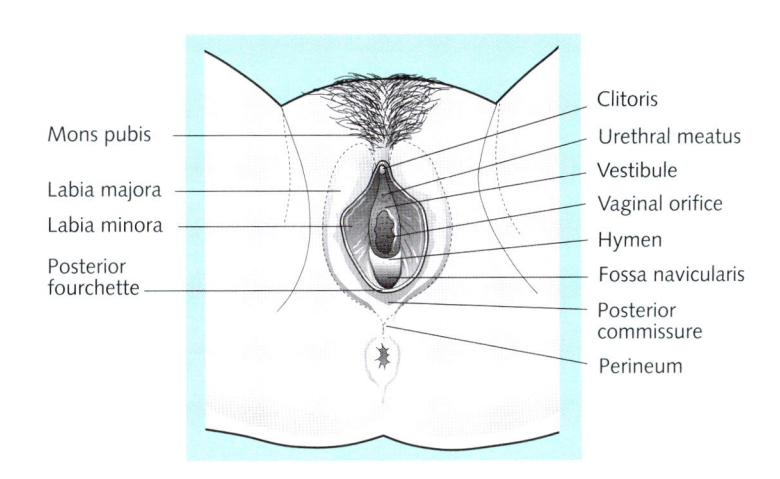

Neoplasia

Fig. 24.3 Vulvar anatomy.

Characteristics of some important vulvar diseases

	Age at presentation	Incidence	Mode of treatment	Recurrence rate	Malignant potential
Vulvar dystrophies					
Lichen sclerosis	Any age but usually postmenopausal	Common	Topical steroids and emollients	Frequent	<5% develop squamous carcinoma of the vulva
Neoplasias					
Vulvar intraepithelial neoplasia	Any age but increasing in the young	Relatively uncommon, but increasing	Usually surgical; more conservative in young women	Up to 80% will recur	Overall low, but higher in the elderly and immunosuppressed
Paget's disease of the vulva	Postmenopausal women	Rare	Surgical	Up to 33% will recur	Associated with adenocarcinoma in 25%. Malignant change in lesion is rare

Fig. 24.4 Characteristics of some important vulvar diseases.

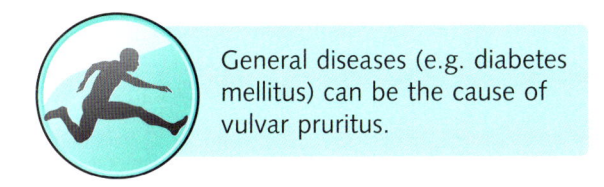

> General diseases (e.g. diabetes mellitus) can be the cause of vulvar pruritus.

Treatment is usually surgical, either by ablating the lesion with laser or cryotherapy or by local excision. VIN will recur in up to 80% of treated women; as the risk of malignant change is small, especially in younger women, major mutilating surgery should be avoided. Surgical treatment is recommended when the risk of malignant change is increased:
- Excessively hyperkeratotic lesions.
- In postmenopausal women.
- In the immunosuppressed.
- If the severity of dysplasia is seen to worsen on serial biopsy.

When conservative treatment is planned, topical steroids may give symptomatic relief.

Squamous carcinoma of the vulva
Squamous carcinoma of the vulva is discussed in Chapter 23.

Paget's disease of the vulva
Paget's disease of the vulva is uncommon; it is usually seen in postmenopausal women. The etiology is unknown, although the lesion is thought to be of glandular origin. In 25% of cases, there is an underlying adenocarcinoma (breast, urinary, genital, or colonic).

Lesions can be unifocal or multifocal and are typically clearly defined, scaly, erythematous plaques with varying degrees of ulceration and leukoplakia. The main symptom is pruritus, and the diagnosis is made histologically. Treatment is surgical using laser ablation or local excision, and up to one-third will recur. Although associated with adenocarcinoma, malignant change within the lesion is rare.

Dermatologic conditions

Many dermatologic conditions can affect the vulva, often with a confusing clinical picture, especially if the vulva is the only area affected.

Psoriasis
The typical raised, erythematous, scaly lesions of psoriasis can occur on the vulva, although here they might appear smooth and without the scaling. The presence of psoriasis elsewhere on the body will suggest the diagnosis, which can be confirmed histologically. Treatment is with topical steroids, but the relapse rate is high.

Eczema
Eczema of the vulva is rare. More commonly, eczematous reactions occur due to contact with irritant substances, such as soaps and detergents. Treatment is by identifying and removing the source of irritation and use of topical steroids.

- What is the most common cause of vulvar pruritus in a postmenopausal woman?
- What are the possible treatments of lichen sclerosis?
- How should the vulvar skin be investigated in the clinic?
- What possible infections could present as vulvar disease?

Further reading
Rock JA, et al. (2003) *Te Linde's Operative Gynecology*, 9th ed. (Lippincott William & Wilkins, Philadelphia).

Wilkinson EJ. (1995) *Atlas of Vulvar Disease*. (Lippincott William & Wilkins, Philadelphia)

25. Pelvic Inflammatory Disease

Definition

PID is defined as the clinical syndrome associated with ascending spread of microorganisms from the vagina or cervix to the endometrium, fallopian tubes, and/or contiguous structures. It usually begins with an acute infection; this might resolve completely or develop a chronic course with repeated acute or subacute episodes.

Incidence

The true incidence of PID is difficult to determine because of the lack of a precise clinical definition or a specific diagnostic test. However, the incidence is strongly correlated with the prevalence of sexually transmitted infections, and has increased in most countries. In the US, the highest annual incidence is among sexually active women in their teenage years; 75% of cases occur in women under the age of 25. Figure 25.1 outlines risk factors for the development of PID.

Etiology

- *Chlamydia trachomatis.*
- *Neisseria gonorrhoeae.*
- Nonspecific.

Chlamydia trachomatis is the most common cause of PID in the US. Along with *Neisseria gonorrhoeae*, this microorganism is responsible for at least 60% of cases of PID. They are thought to act as primary pathogens, causing damage to the protective mechanisms of the endocervix and allowing endogenous bacteria from the vagina and cervix into the upper genital tract as secondary invaders (Fig. 25.2). A variety of endogenous aerobic and anaerobic bacteria have been isolated from women with PID, such as *Mycoplasma* species, but their exact role is uncertain.

Occasionally, PID develops secondary to another disease process, such as appendicitis, or rarely as part of more generalized disease, such as tuberculosis.

Diagnosis

The diagnosis of PID is sometimes a difficult one to make, since it does not rely on one particular sign or symptom or combination of these. However, it is thought that the benefits of early diagnosis and appropriate treatment outweigh the possible overuse of antibiotics in a patient who might seem to have only mild disease.

The differential diagnosis (see Chapter 2) includes:
- Appendicitis.
- Endometriosis.
- Ectopic pregnancy.
- Ovarian cyst rupture.

History

The history might include one or more of the following symptoms:
- Pelvic pain/lower abdominal pain, usually bilateral.
- Deep dyspareunia.
- Dysmenorrhea.
- Increased vaginal discharge.
- Fever.

PID can also be asymptomatic, presenting many years after the acute infection with infertility.

Examination

At least three of the following signs should be present to make the diagnosis of acute PID:
- Raised temperature ≥100.4°F.
- Abdominal tenderness.
- Purulent vaginal discharge.
- Cervical motion tenderness (pain or discomfort on moving the cervix).
- Adnexal tenderness.
- Adnexal swelling.

Pelvic Inflammatory Disease

PID risk factors

Risk factor	Description
Age	75% of patients are below 25 years of age
Marital status	Single
Sexual history	Young at first intercourse
	High frequency of sexual intercourse
	Multiple sexual partners
Medical history	Past history of sexually transmitted disease in patient or partner
	Past history of PID in patient
	Recent instrumentation of uterus, e.g. termination of pregnancy
Contraception	Use of IUD especially insertion within 3 weeks

Fig. 25.1 Risk factors for the development of PID.

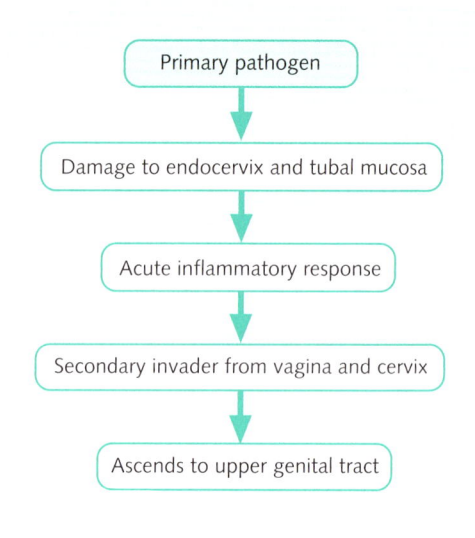

Primary pathogen → Damage to endocervix and tubal mucosa → Acute inflammatory response → Secondary invader from vagina and cervix → Ascends to upper genital tract

Fig. 25.2 Development of PID.

Complications of acute PID

Type of complication	Description
Short term	Pelvic abscess formation
	Septicemia
	Septic shock
Long term	Infertility
	Ectopic pregnancy
	Chronic pelvic pain
	Dyspareunia
	Menstrual disturbances
	Psychological effects

Fig. 25.3 Complications of acute PID.

Work-up

Appropriate work-up includes:
- WBC.
- Blood cultures, depending on the level of the pyrexia.
- Full screen for sexually transmitted infections, including endocervical swabs, possibly urethral swabs, and a urine culture.
- Pregnancy test (urinary β-hCG) depending on date of LMP.
- Ultrasound scan, which might be appropriate to exclude an ovarian cyst complication or tubo-ovarian abscess.
- Laparoscopy may be considered in some cases, e.g. if there is doubt about the diagnosis or if the patient fails to respond to antibiotic therapy.

Complications

The long-term morbidity associated with acute PID is considerable (Fig. 25.3); thus, the need for appropriate treatment, especially to cover chlamydial infection, is important. Moderately severe disease is associated with inflammation and edema in the fallopian tubes, with deposits of fibrin and subsequent adhesion formation between the pelvic and abdominal organs. Thus, tubal morphology and function are affected, resulting in infertility and an increased risk of ectopic pregnancy. Adhesions in the pelvis may lead to chronic pain, either as a sole feature or in relation to menstruation or sexual intercourse.

> Early diagnosis and treatment are important to reduce the risk of long-term complications.

Treatment

- Antibiotic therapy.
- Treatment of sexual partners.
- Surgery.

The aim of treatment is to prevent the long-term sequelae of PID mentioned above. First, administration of broad-spectrum antibiotics is indicated once the diagnosis of PID is suspected and should be started prior to obtaining the results of microbiology specimens (Fig. 25.4).

> Antibiotic therapy must include treatment for Chlamydia because this microorganism is most commonly implicated in PID and its sequelae.

Antibiotic therapy for the treatment of PID

Infecting agent	Therapy
Chlamydia	Tetracyclines (e.g. doxycycline)
	Erythromycin or azithromycin if the patient is pregnant
	Azithromycin if single-dose treatment is preferable
Gonorrhea	Ciprofloxacin
	Ofloxacin
	Ceftriaxone
Anaerobes	Metronidazole

Fig. 25.4 Antibiotic therapy for the treatment of PID.

If a patient resumes sexual intercourse with a partner who is infected but untreated, then there is obviously a high chance of reinfection. Therefore, it is important that the patient notify all sexual contacts so that they can be given treatment, either empirically or as a result of microbiology results.

Apart from diagnostic laparoscopy, there is rarely a need for more invasive surgery in the management of PID. Laparoscopy or laparotomy might be necessary to drain a tubo-ovarian abscess.

Prevention

PID and its sequelae are responsible for a substantial amount of morbidity, both physical and psychological, as well as having considerable financial implications. Therefore, primary prevention of the disease is of great importance and needs the help of both the media and health-care professionals. Government educational programs are currently in progress:

- Educational campaigns to increase awareness of at-risk behavior.
- Opportunistic screening of those at risk (e.g. adolescents, individuals not in monogamous relationships).
- Knowledge of up-to-date treatment regimens with locally agreed protocols.
- Understanding the importance of recommending that sexual partners be notified.

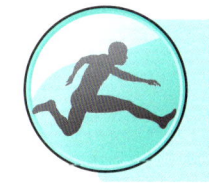

> Effective treatment for PID must include notifying sexual partners and treating appropriately.

- What are the two main causes of PID?
- What are the differential diagnoses of PID?
- What are the studies necessary to exclude PID?
- What are potential sequelae of PID?
- Discuss the treatment options for PID.

Further reading

Hillard PA, et al. (2002) *Novak's Gynecology*, 13th ed. (Lippincott Williams & Wilkins, Philadelphia).

Rock JA, et al. (2003) *Te Linde's Operative Gynecology*, 19th ed. (Lippincott Williams & Wilkins, Philadelphia).

26. Urinary Incontinence

Incidence

Female urinary incontinence is a very common problem, with up to one-quarter of women leaking urine occasionally. The prevalence of regular female urinary incontinence increases with increasing age; 8.5% of women under 65 years of age, rising to 11.6% over 65 years and 43.2% over 85 years.

The most common cause of urinary incontinence is stress urinary incontinence (SUI), also known as GSI, followed by DO, which account for almost 50% and 40% of incontinent women respectively. These and other causes are shown in Fig. 5.1.

Etiology

The bladder has two major roles: the retention of urine and expulsion of urine. Failure to retain urine or loss of normal voiding control gives rise to two distinct etiologies of incontinence.

> Urinary incontinence is often of mixed etiology: stress and urge. In view of this, urodynamic studies are essential before any treatment is instituted.

Stress urinary incontinence

The bladder acts as a low-pressure reservoir. As the volume increases, the bladder pressure rises only slightly. Urethral closure pressure, produced by the passive effect of elastic and collagen fibers and active striated and smooth muscle, causes the urethra to close. Continence requires a positive pressure gradient from the urethra to the bladder. In the resting state the urethral closure pressure is higher than the relatively low bladder pressure and continence is maintained.

Intra-abdominal pressure is transmitted to the bladder, and raised intra-abdominal pressure, such as during coughing or straining, increases the bladder pressure. Intra-abdominal pressure is also transmitted to the bladder neck and that part of the proximal urethra which is intra-abdominal (above the pelvic floor), maintaining the positive pressure gradient and hence continence (Fig. 26.1B). If the bladder neck and proximal urethra are situated below the pelvic floor, then the raised intra-abdominal pressure is no longer transmitted to these structures, the positive pressure gradient is lost and incontinence occurs (Fig. 26.1C).

SUI increases with increasing age, as maximal urethral closure pressure decreases. Also, older women are more likely to be parous and postmenopausal. SUI increases with increasing parity, being associated with the process of vaginal delivery. Prolapse is commonly thought to be associated with SUI, although this is only true if the proximal urethra has descended below the pelvic floor (see above). Atrophic changes associated with the postmenopausal state and vaginal surgery to cure prolapse are also associated with SUI.

Detrusor overactivity

In women with DO, the urethra functions normally, but urinary leakage occurs if the uninhibited detrusor activity increases bladder pressure above maximal urethral closure pressure.

The majority of women with DO have an idiopathic etiology with no demonstrable abnormality to be found. DO can occur following surgery to the bladder neck and proximal urethra, especially following surgery for SUI, during which dissection around these structures occurs. Multiple sclerosis (MS), autonomic neuropathy, and spinal lesions can allow uninhibited detrusor contractions, although those women with neurological lesions are more correctly said to have detrusor hyperreflexia.

Increasing age and a history of nocturnal enuresis are associated with DO, and diuretics will obviously exacerbate this condition.

Urinary Incontinence

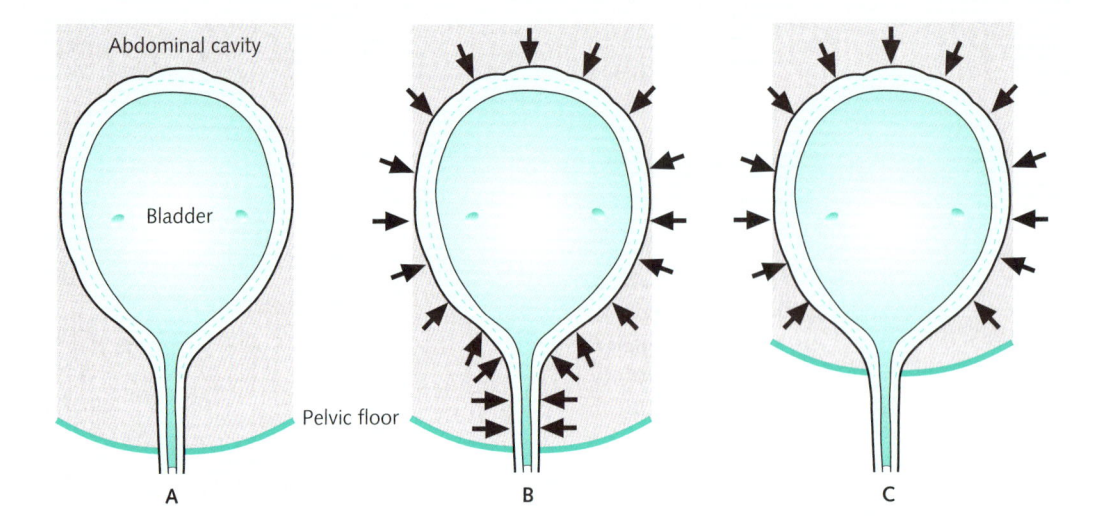

Fig. 26.1 Mechanism of SUI.

Sensory urgency
Irritation of the bladder mucosa, due either to infection (cystitis), bladder stones, or tumors, can cause sensory urgency. The etiology of primary vesical sensory urgency is not well understood, but it accounts for almost 4% of incontinent women.

Voiding disorders
Voiding difficulties can present as acute or chronic urinary retention with overflow incontinence. Chronic overdistention of the bladder is likely to exacerbate and can itself cause voiding difficulties due to detrusor ischemia and denervation.

Central, spinal, and peripheral neurologic lesions can produce voiding difficulties (Fig. 26.2). Approximately 25% of women with MS will present with acute urinary retention. Postoperative pain can cause reflex inhibition of micturition, as can severe inflammation of the bladder, urethra, and vulva.

Drugs can cause voiding difficulties, epidural anesthesia in labor being the most common encountered. Tricyclic antidepressants, anticholinergic agents, α-adrenergic agonists, and ganglion blockers can all cause voiding difficulties.

Voiding difficulties can occur secondary to mechanical obstruction. Impaction of a pelvic mass, e.g. the gravid uterus or fibroids, might obstruct the urethra, as can bladder polyps or

Type of lesion	Neurologic cause of voiding difficulty
Central lesions (suprapontine)	Cerebrovascular accident
	Parkinson's disease
Spinal lesions	Spinal cord injury
	Multiple sclerosis
Peripheral lesions	Prolapsed intervertebral disc
	Peripheral autonomic neuropathies (e.g. diabetic)

Neurologic causes of voiding difficulties

Fig. 26.2 Neurologic causes of voiding difficulties (acute and chronic retention).

malignancy. Edema following bladder neck surgery causes voiding difficulties frequently enough to warrant prophylactic drainage of the bladder following these procedures. Surprisingly, it is rare for prolapse to cause retention.

Fistulas
The most common cause of fistula formation worldwide is obstructed labor. In the US, avoiding prolonged labor has almost eradicated this complication. Although uncommon, fistulas are

likely to be secondary to malignancy, surgery, and radiation to the pelvis, or a combination of these. Fistulas can occur from the ureter, bladder, or urethra to the vagina.

Appropriate work-up

Having excluded UTI, the mainstays of investigation are urodynamic studies. Urodynamic studies are important for diagnosing the causes of incontinence, as symptoms are often multiple and do not correlate well with the underlying disorder (see Chapter 5). Cystoscopy can be helpful by inspecting the anatomy of the bladder and urethra to exclude mechanical causes of incontinence, but it does not allow assessment of their function. Bimanual pelvic examination and pelvic ultrasound will identify pelvic masses. Ureterovaginal fistulas will require radiologic studies. Infusing colored dyes into the bladder and observing vaginal leakage may confirm the presence of vesico- or urethrovaginal fistulas.

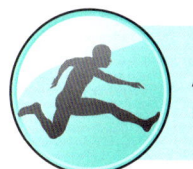

A UTI and neurologic defect must always be excluded.

Complications

Although incontinence itself is not life threatening, it does cause major psychosocial problems. Changes in lifestyle are common, and occasionally the symptoms are so severe as to render the woman housebound. Excoriation and soreness of the vulva occurs secondary to continual dampness, and chronic UTI can lead to long-term damage of renal function. Acute and chronic overdistention of the bladder can cause denervation and necrosis of the detrusor muscle, thereby causing further voiding difficulties.

Treatment

Treatment is determined not only by the underlying condition, but also by the severity of the symptoms. Some women might be happy to undergo a trial of oral medication, but not major abdominal surgery for the same degree of symptoms. Similarly, depending on lifestyle, some women can live with their symptoms, whereas others find the same symptoms intolerable. A sympathetic approach and detailed counseling of the pros and cons of treatment are essential in treating women with incontinence.

Stress urinary incontinence

Kegel exercises are the mainstay of conservative treatment of SUI. Women are taught to use the pelvic floor muscles to achieve better urinary control, and up to 60% will have improvement of symptoms. Techniques include simple pelvic floor exercises or insertion of vaginal cones, which can be retained only by contraction of the relevant pelvic floor muscles. Problems include return of symptoms if exercises are stopped and a spontaneous worsening of symptoms associated with menopause. Estrogen replacement has been shown to improve the symptom of stress incontinence in postmenopausal women, although long-term use is required to maintain the effect.

The majority of women with SUI can be cured by surgery. This is achieved by lifting and supporting the bladder neck and urethra, thereby restoring their intra-abdominal position. This also increases the urethral pressure, by increasing outflow resistance. Abdominal procedures have been shown to be far more effective than vaginal procedures and colposuspension is the surgical procedure of choice, achieving a success rate of up to 90%. Performed through a suprapubic incision, this involves placing sutures from the vagina, adjacent to the bladder neck, to the ligaments at the back of the symphysis pubis. This results in the vagina being elevated and this 'platform' supports the bladder neck in an intra-abdominal position. Slings can be placed under the bladder neck and sutured to the lateral pelvic side wall or rectus muscles to produce a similar effect. Tension-free vaginal tape is a new sling procedure in which a meshlike tape is placed under the urethra and passed through the retropubic space to exit through two suprapubic incisions—initial 5-year results suggest an efficacy approaching that of colposuspension.

Vaginal procedures, such as anterior colporrhaphy, can achieve continence in the short term but will have failed in up to 60% by 5 years. In the presence of poor detrusor activity, the bladder might not produce high enough pressures to overcome the relative outflow obstruction produced by abdominal procedures, so self-intermittent catheterization might be necessary. Urodynamic studies will help to identify this group of women, although all women undergoing abdominal surgery for SUI should be warned of this complication.

Where SUI and DO coexist it is sensible to treat the DO in the first instance. A significant percentage of women will have a satisfactory enough response to simple medical treatment and avoid major surgery.

> The definitive treatment of stress incontinence is surgical: tension-free vaginal tape or colposuspension.

Detrusor overactivity

DO is treated medically except in the uncommon situations where symptoms are severe enough to warrant surgery. Behavioral and drug therapy are the mainstay of medical treatment.

Behavioral therapy

Bladder retraining aims to increase the voiding intervals and may be successful in up to 80% of women with DO, although there is a significant relapse rate. Having explained how the bladder functions, subjects are taught to micturate by the clock rather than desire and are encouraged to increase voiding intervals incrementally. Other techniques include hypnotherapy and acupuncture.

Pharmacotherapy

There is a strong placebo effect in the drug treatment of DO. Drugs that are effective in treating DO rely on their antimuscarinic properties (less correctly termed "anticholinergics"). Antimuscarinic drugs effectively increase bladder capacity by:

Atropine-like side effects	
Type of side effect	Description
Peripheral	Dry mouth
	Reduced visual accommodation
	Constipation
	Glaucoma
Central	Confusion

Fig. 26.3 Atropine-like side effects.

- Delaying initial desire to void.
- Decreasing the strength of detrusor contractions.
- Decreasing the frequency of detrusor contractions.

Although improving symptoms in many women, the use of antimuscarinics is limited by their atropine-like side effects (Fig. 26.3). Oxybutynin is currently widely used, although the recent introduction of a new drug with antimuscarinic properties that are highly selective for the bladder (Tolterodine) has proved popular. Tolterodine shows good efficacy with far fewer antimuscarinic side effects and now can be given as a once daily formulation.

Tricyclic antidepressants also have antimuscarinic properties as well as a central sedative effect. They are useful for incontinent women who suffer from anxiety.

Sensory urgency

Removal of the source of bladder mucosal irritation (infection, bladder stones, tumors) is likely to relieve symptoms.

Voiding difficulties

The symptoms of urinary obstruction can be treated by drug therapy, but catheterization is necessary where retention has occurred.

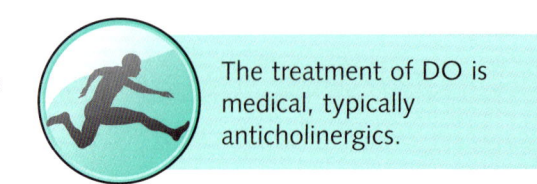

> The treatment of DO is medical, typically anticholinergics.

Pharmacotherapy

Drugs used to treat the symptoms of voiding difficulties are often ineffective or have limited use due to side effects. They work in two ways:
- Relax the sphincter mechanism.
- Inhibit detrusor contractions.

Selective α-blockers, such as terazosin, produce an increase in flow rate and improvement in obstructive symptoms by relaxing the sphincter mechanism. Side effects include sedation, dizziness, tachycardia, and hypotension and must be used with extreme caution in the elderly and in antihypertensive users.

The parasympathomimetics (bethanechol, carbachol, and distigmine) exhibit muscarinic activity, which improves voiding by increasing detrusor contraction. Side effects include sweating, bradycardia, and intestinal colic.

Catheterization

Acute retention of urine requires catheterization. If caused by a gravid uterus, the catheter may need to be left in situ until the uterus has become abdominal. An ovarian cyst or fibroid will need to be removed surgically, although disimpaction from the pelvis is sometimes possible as a palliative measure. Postoperative or postpartum retention usually resolve with bladder drainage. A suprapubic catheter is preferred, as residual volumes can be measured to assess progress. If the bladder has been overdistended, then normal bladder function is unlikely to occur immediately and free bladder drainage is required until normal function returns.

Chronic retention may require long-term indwelling catheters, which has a significant risk of sepsis. Intermittent self-catheterization might be more appropriate in those who are able to perform this technique. Subclinical sepsis is common, although treatment is usually given only if symptoms are present.

Fistulas

Small fistulas might close spontaneously upon provision of a continuous free drainage of urine. This might require stenting of the ureters or catheterization of the bladder. If spontaneous closure does not occur, or if the fistula is large, then surgical closure by a surgeon experienced in such techniques is required.

- What are the main treatments for stress incontinence?
- What are the main treatments for detrusor instability?
- What studies are essential before any surgery is undertaken?

Further reading

Bent AE, et al. (2003) *Ostergard's Urogynecology and Pelvic Floor Dysfunction*, 5th ed (Lippincott Williams & Wilkins).

27. Pelvic Organ Prolapse

Definition

A prolapse is the protrusion of an organ or a structure beyond its normal anatomic site. Pelvic organ prolapse involves weakness of the supporting structures of the pelvic organs so that they descend from their normal positions. The type of prolapse depends on the organ involved and its position in relation to the anterior or posterior vaginal wall (Fig. 27.1). Descent of the uterus is graded according to the position of the cervix on vaginal examination:

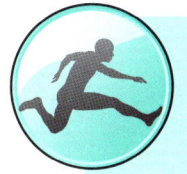

Genital prolapse is common and requires a basic knowledge of pelvic anatomy to help you understand how it develops and how it can be repaired.

- First degree: descent of the cervix within the vagina.
- Second degree: descent of the cervix to the introitus.

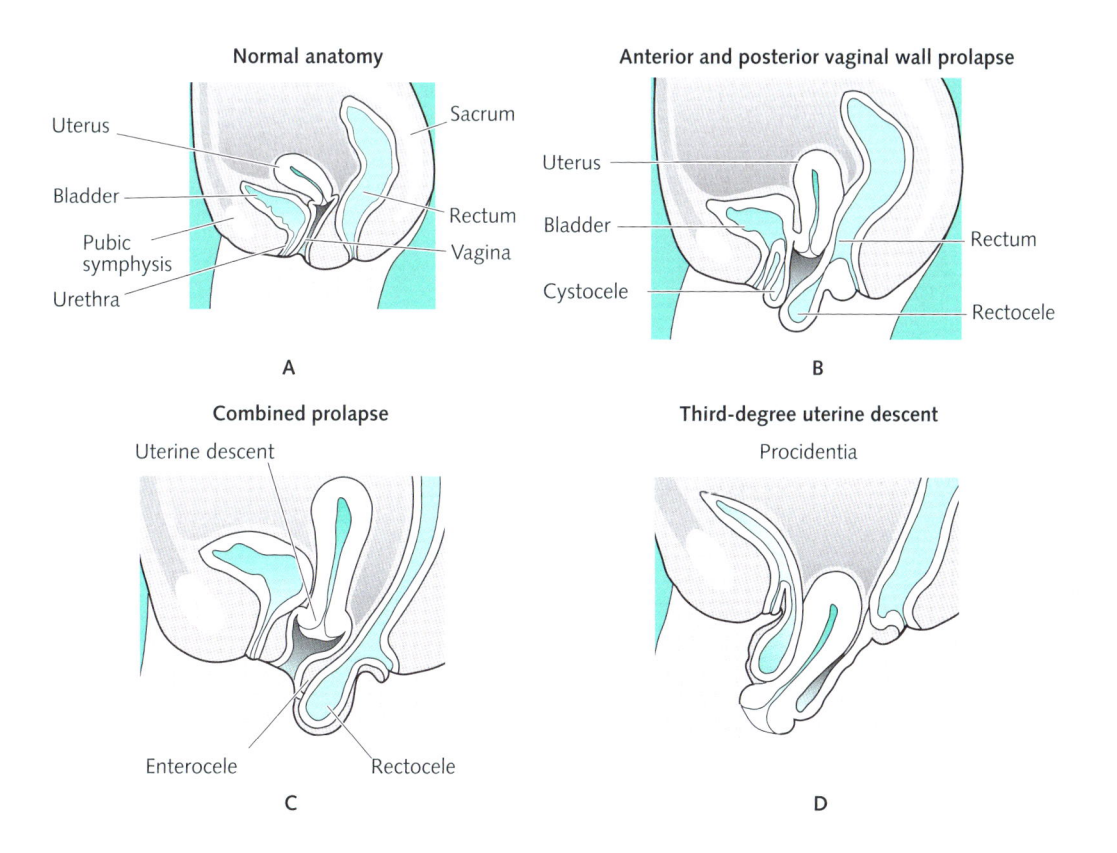

Fig. 27.1 Types of prolapse.

143

- Third degree: descent of the cervix outside the introitus (also known as a procidentia).

Incidence

Pelvic organ prolapse is common; a cystourethrocele is the most common type, followed by uterine descent and then rectocele. The incidence increases with increasing age. Prolapse is seen less commonly in African–American women than in Caucasian women.

Pelvic anatomy

Some knowledge of the pelvic anatomy, with particular reference to the pelvic floor muscles, fascia, and ligaments, is necessary to understand the development of pelvic organ prolapse. Weakness of these tissues, either congenital or acquired, results in descent of the pelvic viscera.

Pelvic floor
The pelvic floor consists of a muscular, gutter-shaped, forward-sloping diaphragm formed by the:
- Levator ani muscles.
- Internal obturator and piriform muscles.
- Superficial and deep perineal muscles.

The levator ani consists of two parts, i.e. the pubococcygeal part anteriorly and the iliococcygeal part posteriorly, and is covered by pelvic fascia. The vagina and urethra pass through the urogenital aperture formed by the medial border of the levator ani. The rectum passes posteriorly, with muscle fibers from the pubic bone uniting behind the anorectal junction. Thus, the muscles provide an indirect support for these structures (Fig. 27.2).

Pelvic ligaments
Condensations of the pelvic fascia form strong ligaments that act to support the upper part of the vagina, the cervix, and the uterus. Those that support the uterus include the:
- Transverse cervical or cardinal ligaments.
- Uterosacral ligaments.
- Round ligaments.

The transverse cervical and uterosacral ligaments consist of smooth muscle and elastic tissue. They support the pelvic side wall and the sacrum respectively. The round ligaments pass from the cornu of the uterus through the inguinal canal to the labium majus. They contain smooth muscle and maintain flexion of the uterus with only minimal role in support.

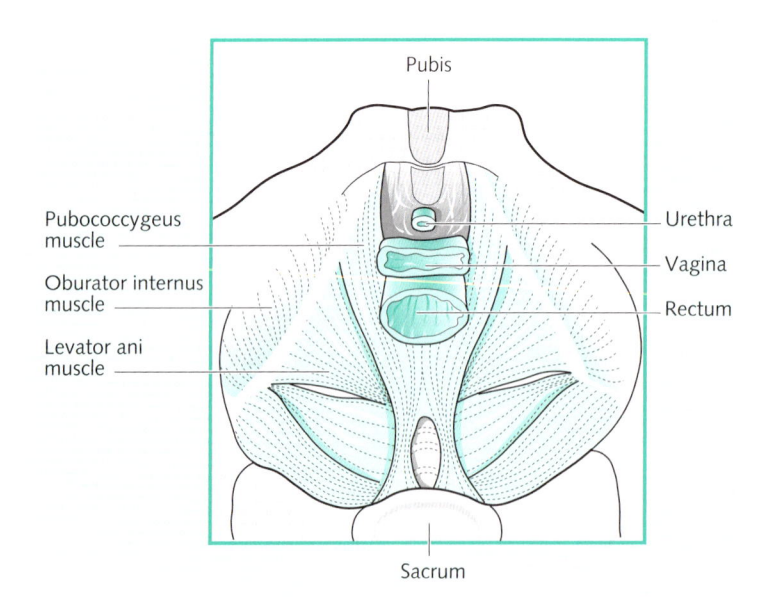

Fig. 27.2 Anatomy of the pelvic floor muscles.

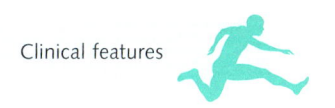

Etiology

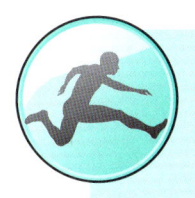

> In terms of etiology, obstetric factors are particularly important; and if prolapse is to be prevented, then good intrapartum management of the patient is essential.

Congenital
Some women are born with a predisposition to pelvic organ prolapse, which is probably secondary to abnormal collagen production. Conditions associated with prolapse include:
- Spina bifida.
- Connective tissue disorder.

Acquired
Although most women with pelvic organ prolapse have a degree of congenital predisposition, the following factors are also important:
- Obstetric factors.
- Postmenopausal atrophy.
- Chronically raised intra-abdominal pressure.
- Iatrogenic.

Obstetric factors
Figure 27.3 lists the factors that can cause prolapse secondary to denervation and muscular trauma of the pelvic floor.

Postmenopausal atrophy
The incidence of prolapse increases with age. This is due to atrophy of the connective tissues secondary to the hypoestrogenic state following menopause.

Chronically raised intra-abdominal pressure
Any factors that raise intra-abdominal pressure in the long term can predispose to prolapse, including:
- Intra-abdominal or pelvic tumor.
- Chronic cough.
- Constipation.

Iatrogenic
Hysterectomy predisposes to future prolapse of the vaginal vault because, in order to remove the uterus, the transverse cervical and uterosacral ligaments have to be divided and the upper vaginal supports are weakened.

Colposuspension predisposes to development of an enterocele because the anterior vaginal wall is lifted anteriorly, which in turn pulls the upper posterior vaginal wall forwards.

Clinical features

History
Most commonly, the patient presents with a history of local discomfort or a feeling of "something coming out," as the prolapsed organ pushes into the vagina and bulges towards the introitus. This can be exacerbated if the intra-abdominal pressure is increased, for example by coughing. It can interfere with sexual function.

Uterine descent often gives symptoms of backache, although other causes of backache must be excluded, especially in this older patient group. A procidentia causes discomfort, as it rubs on the patient's clothing; this can cause a bloody, sometimes purulent, discharge.

Other symptoms depend on the organ/organs involved. Urinary symptoms occur with a cystocele or a cystourethrocele, such as frequency of micturition. The patient might notice incomplete emptying of the bladder, which predisposes her to urinary infection and even possibly overflow incontinence. Stress incontinence might be present if there is descent of the urethrovesical junction (bladder neck).

A rectocele can cause incomplete bowel emptying. This can be relieved if the patient pushes back the prolapse digitally.

Obstetric factors that may predispose to pelvic organ prolapse	
• Prolonged labor	• Fetal macrosomia
• Precipitous labor	• Increasing parity
• Instrumental delivery	

Fig. 27.3 Obstetric factors that may predispose to pelvic organ prolapse.

Examination
- General examination.
- Abdominal palpation.
- Speculum examination.
- Bimanual pelvic examination.

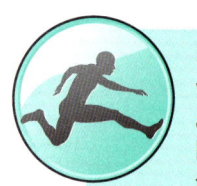

> Examination of the patient with a prolapse must include abdominal palpation and bimanual pelvic examination to exclude an abdominal or pelvic mass as the cause of the prolapse.

A general examination should be performed, particularly if the patient's medical history might influence future management options. Abdominal palpation is essential to exclude a mass that might be causing the pelvic organs to prolapse.

Inspection of the vulva might reveal an obvious pelvic organ prolapse. The patient should be examined in the left lateral position using a Sims' speculum. With the posterior vaginal wall retracted, any anterior wall prolapse will be demonstrated if the patient is asked to bear down. This can extend anteriorly as far as the urethral orifice, distinguishing between a cystocele and a cystourethrocele. Conversely, if the anterior vaginal wall is retracted, then an enterocele or rectocele will be seen. A bulging rectocele can be reduced digitally to exclude an enterocele.

Uterine descent can be assessed using the Sims' speculum but this might be difficult in the outpatient setting; unless the cervix is at or protruding through the introitus, then the degree of uterine prolapse might be better determined under general anesthesia, when traction can be applied to the cervix. There might be combined prolapse, most commonly uterine descent associated with anterior vaginal wall prolapse.

If the patient has a full bladder, then stress incontinence can be demonstrated by asking her to cough. A bimanual pelvic examination is mandatory to exclude a pelvic mass as the cause of the prolapse.

Management

The aim is to replace the prolapsed organs to their normal anatomical site. The options can be categorized into:
- Prevention.
- Conservative measures.
- Surgery.

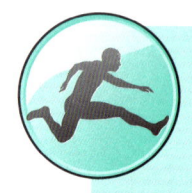

> Always remember to consider the patient's general health and other conservative measures, such as HRT, as well as the need for surgery.

Prevention
Because obstetric factors are most commonly involved in the development of a pelvic organ prolapse, it is important that damage to the supporting structures of the pelvis is minimized. Appropriate management of labor should include:
- Avoid prolonged first and second stages.
- Postnatal pelvic floor exercises.

The current decline in parity, as well as the increasing use of cesarean section, might reduce the incidence of prolapse.

Conservative measures
Improvement in general health should aim to treat the underlying cause of chronically raised intra-abdominal pressure, including:
- Weight loss.
- Advising the patient to stop smoking to reduce cough.
- Treat constipation.

Pelvic floor exercises
Pelvic floor exercises can improve symptoms of minor degrees of pelvic organ prolapse sufficiently to avoid surgery. However, their use is probably more important in prevention.

Hormone replacement therapy
In the presence of atrophic pelvic tissues, HRT can help in minor degrees of prolapse by increasing skin collagen content. Preoperative use of HRT reduces

the friability of atrophic tissues, making tissue handling easier during surgery.

Vaginal pessaries

The most commonly used pessary is a ring pessary made of inert plastic. The diameter is measured in millimeters and the appropriate size is assessed by vaginal examination. The pessary is passed into the vagina so that it sits behind the pubic bone anteriorly and in the posterior fornix of the vagina posteriorly, enclosing the cervix. The other less common types of pessary include the cube, Gellhorn, or donut pessaries.

The indications for the use of a vaginal pessary include:
- The patient has not completed her family.
- The patient prefers conservative management.
- The patient is medically unfit for surgery.
- While the patient is awaiting surgery.

With major degrees of prolapse, especially where the introitus is lax and the perineal body deficient, the pessary might not stay in situ. The main complications of a pessary are vaginal discharge or bleeding, particularly if the pessary is not replaced every 6 months. Vaginal ulceration can occur if the ring is too large and the pessary might simply fall out if it is too small. Granulation tissue might develop, incarcerating the pessary, if it is not changed regularly.

Surgical treatment

Surgery should be considered with a severe degree of prolapse or if conservative management fails. Prior to surgery it is important to know whether a woman is sexually active, because the vagina might be narrowed and shortened, potentially causing dyspareunia.

Surgery is not recommended in a woman who has not completed her family. Cesarean section is indicated following pelvic floor repair due to prolapse; vaginal delivery is likely to result in soft tissue trauma and recurrence of prolapse.

Anterior colporrhaphy

This operation, also known as an anterior repair, is indicated for the repair of a cystocele or a cystourethrocele. A portion of redundant anterior vaginal wall mucosa is excised and the exposed fascia is plicated to support the bladder.

Posterior colporrhaphy

Also known as a posterior repair, this operation is used to repair a rectocele or a rectocele combined with an enterocele. Using a similar technique to the operation described above, a triangle of posterior vaginal wall mucosa (its apex behind the cervix and the base at the introitus) is removed. The underlying levator ani muscles are plicated to support the perineum. If an enterocele is present, then the pouch of Douglas is opened and the enterocele sac of redundant peritoneum is excised.

Vaginal hysterectomy

This operation is performed for uterine prolapse, although it might be indicated for other gynecologic pathology. It can be combined with one or both of the operations mentioned above.

Manchester repair (Fothergill procedure)

This operation is no longer commonly performed for uterine prolapse—in cases where there is a reason to preserve the uterus. It consists of amputation of the cervix and then apposing the cardinal ligaments to lift the uterus, followed by anterior and posterior colporrhaphy if necessary.

Sacrospinous fixation

Using the transvaginal approach, the prolapsed vaginal vault is fixed to sacrospinous ligament, which runs from the ischial spine to the lower lateral aspect of the sacrum. Care must be taken to avoid the pudendal nerve and vessels, as well as the sacral plexus and the sciatic nerve.

Sacral colpopexy

This abdominal procedure involves suspending the vaginal vault from the sacrum or from the sacral promontory, using either strips of fascia or synthetic mesh. The main complications are intraoperative hemorrhage and infection of the mesh.

- What are the common presenting symptoms of pelvic organ prolapse?
- What are the different types of prolapse?
- Describe how a patient complaining of prolapse should be examined.
- Discuss the conservative management of prolapse.
- For which patients is conservative management appropriate?

Further reading

Bent AE, et al. (2003) *Ostergard's Urogynecology and Pelvic Floor Dysfunction*, 5th ed. (Lippincott Williams & Wilkins).

28. Infertility

If a cause for a couple's infertility is discovered (see Chapter 8), then treatment can be aimed at the problem, but many couples suffer unexplained infertility. They can still be helped by the methods described below.

Anovulation

The absence of ovulation should be suspected if a woman's cycle is irregular and is confirmed if there is no rise of progesterone in the luteal phase of the cycle. If the woman is not ovulating:
- Maximize general health (correct thyroid disease, diabetes, etc.).
- Consider BMI (ovulation is less likely at the extremes of weight).
- Discuss psychological stress levels.
- Prescribe clomiphene (see below) to induce ovulation.

> There is no evidence that the use of temperature charts or LH "ovulation predictor" kits to time intercourse around ovulation improves the chance of conception; body temperature is a poor predictor of ovulation, and LH kits, although better, are expensive. Also, timing intercourse is psychologically stressful and can be counterproductive.

Clomiphene is an antiestrogen that occupies estrogen receptors in the hypothalamus, thereby increasing GnRH release, which leads to increased release of LH and FSH. This induces follicular development and ovulation. It is given on days 2–6 of the cycle. Ovulation should be confirmed by a raised progesterone level. If ovulation does not occur, then the dose can be increased the next month.

The patient must be warned of the risk of multiple pregnancy. Some practitioners arrange to scan the ovaries during the cycle to see whether follicles are developing and, when there are many follicles, to advise couples to use barrier contraception for that month.

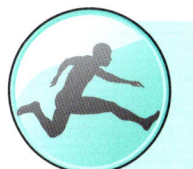

> All procedures that involve ovarian stimulation will lead to a risk of multiple birth. Why worry? Miscarriage is more common, cerebral palsy is three times more common, perinatal mortality is five times more common, and the mother is more likely to suffer from hyperemesis, pre-eclampsia, and premature labor.

Uterine and pelvic problems

Submucous fibroids, polyps, and uterine septums, which all distort the uterine cavity, do not cause infertility, but they are thought to impair fertility and cause miscarriage. They should be removed prior to in vitro fertilization (IVF) to maximize the chances of success. Hydrosalpinges reduce the implantation rate and can be removed or drained for this reason. Endometriosis is associated with infertility. Surgical treatment of mild endometriosis (i.e. cauterization/ablation or laser at time of laparoscopy) has been shown to improve fertility temporarily.

Tubal problems

Tubal problems can be diagnosed on a hysterosalpingogram, but blocked tubes are usually confirmed at laparoscopy, using the dye test. If the tubes are not patent, then the choice is between tubal surgery and IVF.

Tubal surgery
Some centers perform tubal surgery, usually using microsurgical techniques, for selected patients. The patient must be aware that her risk of ectopic

pregnancy will be increased, as the tubes are scarred. Success rates vary, with the best results being seen where tubal damage was proximal. Distal damage can be treated by laparoscopic salpingostomy. Midtubal damage has the poorest prognosis, unless it is due to Filshie clip sterilization, in which case there is a relatively good prognosis.

In vitro fertilization

Some patients are referred directly for IVF. As the success of IVF is influenced by age, if the woman is older it might be better not to wait for tubal surgery and then wait to see if it works, because by the time she gets to IVF her chance of conception will be lower. If there is severe tubal damage, or tubal blockage in association with other pathology (e.g. adhesions), then referral for IVF is more sensible. IVF involves several steps:

- Down-regulation of the woman's own hormones using nafarelin acetate or leuprolide acetate, which are GnRH agonists. They initially stimulate LH and FSH, but they then cause down-regulation, leading to reduction in estrogen production and "menopausal" side-effects. These drugs are given by nasal spray or subcutaneous injection.
- Induction of multiple follicular development using gonadotrophins, such as human menopausal gonadotrophin, which contains FSH and LH and is prepared from the urine of menopausal women, hCG, which is obtained from the urine of pregnant women and has a similar action to LH, or recombinant FSH, an expensive but pure form of FSH.
- Egg collection: performed transvaginally using ultrasound, under sedation (Fig. 28.1).
- Sperm preparation.
- IVF of the oocytes with sperm.
- Transfer of the healthy embryos (maximum of three) back into the uterine cavity (Fig. 28.2).

New techniques making IVF more specialized are being developed all the time. If a couple is affected by a hereditary disorder that can be detected using gene probes, then the embryos can be subjected to preimplantation diagnosis. Cells from each embryo are removed and analyzed so that only unaffected embryos are replaced. In some cases of genetic abnormality or advanced maternal age, eggs can be collected from a healthy donor, then mixed with the man's sperm in vitro. New techniques of "assisted hatching," where the zona pellucida of the embryo is breached before reimplantation, are said to improve the chances of successful implantation.

Male infertility

If the semen analysis is persistently abnormal despite advice regarding loose underwear and reduction of alcohol and nicotine intake, assisted fertility can be considered. Intrauterine insemination (IUI) may be tried before IVF or

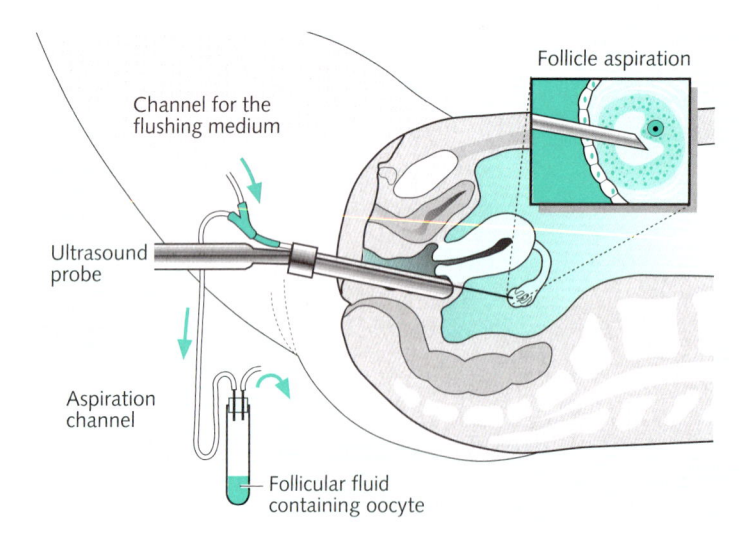

Fig. 28.1 Egg collection.

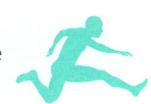

Fig. 28.2 Embryo transfer.

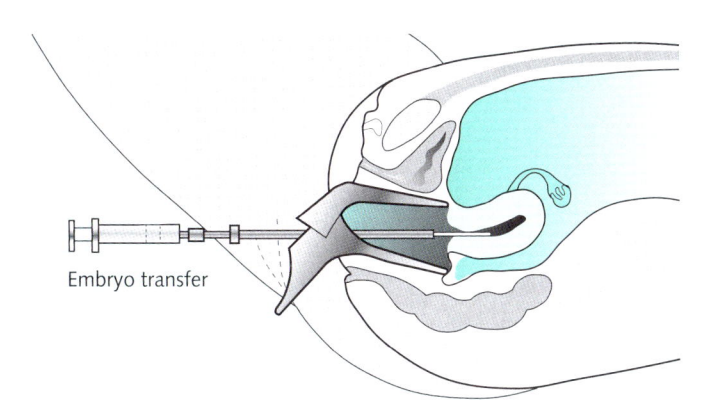

intracytoplasmic sperm injection (ICSI) because it involves less intervention.

Intrauterine insemination

IUI usually involves inducing follicular development and ovulation in the woman as for IVF. The process can be carried out with spontaneous ovulation, but the success rate is lower. However, the incidence of multiple pregnancy is also lower. At 36 h after ovulation, prepared sperm is placed into the uterine cavity using an intrauterine catheter.

Donor insemination (DI) is an option for couples where the sperm is of poor quality. Its use has fallen since the advent of ICSI (see below), but ICSI is not always successful.

Intracytoplasmic sperm injection

ICSI is an advanced form of IVF where one sperm is injected into the egg (Fig. 28.3). This technique has revolutionized treatment for couples where the man's sperm count is very low or showing many abnormal forms. If there are no sperm in the semen at all (due to obstruction or to congenital absence of the vas deferens), sperm can sometimes be extracted from the vas, the epididymis, or even from a testicular biopsy.

Surgical options for male infertility

If the sperm count is suboptimal because of epididymal blockage, surgery can be performed to restore patency. A varicocele, if present, can be repaired. This has not been proven conclusively to improve spermatogenesis, but it is known that the incidence of varicocele in the male partner of

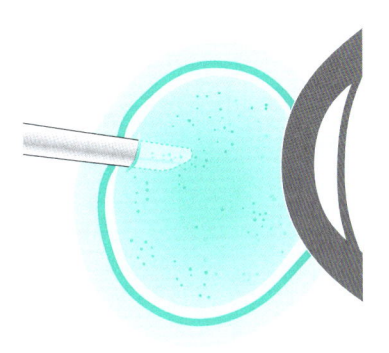

Fig. 28.3 Sperm injection into an egg.

couples with infertility is 40% compared with 15% in the general population.

Unexplained infertility

Couples with unexplained infertility are helped by IUI with controlled ovarian stimulation, and if this is unsuccessful may try IVF.

Ovarian hyperstimulation syndrome

Gonadotrophin therapy can lead to ovarian hyperstimulation syndrome (OHSS). This is a serious condition in which the ovaries are enlarged with cysts, related to multiple follicular development. In its mild form the patient suffers only mild abdominal discomfort. In worse cases, however, nausea and vomiting develop, there is pronounced, painful abdominal distention, and fluid shifts, resulting in ascites and pleural effusions. Hepatorenal failure and adult respiratory distress syndrome can ensue and the patient is at greatly increased risk of thromboembolism. Hospitalization and careful fluid balance are necessary. There is no real treatment for OHSS, which is why its prevention by careful ultrasound monitoring of the ovaries and serial blood tests for serum estradiol is so important.

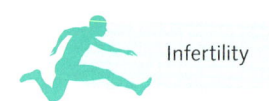

Prognosis for the infertile couple

As a result of developments in infertility treatment, couples have a 30% greater chance of a live birth than they did at the beginning of the 1990s. However, the reality is that the majority of couples undergoing a cycle of fertility treatment will not have a baby, which is why the role of the counselor in the infertility team is so important.

IUI and DI with ovarian stimulation give around a 9.5% chance of live birth per treatment cycle. The results are age dependent.

IVF success rates (i.e. live birth) are around 15–20%. The results are better if the mother is under 30; once over 35 there is a marked decrease, and over 40 the chance is around 12%. ICSI improves the chances of live birth to around 21%.

- What is the desired effect of clomiphene and which blood test can be used to look for this effect?
- Pregnancies conceived after tubal surgery are more at risk for which complication?
- Prior to egg collection for IVF, what treatment is given to the woman?
- Which factor most affects the likelihood of live birth following IVF?
- What are the two options available when the man has a low sperm count that is not due to a cause that can be treated surgically?

Further reading
Speroff L, et al. (2005) *Clinical Gynecologic Endocrinology and Infertility*, 7th ed. (Lippincott Williams & Wilkins).

29. Early Pregnancy Failure

Miscarriage

Miscarriage is the most common complication of pregnancy and will be experienced by 1 in 4 women at some point in their lives. It is defined as the loss of a pregnancy before 20 weeks.

Etiology
It is often difficult to identify the cause of a miscarriage, but factors that have contributed can be noted. These include:
- Fetal abnormality: 50% of miscarried fetuses are genetically (e.g. trisomy, monosomy) or structurally (e.g. neural tube defect) abnormal. Multiple pregnancies are more likely to be affected in these ways.
- Infection: Toxoplasma species, the rubella virus, tuberculosis, Listeria species, malaria, Salmonella species, and CMV are just a few of the potential causes. Bacterial vaginosis, where there is a change in the natural flora of the vagina, has been linked to second-trimester miscarriage.
- Maternal age: the miscarriage rate begins to increase when the mother reaches the age of 35.

Risks of miscarriage in relation to mother's age:
- under 35: 6.5%
- 35–40: 15%
- over 40: 23%

- Abnormal uterine cavity: the presence of an IUD, submucous fibroids, a congenital septum, or adhesions (Ashermann's syndrome).
- Maternal illness: e.g. Wilson's disease, poorly controlled diabetes, and thyroid or renal disease.
- Intervention: e.g. amniocentesis, CVS.
- Antiphospholipid antibodies and cervical insufficiency ("incompetence") can result in second-trimester loss (see the section "Recurrent miscarriage," below).

Investigation of the cause of miscarriage is usually delayed until the woman has had three miscarriages (see the section "Recurrent miscarriage," below).

Investigation of miscarriage
Ultrasound is used to aid diagnosis where women present with bleeding and the os is closed on examination. If the os is open then a miscarriage is inevitable and a scan is unnecessary, but is sometimes performed at the request of the patient.

Management of miscarriage
Once the fetus has died, the uterus will expel the products of conception. This process can take some weeks if left to happen spontaneously. Because of the fear of infection of retained products women have traditionally been advised to have a surgical evacuation to empty the uterus (a procedure that many women still think of as a "D&C"). Studies comparing the operative route with expectant management have now confirmed no difference in infection rates. Evacuation of retained products of conception is a simple operation that takes 5–10 min; the cervix is dilated to allow suction or sharp curettage. The pregnant uterus is easily perforated, so curettage must be gentle. Oxytocin can be given intravenously during the procedure to encourage uterine contraction and to minimize blood loss. Products of conception are sent for pathology.

If the patient is offered the choice of expectant management, then she should have follow-up scans to confirm that the uterus is empty. They, and women who have had a D&E, should be warned of the possibility of endometritis and told of the symptoms and signs to watch out for. These are: fever, feeling unwell, lower abdominal pain, and a change in vaginal bleeding, which can become offensive smelling and suddenly heavy.

If the woman is rhesus negative she will need Rhogam.

Unless work-up for recurrent miscarriage is needed, no follow-up in hospital is necessary. Before going home the woman should be given a

153

Early Pregnancy Failure

Why has this happened?

She should be reassured that she has done nothing wrong and is not to blame, but told that in most cases we do not find the cause for early miscarriage. Flying, working, having Pap smear tests, using mobile phones and having intercourse when pregnant do not cause miscarriage.

Will it happen again?

Many women who have had a miscarriage will go on to have a healthy term pregnancy. Realizing how common early miscarriage is may reassure her.

When can I start trying to get pregnant again?

Physically there is no reason why she cannot conceive with her next cycle, and this has no adverse effects on a resulting pregnancy, but mentally it may be better to have a few months to recover from the miscarriage. Couples can be advised to use condoms if they wish to wait for this time, as condoms are an instantly reversible form of contraception.

When will my next period come?

The next period may be early or late, but should be expected in roughly one month (or sooner or later depending on her usual cycle length). If she does not use contraception after the miscarriage and the next period is late she should seek a pregnancy test.

Fig. 29.1 Common questions asked by women who have suffered a miscarriage.

contact number for a local support group that can help her answer the questions that will arise after the miscarriage (Fig. 29.1). If she is not going to try to get pregnant again in the near future, then methods of contraception should be discussed.

Recurrent miscarriage

This is currently defined as three or more consecutive miscarriages and affects 1 in 100 women. In many cases no specific cause will be found, but the causes below can be used to guide the treatment of other women, leading to a positive outcome.

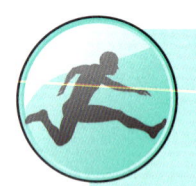

Incidence of miscarriage:
- Overall, any pregnancy: 15%
- After one miscarriage: 20%
- After two miscarriages: 30%
- After three miscarriages: 40%

Etiology of recurrent miscarriage

- Parental genetic abnormality (e.g. balanced translocation): found in 3–5% of partners in couples affected by recurrent loss. Those diagnosed are referred to a clinical geneticist.
- Uterine abnormality (e.g. septum, submucosal fibroid): the incidence of these in women with recurrent miscarriage has not been shown to be significantly different from women with normal pregnancies, but once diagnosed it may be difficult to dissuade the woman from seeking surgery.
- PCOS: the higher rate of miscarriage in these women has been attributed to their higher levels of LH. Unfortunately, suppression of LH does not improve the live birth rate.
- Antiphospholipid antibodies: this family of autoantibodies includes lupus anticoagulant and anticardiolipin antibodies. Their presence impairs trophoblast function, partly by causing thrombosis of the uteroplacental vessels. Some affected patients might have only a 10% chance of a live birth if untreated.
- Thrombophilic defects (e.g. factor V Leiden mutation): women who have thrombophilia due to protein C resistance (most commonly due to a mutation of the factor V Leiden gene), or abnormalities of protein S or antithrombin, are more prone to recurrent miscarriage.
- Cervical insufficiency ("incompetence"): this is usually secondary to cervical trauma caused by damage in childbirth or from surgical procedures (e.g. LEEP or cone biopsy), but in some cases can be congenital. It causes mid-trimester miscarriage.

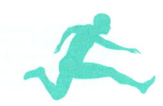

- Bacterial vaginosis: an imbalance in vaginal flora—with a lack of lactobacilli, which are usually commensal—results in bacterial vaginosis. The cause of this change is unknown. It is not linked to early miscarriage, but it does predispose to mid-trimester miscarriage.

Treatment of recurrent miscarriage

The treatment must be aimed at the cause. If no cause is found (as is the case for a significant proportion), then support and reassurance should be offered:
- Couples affected by genetic abnormality might opt for prenatal diagnosis, or even IVF with preimplantation testing (see Chapter 28).
- Uterine septae and submucous fibroids are best treated hysteroscopically, but treatment does not always improve the chances of a successful pregnancy.
- Maintaining a normal BMI in PCOS has been shown to improve pregnancy outcome, whereas hormonal manipulation has not.
- Women with antiphospholipid antibodies are given 81 mg aspirin daily as soon as the pregnancy test is positive and 5000 units subcutaneous heparin twice daily once fetal heart activity is seen on scan (around 6.5 weeks). The treatment is stopped at 38 weeks. The same treatment for women with thrombophilias has yet to be proven to be effective in trials.
- Cervical cerclage (suture) for insufficiency can be performed in pregnancy using the transvaginal route at around 14 weeks, or before conception by the transabdominal route (see Chapter 38). With the former the suture is removed at around 36 weeks to allow vaginal delivery. Abdominal sutures are left in situ and the woman is delivered by cesarean section.
- Bacterial vaginosis is simply treated with metronidazole or intravaginal antibiotic cream.

Treatments not proven to be effective include progesterone pessaries/tablets/injections in the first trimester, LH suppression, immunotherapy for women said to be "allergic" to their fetus, oral/systemic steroids for women with antiphospholipid antibodies, and hCG supplementation.

Ectopic pregnancy

This is a pregnancy that has implanted outside the uterine cavity (see Fig. 29.2 for likely sites). The incidence of ectopic pregnancy is increasing due to the rising number of cases of PID and as IVF pregnancies increase in number. Currently in the US the incidence is around 1 per 150 term deliveries; 10–15% of ectopics occur after IVF.

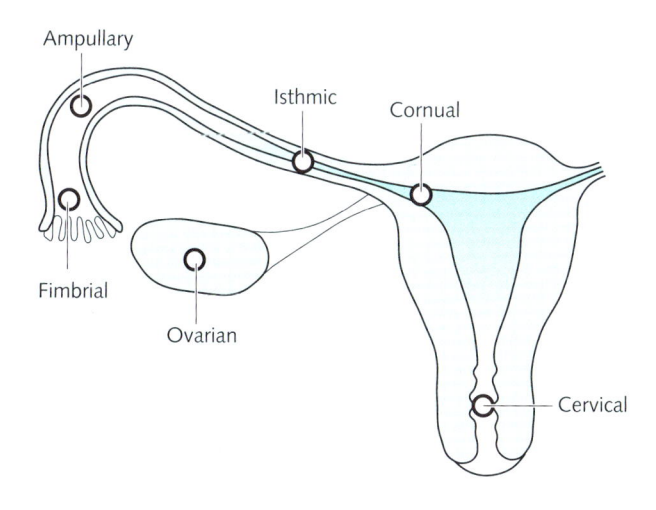

Fig. 29.2 Implantation sites of ectopic pregnancy.

Early Pregnancy Failure

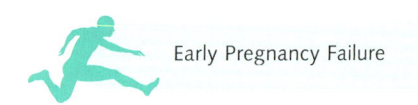

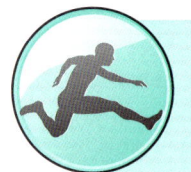

If a woman has a positive pregnancy test with bleeding or pain, then ectopic pregnancy must be ruled out.

Etiology of ectopic pregnancy

Ectopic pregnancy is caused by conditions that damage the uterine tubes or their ciliary lining, thus hindering the passage of the fertilized egg towards the uterine cavity, and anything that distorts the cavity itself or predisposes to abnormal implantation. These include:

- PID.
- Tubal surgery, e.g. sterilization, reversal of sterilization, previous ectopic pregnancy.
- Peritonitis or pelvic surgery in the past (e.g. appendicitis).
- IUD in situ.
- IVF.
- Endometriosis.
- Progesterone-only ("mini") pill; this does not cause ectopic pregnancy, but if a woman conceives when using it then the pregnancy is more likely to be ectopic than if she is using no contraception at all.

Clinical evaluation of ectopic pregnancy

In a few cases the patient will require immediate resuscitation and, as soon as possible, laparotomy. Those who have an acute abdomen but who are stable can have a laparoscopy to confirm the diagnosis. Treatment can then be performed laparoscopically or at laparotomy, depending on the surgeon's skill.

If, as in most cases, the presentation is subacute, then it is not necessary to head straight for the operating room. An ultrasound can be arranged; this may not identify the ectopic pregnancy, but it will demonstrate the fact that the uterus is empty. If there has been bleeding from the ectopic then the ultrasound will show free fluid in the pelvis. In some cases a mass in the adnexa can be visualized, and, uncommonly, this might contain a live ectopic, with a fetal heartbeat present.

The appearance of an empty uterus on scan in the presence of a positive pregnancy test should always raise the strong suspicion of ectopic pregnancy, which can be confirmed at laparoscopy.

However, in some cases there might be uncertainty about the dates of LMP, meaning that the pregnancy could still be a very early gestation, which might account for the 'empty' appearance of the uterus.

In other cases the history might not be clear cut and there could be suspicion that the woman has had a complete miscarriage, which also gives the appearance of an empty uterus on scan, and, as β-hCG does not return to a nonpregnant level immediately, this can cause confusion. In these cases, if the patient is stable and there is doubt about the diagnosis then it is reasonable to delay laparoscopy by performing two blood tests for β-hCG 48 h apart. If the pregnancy is viable then the level will double. In the case of miscarriage it will fall significantly. With an ectopic the level will plateau or rise, but not as much as double; the patient can then be set up for laparoscopy.

Treatment of tubal pregnancy

The aim is to eliminate the ectopic pregnancy in such a way as to minimize the risk of future pregnancies being ectopic. Various methods are used.

Surgical management

These techniques can all be performed at laparotomy, through a low transverse incision, or at laparoscopy. The skill of the operator will dictate the choice (Fig. 29.3).

Salpingectomy, complete or partial

Where the affected tube, or part of it, is removed. This might be the only option if the ectopic has ruptured, because the tubal anatomy will have been destroyed. In the event that an ectopic has occurred following IVF where the tubes are scarred, then the patient and surgeon might decide that it would be wise to remove both tubes at operation so that future IVF attempts do not lead to further tubal pregnancies.

Salpingotomy

An incision is made over the ectopic, which is removed, and the tube is usually allowed to heal.

Salpingostomy

An incision is made over the ectopic, which is removed, and the tube is left open and will heal by secondary intention.

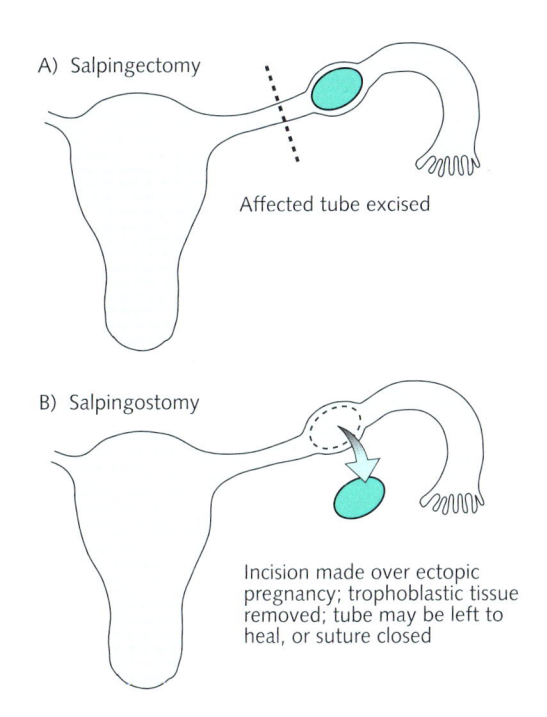

Fig. 29.3 Surgical options for treatment of tubal ectopic pregnancy.

"Milking" the tube
When the ectopic is near the ampulla it is sometimes possible to squeeze it out of the end of the tube without needing to cut the tube at all.

Medical treatment
The use of the cytotoxic drug methotrexate to treat ectopic pregnancy is increasing, but it is not available in all hospitals. It can be given as intramuscular injections or by injection directly into the ectopic pregnancy, either at laparoscopy or transvaginally under ultrasound control.

Patients are carefully selected for medical management: it is only suitable if the pregnancy is small and the tube is intact. The sac is measured on ultrasound scan as less than 4 cm in size and the β-hCG level should be less than 6000 iu/L.

Follow-up of ectopic pregnancy
Patients treated with methotrexate or by conservative surgery (i.e. salpingostomy, salpingotomy, or milking out the ectopic) must have serial β-hCG levels performed to ensure the resolution or removal of all trophoblastic tissue. Around 5% of patients treated medically will require further treatment with either methotrexate or a surgical procedure.

Prognosis after ectopic pregnancy
The chance of a repeat ectopic pregnancy is dependent on the health of the remaining tubal tissue. If management was conservative then the affected tube will have been scarred by the ectopic pregnancy. Rates of ectopic implantation in future pregnancies are around 11% after medical treatment, 12% after "conservative" surgery, and 9% after salpingectomy. The chance of conception after salpingectomy is obviously lower, so the risks must be weighed when deciding on management.

Other sites of ectopic pregnancy
These have high rates of maternal mortality and morbidity. Cervical, interstitial, and intramural pregnancies are best treated with methotrexate. The hemorrhage that can ensue from rupture or from attempted surgical treatment can be severe, necessitating hysterectomy and sometimes proving fatal. Cornual pregnancy is treated surgically, to remove the rudimentary horn in which the pregnancy has implanted and the tube on the affected side. Ovarian pregnancy can be treated surgically, performing wedge resection of the ovary, or medically. Abdominal pregnancy, if the fetus survives, should be delivered as soon as the fetus is viable.

Heterotopic pregnancy
The extremely rare combination of intra- and extrauterine pregnancy is becoming more common with the increase in IVF pregnancies where at least two embryos are replaced. The incidence is 1/10,000 pregnancies. Treatment is usually surgical, with the procedure being performed laparoscopically, but avoiding instrumentation of the uterus. There is an increased risk of miscarriage for the intrauterine pregnancy, this being around 25%.

Trophoblastic disease

This term covers partial and complete molar pregnancies and the choriocarcinoma that can follow them.

Definitions

Incidence of molar pregnancy
In the US, complete mole occurs around 1 per 1000 normal pregnancies. Partial mole is more common, but the exact incidence is harder to calculate as many go unreported. Three percent of molar pregnancies do not regress spontaneously and, therefore, require chemotherapy; this is more common with complete moles than partial moles.

Some ethnic groups are more prone to molar pregnancy. It is more common in the Far East, but the incidence there is decreasing, prompting the suspicion that there is a nutritional element.

Women at the extremes of reproductive age are more likely to experience trophoblastic disease.

Diagnosis and clinical evaluation of molar pregnancy
There is likely to be bleeding early in the pregnancy, so the diagnosis can be made on ultrasound or perhaps picked up first by the histopathologist after the study of retained products of conception. The trophoblastic tissue secretes hCG, so serum levels are very high and might lead to exaggerated symptoms of pregnancy (e.g. hyperemesis).

Management of molar pregnancy
Molar pregnancies are treated with surgical evacuation in the same way as miscarriage. The products of conception are sent for pathology. The patient must then be followed up with weekly serum samples for β-hCG to ensure that levels are falling, as this will confirm that the trophoblastic tissue is regressing. Once the levels are normal, serum samples are tested every month for β-hCG in case of reactivation of trophoblast tissue.

If hCG levels return to normal within 8 weeks, follow-up is limited to 6 months. All other cases are followed for 1 year. Women are advised to use hormonal contraceptives and not to become pregnant until levels have been normal for 6 months. In future pregnancies, serum β-hCG will be measured at 6 and 10 weeks postpartum because of the possibility of choriocarcinoma occurring.

If hCG levels rise, plateau, or are still abnormal 6 months after surgical evacuation,

- Complete mole: a pregnancy within the uterus consisting of a multivesicular mass of trophoblastic tissue with hydropic change (looking like a bunch of grapes on ultrasound), and no evidence of a fetus, formed by mono or dispermic fertilization of an oocyte which has deleted all maternal genetic material, i.e. all genes are paternal (see below)

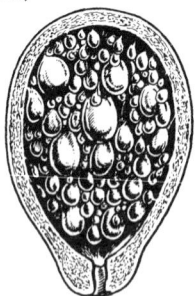

- Partial mole: a pregnancy within the uterus consisting of some trophoblastic proliferation and some hydropic change, where a fetus (usually nonviable) may also be seen. Formed by dispermic fertilization of an oocyte resulting in triploidy i.e. maternal and paternal genes
- Choriocarcinoma: a tumor of trophoblastic cells which secrete hCG occurring when molar pregnancies do not regress after surgical evacuation or, more rarely, after a nonmolar pregnancy

Fig. 29.4 Definitions. (Reproduced with kind permission from *Gynaecology Illustrated* (5th edn), published by Churchill Livingstone.)

Trophoblastic disease

then chemotherapy is started. Most are given methotrexate and folic acid, although some with adverse prognostic factors might need different combinations of other chemotherapies.

The current survival rate of patients requiring chemotherapy is 94%. Metastases from choriocarcinoma are seen in the lung, liver, and brain.

- What is the definition of recurrent miscarriage? How common is this condition?
- Which hormone is measured when investigating the possibility of ectopic pregnancy? After what interval should a repeat sample be sent?
- What are the surgical and medical options for treatment of ectopic pregnancy?
- What is the difference between the genetic make-up of complete and partial moles?
- How is choriocarcinoma treated?

Further reading

Gabbe SG, et al. (2002) *Obstetrics: Normal and Problem Pregnancies*, 4th ed. (Churchill Livingstone), Chapter 38.

Speroff L, et al. (2005) *Clinical Gynecologic Endocrinology and Infertility*, 7th ed. (Lippincott Williams & Wilkins).

30. Menopause

Definitions

The term "menopause" specifically refers to the last menstrual bleed that a woman experiences. It is a retrospective diagnosis, generally considered to have occurred after 1 year of amenorrhea. The range of age at menopause is 45 to 55 years, with an average of 51 years; factors that affect this include cigarette smoking, which lowers the age, and an inherited genetic predisposition. A premature menopause is one that occurs before the age of 40–45 years. This can occur naturally, by surgery (bilateral oophorectomy), or by chemotherapy or radiotherapy.

The term "climacteric" is used to describe the perimenopausal period, i.e. the transitional phase around the time of a woman's last menstrual bleed when endocrine changes occur as ovarian follicular activity ceases.

With the average life expectancy of women today at 78 years, a woman can spend up to a third of her life in the postmenopausal phase. Therefore, an understanding of the physiologic and psychologic changes that take place is important.

Pathophysiology

The total number of oocytes is at a maximum at 20 weeks of in utero fetal development and progressively decreases to about 750,000 at the time of birth. From childhood through to adult life, the number of oocytes becomes further depleted by ovulation and atresia. Eventually, at the time of the climacteric, the remaining oocytes are increasingly resistant to stimulation by the gonadotrophins FSH and LH, and the Graafian follicles that form do not secrete sufficient estrogen and progesterone to cause regular menstruation.

The endocrine changes that occur at the climacteric are:

- Hypothalamic–pituitary hyperactivity (raised FSH and later LH).
- Decreased or absent progesterone levels.
- Unopposed estrogen secretion.

These changes result in DUB secondary to anovulatory cycles as menopause approaches. In time, insufficient follicles develop with subsequent inadequate estrogen to stimulate the endometrium; therefore, menstruation ceases.

Clinical features of menopause

Figure 30.1 illustrates the clinical features of menopause.

Immediate symptoms

The more short-term symptoms associated with the climacteric can begin prior to menopause (Fig. 30.2).

Vasomotor symptoms

These include those characteristically associated with menopause, i.e. hot flashes and night sweats, which are the result of poor peripheral vascular control secondary to estrogen deficiency. Night sweats can result in insomnia, with lethargy and loss of concentration during the day.

End-organ atrophy

The genital tract and the lower urinary tract have the same embryological origin, and thus both systems will be affected by loss of estrogen.

The vulva and vagina become atrophic and the thinner epithelium is more susceptible to infection or trauma.

Vaginal dryness causes dyspareunia, which can contribute to the psychosexual symptoms that are another factor associated with menopause.

The supporting tissues of the pelvic organs (see Chapter 27) become thinner and weaker, resulting in the development of vaginal and uterine prolapse. The epithelium of the urethra and the trigone also become atrophic, with weakening of the connective and elastic tissue of the lower urinary tract. Thus, postmenopausal women may complain of dysuria, frequency, and urgency.

Menopause

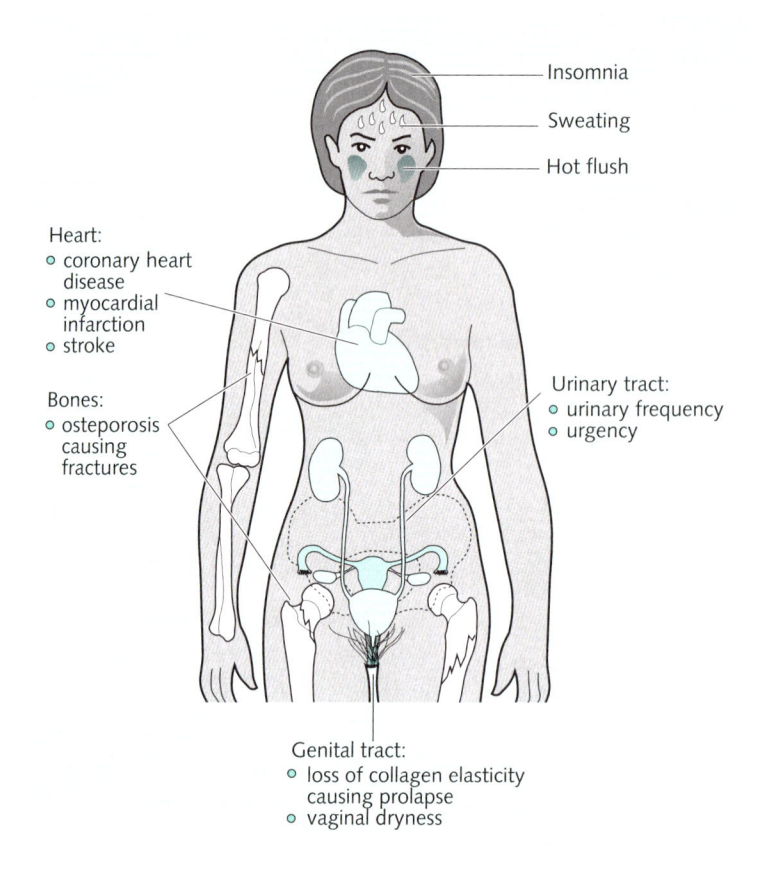

Fig. 30.1 The clinical features of menopause.

Labels on figure:
- Insomnia
- Sweating
- Hot flush
- Heart:
  - coronary heart disease
  - myocardial infarction
  - stroke
- Bones:
  - osteoporosis causing fractures
- Urinary tract:
  - urinary frequency
  - urgency
- Genital tract:
  - loss of collagen elasticity causing prolapse
  - vaginal dryness

The immediate effects of menopause

- Vasomotor symptoms
- End-organ atrophy
- Psychological symptoms

Fig. 30.2 The immediate effects of menopause.

Psychologic symptoms
These include depression, irritability, poor memory, and loss of libido, which are particularly common prior to the woman's last period. It is thought that fluctuating hormone levels are important, as opposed to simply low hormone levels. Social and environmental factors can play a part in these symptoms, but should not necessarily be taken as the diagnosis.

Long-term symptoms
With an increasingly elderly population, the long-term consequences of menopause carry a high morbidity and mortality, as well as being important social and economic factors.

Osteoporosis
Osteoporosis is a skeletal disease characterized by low bone mass and disruption of the normal bone architecture; this results in increased bone fragility and, thus, susceptibility to fractures. Bone mass in both men and women reaches a peak at 30–40 years of age and then starts to decline. However, in women, there is an acceleration in this decline immediately after menopause. As a result, this increased bone loss, combined with the lower peak bone mass prior to menopause, predisposes women to a greater risk of fracture compared with men.

Postmenopausal osteoporosis is caused by changes in bone remodeling, such that the rate of

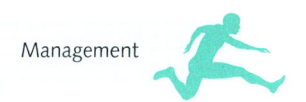

Factors which predispose to the development of osteoporosis
• Family history • Nulliparity • Late menarche and/or early menopause • Small build • Lack of exercise • Smoking • Drugs including corticosteroids and heparin

Fig. 30.3 Factors which predispose to the development of osteoporosis.

osteoclast bone resorption exceeds that of osteoblast bone formation. Other factors can contribute to this (Fig. 30.3), particularly a family history of osteoporosis. It is important that postmenopausal women with any of these associated risk factors should be counseled about treatment, such as HRT, to reduce their risk of fractures. The three most common sites for fractures in this group are the spine, the hip, and the distal radius. In the US, 130,000 vertebral fractures and over 50,000 hip fractures occur each year.

Cardiovascular disease
Ischemic heart disease is about five times less common in a premenopausal woman than in a man. However, following menopause, the incidence rises so that, by the age of 70, there is no longer any sex difference. This is thought to be caused by a shift in lipoprotein metabolism with an increase in the serum low-density lipoprotein (LDL) level, so that the high-density lipoprotein (HDL) to LDL ratio is altered.

A similar pattern is seen in the incidence of strokes (cerebrovascular accidents). At the time of menopause, there is a small rise compared with premenopausal women, but this is much less marked than in ischemic heart disease.

Management
History
Presenting symptoms include:
- Vasomotor symptoms and mood changes.
- Menstrual history.
- Sexual history, including contraception.
- Gynecologic history, including recent Pap smear.
- Family history, in particular of osteoporosis.

Examination
This should include blood pressure and a breast examination, as well as abdominal and pelvic examination.

Evaluation
Plasma gonadotrophins and estrogen levels vary markedly in the climacteric; thus, the diagnosis of menopause is usually made on clinical grounds, although it is confirmed by a raised serum FSH concentration.

Other investigations should be performed according to the patient's age and presenting symptoms, including:
- Cervical Pap smear.
- Mammogram.
- Pelvic ultrasound.
- Endometrial sampling.
- Bone mineral density measurement.

Treatment
General measures include:
- Diet, exercise, and weight control.
- Treat any medical condition, such as hypertension or diabetes.
- Psychologic support if appropriate.

Hormone replacement therapy
Both the immediate and the long-term effects of menopause have been shown to be improved by administering estrogen and progesterone. Estrogen therapy has been proven to improve the bone mineralization of osteoporosis and to reduce substantially the risk of fractures. With respect to cholesterol metabolism and the associated risk of vascular disease, giving oral estrogen lowers total cholesterol and LDL levels and raises the HDL fraction. This effect might be negated somewhat by the concomitant administration of progesterone.

> If the patient has a uterus and wishes to start HRT, then therapy with both estrogen and progesterone should be initiated.

Menopause

All patients should be fully informed about the benefits and risks of HRT, so that they can decide whether to commence treatment. In particular, women in menopause who are below 45 years of age and women with osteoporosis or with a combination of risk factors for the disease must discuss HRT thoroughly. Figure 30.4 lists the contraindications to HRT. Particular controversy exists over the risk of HRT in the development of breast cancer; recently, it has been proven that there is a slight increased risk, but this is likely to be offset by the improved morbidity from osteoporosis.

The most important point to remember in prescribing HRT is that giving a woman with an intact uterus long-term unopposed estrogen will cause stimulation of the endometrium, which puts her at risk of endometrial hyperplasia or even endometrial carcinoma. She must, therefore, also be given concomitant progesterone therapy to prevent this.

The next decision in prescribing is whether the patient finds a monthly withdrawal bleed acceptable. If she does, then she can be given estrogen with cyclical progesterone to protect the uterus. If she prefers not to have a regular bleed and has not had any bleeding for more than 1 year, then the woman might be suitable for continuous combined estrogen and progesterone therapy, which should avoid monthly bleeds.

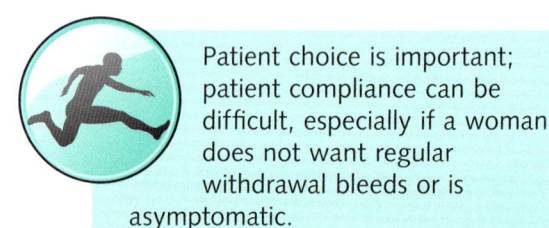

> Patient choice is important; patient compliance can be difficult, especially if a woman does not want regular withdrawal bleeds or is asymptomatic.

Finally, the route of administration of the treatment must be discussed with the patient (Fig. 30.5).

Nonhormonal drug treatment

Clonidine is a central α-adrenergic stimulator that has been used in the past for the treatment of hot flashes and night sweats.

Other drug treatments are appropriate to offer protection against long-term consequences of menopause, in particular osteoporosis, in those postmenopausal women for whom estrogens are neither contraindicated nor desired.

Contraindications to hormone replacement therapy

- Endometrial carcinoma
- Breast carcinoma
- Undiagnosed vaginal bleeding
- Undiagnosed breast lump
- Suspected pregnancy
- Liver disease with impaired liver function
- Previous TED associated with hormonal contraception, pregnancy or estrogen replacement

Fig. 30.4 Contraindications to HRT.

Routes of administration of hormone replacement therapy

Route	Advantages	Disadvantages
Oral	Cheap	Partial metabolism in gut
	Effective	Peaks and troughs in plasma levels
Transdermal	Avoids liver	Cost
	Continuous absorption	Skin reactions
Topical gel	Continuous absorption	Estrogen-only preparation
		Messy
Vaginal cream	Specific local effect	Estrogen-only preparation
		Long-term endometrial stimulation because of systemic absorption

Fig. 30.5 Routes of administration of HRT.

Raloxifene (Evista) is a newly developed selective estrogen receptor modulator with a similar structure to tamoxifen, a drug used to treat breast cancer. It has no effect on menopausal symptoms such as hot flashes, but it offers long-term protection against osteoporosis.

Other drug treatments, such as bisphosphonates, are also effective for osteoperosis treatment in asymptomatic woman. Increasing dietary calcium and vitamin D are also recommended.

- What is the definition of menopause? How can it be diagnosed?
- What are the short-term symptoms of menopause?
- What are the possible long-term sequelae of menopause?
- Describe the various types and routes of administration of HRT.
- What are the potential risks of HRT?
- Describe some of the alternatives to HRT in the treatment of menopausal problems and compare their relative merits and risks.

Further reading

Rossouw JE, et al. (2002) Risks and benefits of estrogen plus progestin in healthy postmenopausal women: principal results from the Women's Health Initiative randomized controlled trial. *JAMA* 288(3):321–33. http://www.whi.org

31. Contraception, Sterilization, and Unwanted Pregnancy

Introduction

The ideal contraceptive is one that is 100% effective, with no side effects, is readily reversible, and does not need medical supervision; this does not exist. Hence, it is important that the doctor assesses the patient's requirements at the particular time in her life that she requests contraception, and reviews the advantages and disadvantages so that the patient can make an informed choice (see *Crash Course in Endocrinology*).

> Informed choice as to the method of contraception used by every individual patient is important.

The effectiveness of a particular method is measured by the number of unwanted pregnancies that occur during 100 women years of exposure; this is known as the Pearl Index (Fig. 31.1).

Natural family planning methods

Rhythm method

The rhythm method involves predicting the time of maximum fertility (3 to 4 days around ovulation) by:
- Using a menstrual calendar.
- Charting the basal body temperature, which rises 0.2–0.4°C when progesterone is released from the corpus luteum.
- Recognizing changes in cervical mucus.
- Using an ovulation predictor kit (e.g. Clear Plan or Clear Blue).

Advantages
The rhythm method might be useful if other methods are unacceptable to the couple, such as in certain religious groups or because of unwanted side effects.

Disadvantages
The method relies on a regular menstrual cycle, lengthy instruction, and commitment. In addition, it has a high failure rate.

Coitus interruptus

Advantages
Still widely practiced, this method is free and without side effects.

Disadvantages
The failure rate is high due to variable ejaculatory control and the fact that pre-ejaculatory fluid contains some sperm. There is no protection against sexually transmitted infections.

Barrier methods

These methods include the male condom and, for women, the diaphragm, the cervical cap, and the female condom. Their effectiveness increases with concomitant use of a spermicide, such as nonoxynol-9, which alters sperm membrane permeability, resulting in sperm death (use of spermicides alone as contraception is not recommended).

Advantages
When used properly, these are effective, free from side effects, and widely available. They offer protection against sexually transmitted infections, in particular the male condom, which protects against HIV.

Disadvantages
They must be applied before penetration and can reduce the level of sensation. The diaphragm and the cap have to be fitted and checked regularly by a trained professional. In all methods, effectiveness is dependent on correct use and sustained motivation.

Contraception, Sterilization, and Unwanted Pregnancy

The relative effectiveness of contraception methods	
Method	Relative effectiveness
Sterilization: female	0–0.2
Sterilization: male	0–0.5
Combined OCP	0.2–3.0
Progesterone-only contraception	0.3–4.0
Depot injection	0–1.0
IUD	0.3–2.0
Mirena IUD	0–0.2
Condoms: male	2.0–15.0
Diaphragm	2.0–15.0

Fig. 31.1 Methods of contraception and their relative effectiveness as measured by the Pearl Index.

Contraindications to the combined oral contraceptive pill	
Degree of contraindication	Description
Absolute	Pregnancy
	Arterial or venous thrombosis
	Liver disease
	Undiagnosed vaginal bleeding
	History of estrogen-dependent tumor
Relative	Family history of thrombosis (consider investigations for thrombophilia)
	Hypertension
	Migraine with aura
	Varicose veins

Fig. 31.2 Contraindications to the combined OCP.

Hormonal contraception

Oral contraceptive pill
Since their introduction in 1961, various combinations of different estrogens and progestins have been used to prevent pregnancy. OCPs have the following modes of action:
- Inhibiting ovulation by:
  - Inhibiting FSH release.
  - Preventing follicular ripening.
  - Preventing the LH surge.
- Altering the endometrium.
- Altering the cervical mucus.

Contraindications
Figure 31.2 lists the contraindications to OCPs.

Advantages
This method is reliable if taken correctly, convenient, and not intercourse related. Its use reduces dysmenorrhea, menorrhagia, and premenstrual syndrome symptoms. It also controls functional ovarian cysts and is associated with a reduced incidence of carcinoma of the ovary and endometrium.

Disadvantages
The main risks of OCPs are thromboembolism and cardiovascular complications; these are exacerbated by:

- Age.
- Obesity.
- Cigarette smoking.
- Diabetes.
- Hypertension.
- Familial hyperlipidemia.

Other more minor side effects include weight gain, decreased libido, breast discomfort, mood disturbance, and breakthrough bleeding. The effectiveness of OCPs is limited by some antibiotics, by hepatic enzyme-inducing drugs, and by vomiting and diarrhea. Use is associated with an increase in CIN and carcinoma of the cervix; the effect on breast cancer is uncertain.

Progesterone-only pill
Although slightly less effective than combined OCPs, the progesterone-only pill ("mini-pill") is used in women in whom estrogens are contraindicated or who cannot tolerate the side effects. This includes women aged over 35 who smoke and those who are breast-feeding.

The mode of action differs from the combined OCP in that ovulation is suppressed in only 50–60% of cycles, but with similar changes in cervical mucus and in the endometrium, as well as reduced tubal motility.

Advantages
Without estrogen, few serious side effects occur.

Disadvantages
Efficacy is reduced if the time of pill taking is delayed by more than 3 h. The main problem is a change in menstrual pattern, with spotting or breakthrough bleeding that does not settle despite continued use.

Injectable progestins
Intramuscular injection of medroxyprogesterone acetate given every 3 months ensures that high-dose progesterone is gradually released into the circulation and inhibits ovulation; it is almost as effective as the combined OCP.

Advantages
This method of contraception is highly effective and not intercourse related; it also does not require daily motivation.

Disadvantages
- Because it is injected, it cannot be removed and any side effects must be tolerated for 3 months.
- Most women become amenorrheic, but heavy, unpredictable bleeding patterns can sometimes occur.
- Being a slow-release depot preparation, there might be a delay in return to fertility of 12 to 18 months.

Postcoital contraception/emergency contraception
Since 1984, the Yuzpe method has been used to reduce the risk of pregnancy by administering two doses of the following medication 12 h apart and within 72 h of unprotected intercourse:
- 100 µg ethinylestradiol *plus*
- 500 µg levonorgestrel.

The endometrium is made unfavorable for implantation and there is interference with normal corpus luteum function. If taken before the preovulation estrogen surge, then ovulation can be inhibited.

The medication is often administered with an antiemetic to reduce nausea and vomiting, which occurs in up to 50% of patients.

The failure rate is 2–5%, depending on the time in the cycle at which it is taken.

Counseling is essential, so that the patient understands the implications of the failure rate and so that she makes sure she is followed up, especially if she has not had a period, but also to decide on future long-term contraception.

More recently, this method has been superseded by Plan B (two tablets of 0.75 mg levonorgestrel) taken 12 h apart. This requires a prescription from a physician.

Another method of emergency contraception is to insert an IUD within 5 days of unprotected intercourse (see below for more details); this can be removed after the patient's next period or left in situ to provide ongoing contraception.

> Postcoital or emergency contraception is not for routine use:
> - High-dose OCP within 72 h.
> - Insert an IUD within 5 days.

Intrauterine devices

Insertion of one of a variety of synthetic devices into the uterine cavity (Fig. 31.3) is likely to ensure that blastocyst implantation is prevented. There is also some foreign-body reaction to the IUD in the endometrium, resulting in altered cell numbers and fluid compositions, which might affect gamete viability. There might also be changes in the cervical mucus; these reduce sperm penetration.

Contraindications
Figure 31.4 lists the contraindications to IUD use.

Advantages
Once in situ, IUDs can remain in place for 5 to 10 years and their effect on preventing conception is almost immediately reversible. The progesterone-containing IUD, the Mirena, has the extra advantage related to local secretion of progesterone, which acts on the endometrium; this results in amenorrhea in up to 85% of patients at 6 months. Hence, this type of IUD has various gynecologic indications, such as treating menorrhagia and dysmenorrhea.

169

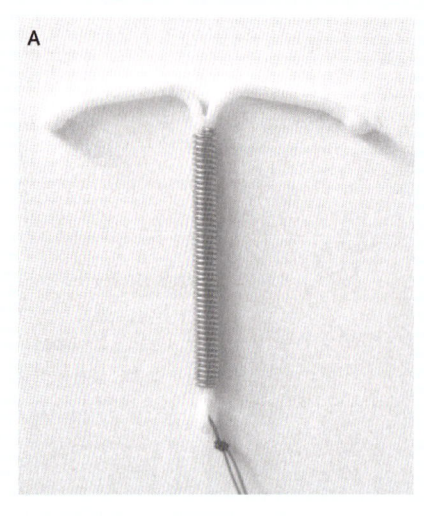

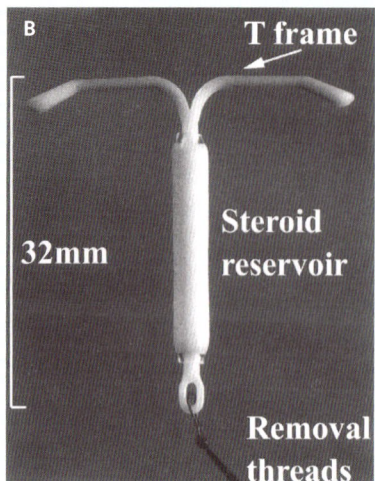

Fig. 31.3 Types of IUD: (A) Copper T; (B) Mirena IUD.

Contraindications to the intrauterine device

- Pregnancy
- Undiagnosed uterine bleeding
- Active and/or past history of PID
- Previous ectopic pregnancy
- Previous tubal surgery

Fig. 31.4 Contraindications to the IUD.

Disadvantages
- Infection.
- Uterine perforation.
- Expulsion of IUD.
- Menorrhagia and/or abdominal pain.
- Ectopic pregnancy.

Introduction of infection at the time of insertion of the IUD is one of the main risk factors for using this form of contraception; for this reason, it is usual to take a Gonorrhea and Chlamydia swab from the patient and/or give prophylactic antibiotics. The possibility of developing PID means that an IUD is less commonly used in nulliparous women, especially if they have multiple partners.

Other disadvantages that the patient should be told about include risk of uterine perforation at the time of coil insertion or possibly at a later date. The woman should be taught to check that she can feel the strings of the coil to ensure that it has not fallen out. If either of these situations arises, attempts to locate the IUD should be made by X-ray, ultrasound, or possibly hysteroscopy and/or laparoscopy.

The most common reasons for a patient requesting removal of the IUD are menorrhagia and abdominal pain; these symptoms are much less common with a Mirena™ than with other IUDs. If a pregnancy does occur with a coil in situ, then the risk of an ectopic pregnancy is higher than with other forms of contraception.

Female sterilization

The more commonly used techniques include the application of Falope rings or Filshie clips to each tube laparoscopically (or electrocautery and fulguration of the tubes) as a same-day procedure. At laparotomy, a modified Pomeroy tubal ligation is usually performed, e.g. at cesarean section. Rarely, in the presence of pelvic pathology, a hysterectomy is appropriate. It is now possible to perform sterilization hysteroscopically by insertion of microcoils into the fallopian tubes.

Counseling
Sterilization should be regarded as an irreversible procedure; therefore, the patient must be sure that she has completed her family and that she has

considered all other methods of contraception. The issues are particularly emotional if the patient makes the request at the time of termination of pregnancy or cesarean section.

Although the most successful form of contraception (see Fig. 6.1), there is still a failure rate of about 2 per 1000; this might be due to failure to exclude pregnancy preoperatively, incorrect application of a clip or ring, or incomplete fulguration of the tubes. If a pregnancy does occur, the risk of an ectopic pregnancy is higher than with other forms of contraception.

Male sterilization

Compared with female sterilization, a vasectomy is a relatively easy operation, avoiding the risks of a general anesthetic. The vas deferens is ligated via bilateral incisions in the scrotum. Another method of contraception must be used until two azoospermic samples have been obtained 3 and 4 months after the procedure. The failure rate is similar to the female operation.

Termination of pregnancy

Since *Roe v. Wade*, which was decided on January 22, 1973, a woman has been legally able to make the decision to terminate her pregnancy with her health-care providers' assistance. The procedure is legal in all 50 states until a gestational age of 14 weeks and is legal in a few select states until 24 weeks.

Counseling

Alternatives to abortion should be discussed with the woman, including support if she continues the pregnancy or adoption. If she decides to proceed with the termination, then the appropriate method must be agreed (see below) and future contraception should be arranged.

Surgical methods

Up to 14 weeks of pregnancy, suction aspiration is the most commonly used method. Preoperative prostaglandin to ripen the cervix is often used, especially in nulliparous women, followed by cervical D&E of the uterus using a plastic cannula.

After 14 weeks, D&E can be used; the uterine contents must be crushed as well as using curettage.

Medical methods

Increasingly, medical termination can be offered with up to 63 days of amenorrhea. Mifepristone, an antiprogesterone, is given orally 36–48 h before vaginal insertion of a prostaglandin E1 analog; complete abortion occurs in 95% of patients.

In the second trimester, synthetic prostaglandin tablets are placed in the posterior fornix every 3–4 h; incomplete abortion is not uncommon, and surgical evacuation must be performed.

Complications

- Infection: screen for chlamydia preoperatively and/or give prophylactic antibiotics.
- Trauma: to cervix or uterus, including perforation (cervical incompetence may occur with repeated procedures).
- Hemorrhage: might be secondary to the above or the result of incomplete evacuation.

- How are contraceptive failure rates described?
- What are the contraindications to using the combined OCP?
- What are the noncontraceptive benefits of the combined OCP?
- Name the progesterone-only methods of contraception and describe their mechanism of action.
- Describe the mechanism of action of the levonorgestrel IUD.
- What are the possible options for emergency contraception and how long after intercourse can they be used?
- Describe the possible options for sterilization.

Further reading

Hillard PA, et al. (2002) *Novak's Gynecology*, 13th ed. (Lippincott Williams & Wilkins, Philadelphia).

Speroff L, et al. (2005) *Clinical Gynecologic Endocrinology and Infertility*, 7th ed. (Lippincott Williams & Wilkins, Philadelphia).

32. Gynecologic Endocrinology

Amenorrhea: primary and secondary

Delayed puberty
This is discussed in Chapter 19.

Precocious puberty
Precocious puberty is said to have occurred when sexual maturation takes place before the age of 9 years.

Etiology
The possible etiologies for precocious puberty are summarized in Fig. 32.1 and an algorithm for identifying the most common causes is shown in Fig. 32.2. Although it is important to exclude androgen-secreting tumors in the ovary and adrenal glands, most cases are constitutional.

Work-up
- Full history and physical examination.
- Full endocrine profile (estradiol, FSH, LH, testosterone, sex hormone binding globulin (SHBG), androstenedione, dehydroepiandrosterone sulfate, 17-OH progesterone).
- Bone age studies.
- Imaging: ultrasound scanning of the gonads and adrenals should be performed as a first line, but CT or MRI are the gold-standard investigations for excluding tumors.

Management
- Endocrine: the mainstay of endocrine support is suppression of estrogen and androgen production by GnRH analogues to reverse the physical changes. This can either be given as a daily nasal spray or monthly depot preparation.
- Psychologic support: this is vital, and counseling important, because the affected girl will see herself as being different from her friends.
- Surgical: if a tumor is discovered then this must be dealt with, usually surgically.

Hirsutism and virilism

Hirsutism, i.e. excessive facial and body hair growth, can be either genetic (idiopathic) or due to increased androgen levels, or sometimes both. Virilism occurs secondary to high circulating levels of androgens and is diagnosed when clitoral hypertrophy, breast atrophy, deepening of the voice, and male-pattern balding occur either alone or together. Approximately 10% of healthy normal women can be said to have some degree of hirsutism without signs of virilism; however, virilism rarely occurs in the absence of hirsutism (except in the newborn). The causes of hirsutism and virilism are shown in Fig. 32.3.

- The mainstay of treatment for PCOS is weight loss.
- Although the most common cause of hirsutism in women is PCOS, it is vital to exclude an androgen-secreting tumor.
- The psychological effects of precocious and delayed puberty can be profound and should not be neglected.
- Virilism is never idiopathic, whereas hirsutism can be.
- Rapid-onset hirsutism and virilism is suggestive of an androgen-producing tumor.

History
The timing of onset and the speed of progression of symptoms need to be elicited from the history. For instance, women with PCOS typically have mild symptoms that have been present since menarche, whereas androgen-secreting tumors of the ovary characteristically produce high levels of androgens, which cause severe symptomatology

173

Gynecologic Endocrinology

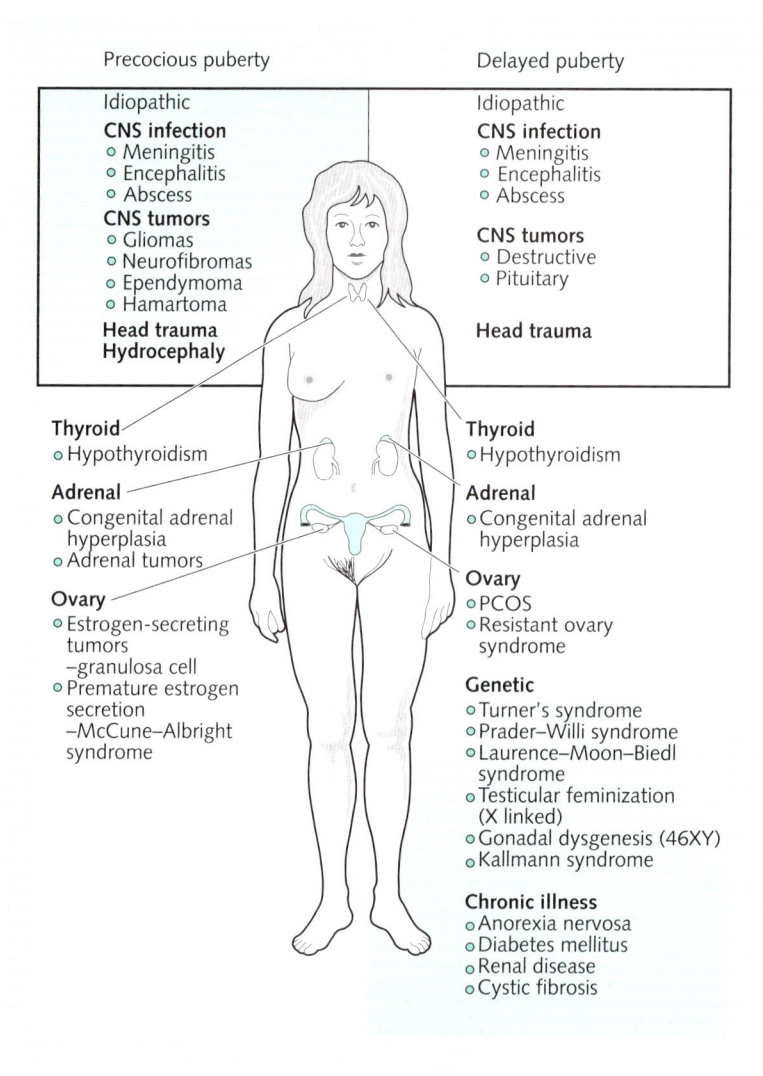

Fig. 32.1 Causes of precocious puberty and delayed puberty.

Precocious puberty

Idiopathic
CNS infection
- Meningitis
- Encephalitis
- Abscess

CNS tumors
- Gliomas
- Neurofibromas
- Ependymoma
- Hamartoma

Head trauma
Hydrocephaly

Thyroid
- Hypothyroidism

Adrenal
- Congenital adrenal hyperplasia
- Adrenal tumors

Ovary
- Estrogen-secreting tumors
  – granulosa cell
- Premature estrogen secretion
  – McCune–Albright syndrome

Delayed puberty

Idiopathic
CNS infection
- Meningitis
- Encephalitis
- Abscess

CNS tumors
- Destructive
- Pituitary

Head trauma

Thyroid
- Hypothyroidism

Adrenal
- Congenital adrenal hyperplasia

Ovary
- PCOS
- Resistant ovary syndrome

Genetic
- Turner's syndrome
- Prader–Willi syndrome
- Laurence–Moon–Biedl syndrome
- Testicular feminization (X linked)
- Gonadal dysgenesis (46XY)
- Kallmann syndrome

Chronic illness
- Anorexia nervosa
- Diabetes mellitus
- Renal disease
- Cystic fibrosis

Precocious and delayed puberty

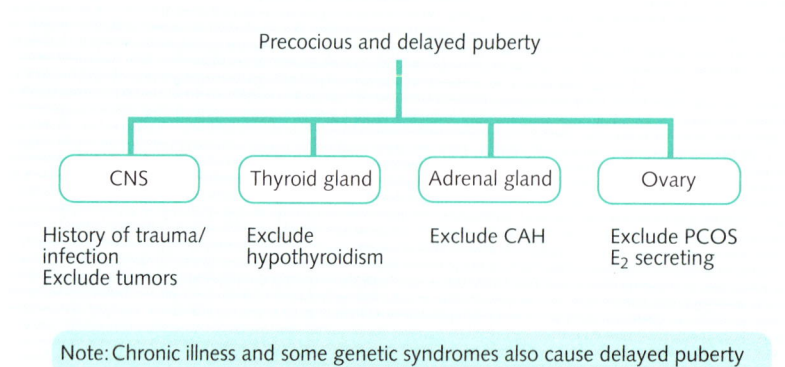

- **CNS**: History of trauma/infection; Exclude tumors
- **Thyroid gland**: Exclude hypothyroidism
- **Adrenal gland**: Exclude CAH
- **Ovary**: Exclude PCOS; E_2 secreting

Note: Chronic illness and some genetic syndromes also cause delayed puberty

Fig. 32.2 Algorithm for precocious and delayed puberty.

Hirsutism and virilism

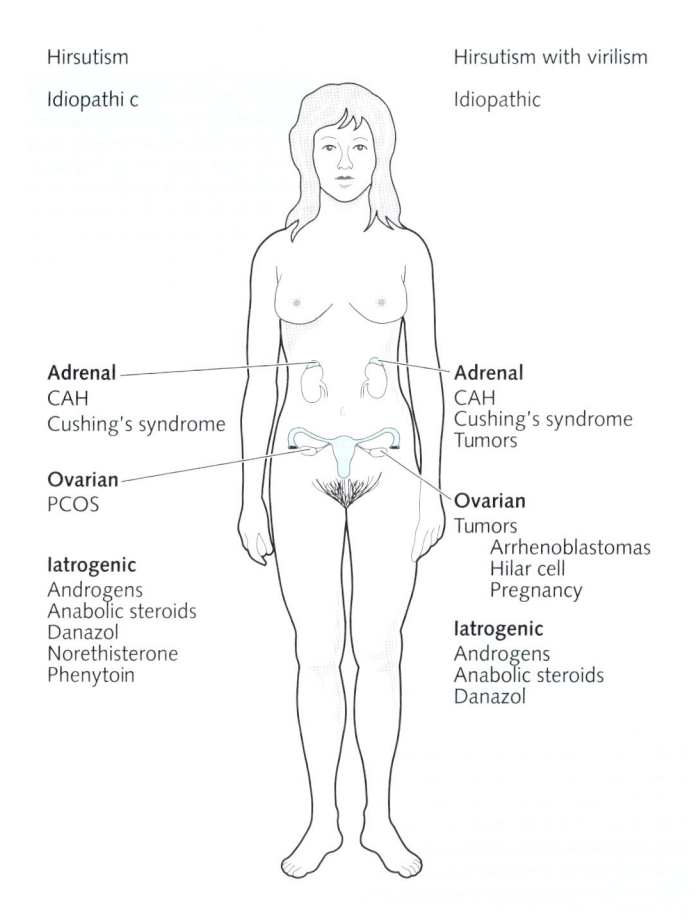

Fig. 32.3 Causes of hirsutism and virilism.

Hirsutism
Idiopathic

Hirsutism with virilism
Idiopathic

Adrenal
CAH
Cushing's syndrome

Ovarian
PCOS

Iatrogenic
Androgens
Anabolic steroids
Danazol
Norethisterone
Phenytoin

Adrenal
CAH
Cushing's syndrome
Tumors

Ovarian
Tumors
 Arrhenoblastomas
 Hilar cell
Pregnancy

Iatrogenic
Androgens
Anabolic steroids
Danazol

over a short period of time. A detailed menstrual history is important, because oligomenorrhea (infrequent periods) is associated with PCOS and amenorrhea is often associated with virilism. A family history of hirsutism is often present with idiopathic hirsutism and the menstrual history is usually normal.

PCOS typically presents with oligomenorrhea and hirsutism from the time of menarche. There might be a history of infertility secondary to chronic anovulation or a history of glucose intolerance. Although acne and seborrhea occur relatively commonly, the androgen levels are not usually high enough to produce symptoms of virilism.

CAH usually presents in infancy with ambiguous genitalia, but milder cases might not present until puberty and might have a history similar to women with PCOS.

Cushing's syndrome (excess cortisol) presents commonly with a gradual change in appearance associated with a host of other symptoms, including central obesity, muscle wasting and weakness, hypertension, and purple striae.

A careful drug history is imperative, as not only do many of the hormonal therapies used in gynecology have androgenic properties, but there is an increase in the use of anabolic steroids even amongst women.

Examination
- Grading of hirsutism can be made objectively with detailed scoring systems, but simple descriptive assessments are more practical. Signs of virilism should be looked for.
- Women with PCOS are often obese, although not always so. Acanthosis nigricans (pigmented raised patches found on the neck and skin

flexures) is sometimes present in women with PCOS associated with insulin resistance.
- Severe CAH will have been diagnosed during childhood due to ambiguous external genitalia or salt-losing conditions. Women with milder, late-onset forms of CAH have little to distinguish them from those with PCOS, i.e. obese, hirsute, and with some menstrual disorder.
- Women with Cushing's syndrome will have the typical appearance of central obesity, peripheral muscle wasting, hypertension, and striae.
- Androgen-producing tumors cause little in the way of systemic upset, apart from marked signs of virilism. They are usually too small to cause palpably enlarged ovaries.
- Women with idiopathic hirsutism usually have no abnormal findings on examination.

Etiology

Hirsutism and virilism occur due to excess circulating endogenous or exogenous androgens. Endogenous production by the ovary is the most common source.

Ovarian androgens

PCOS is the most common cause of hirsutism (90%) and occurs in about 20% of women. Raised levels of circulating LH and sex steroids are characteristic of this syndrome and occur through different pathways (Fig. 32.4). Pituitary production of LH is raised in PCOS, causing increased ovarian androgen production. This leads to a reduced production of SHBG by the liver and, as SHBG binds to circulating androgens, increased free testerone levels. Androgens are converted to estrogens in adipose tissue, raising estradiol levels, which further stimulate pituitary production of LH. Obesity not only increases insulin levels, which stimulates further ovarian androgen production, but also reduces SHBG levels and increases the peripheral conversion of androgens to estrogens.

Androgen-secreting tumors of the ovary are rare and include arrhenoblastomas and hilar cell tumors. Pregnancy luteomas are a rare source of excess ovarian androgen secretion. They develop due to an exaggerated response by the ovarian stroma to hCG.

Adrenal androgens

CAH is the term used to describe a group of rare disorders caused by defects in hydroxylation of cortisol precursors, most commonly 21-hydroxylase deficiency. The net effect is increased circulating levels of cortisol precursors and androgens. Excessive stimulation of the adrenal cortex produces raised cortisol levels and is often associated with excess androgen production (Cushing's syndrome). Adenomas and adenocarcinoma of the adrenal gland produce high levels of androgens and are rare.

Exogenous androgens

Androgens and anabolic steroids will cause hirsutism and virilism, depending on the amount and length of time taken. Certain drugs prescribed for medical disorders have androgenic properties and, if taken in high enough doses and for long

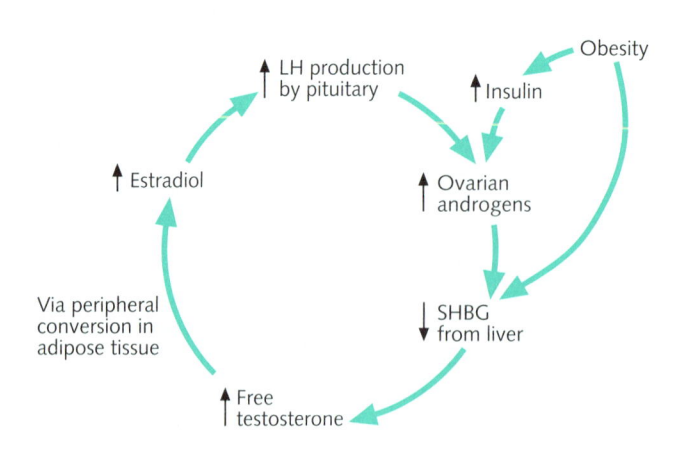

Fig. 32.4 Mechanism of increased androgen production in PCOS.

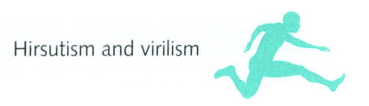

periods of time, can cause hirsutism (a type of progesterone, phenytoin) and virilism (danazol).

Appropriate work-up

Work-up is determined somewhat by the degree of symptoms (Fig. 32.5). Having excluded a history of exogenous androgens, if hirsutism is the only presenting complaint then PCOS is the likely cause, accounting for 90% of cases. Diagnosis is made from the history, biochemical tests, and ultrasound imaging of the ovaries. A rapid onset of symptoms, especially where virilism is present, would suggest high circulating levels of androgens secondary to more serious pathology. Testosterone levels more than twice the upper limit of normal suggest an ovarian or adrenal androgen-secreting tumor, which could be identified by imaging tests such as ultrasound or CT scanning. Small tumors might be missed, so a high level of suspicion is needed. Investigations for CAH and Cushing's syndrome should be performed if symptoms and clinical signs suggest these diseases. Idiopathic hirsutism is a diagnosis made by excluding other pathologies.

Complications

The main complication of hirsutism is psychosocial and this complaint should, therefore, be dealt with sympathetically. Some signs of virilism, such as deepening of the voice and clitoromegaly, might be irreversible. Complications associated with PCOS include obesity, insulin resistance, and glucose intolerance. Chronic anovulation affects fertility and can cause endometrial hyperplasia and adenocarcinoma as a result of the unopposed effect of estrogens.

Treatment

Idiopathic hirsutism can be treated cosmetically using techniques such as bleaching or electrolysis. The effects of obesity in women with PCOS have been described above, and encouraging weight loss is important in PCOS. Medical treatment of women with PCOS is most effective using OCPs, especially Yasmin®, since it contains drospirenone, a progesterone with anti-androgenic properties. Although improvement of hirsutism can take many months, the progestogenic effect of drospirenone will protect the endometrium from the effects of unopposed estrogen. Recent data suggest that PCOS might be driven by insulin resistance; as such, good results have been obtained by the use of the oral hypoglycemic agent metformin.

Androgen-secreting ovarian and adrenal tumors should be surgically removed, with preservation of the ovaries in younger women.

Glucocorticoid and often mineralocorticoid replacement is the mainstay of treatment in CAH. Hirsutism and virilism should improve with therapy, but it is sometimes necessary to perform surgical reconstructive procedures to the external genitalia.

Treating the cause of excessive cortisol production in Cushing's syndrome should result in normal circulating levels of adrenal androgens.

Women with gynecologic conditions requiring treatment with drugs that have androgenic properties should be forewarned of the potential virilizing side effects. Immediate cessation should be advised. Phenytoin should not be stopped suddenly, because this could precipitate status epilepticus.

Hirsutism/virilism

- Adrenal gland
  Exclude:
  CAH
  Cushing's syndrome
  Tumors
- Ovary
  Exclude:
  PCOS
  Androgen-secreting tumors
- Iatrogenic causes
  Exogenous androgenic drugs
- Idiopathic
  Hirsutism only

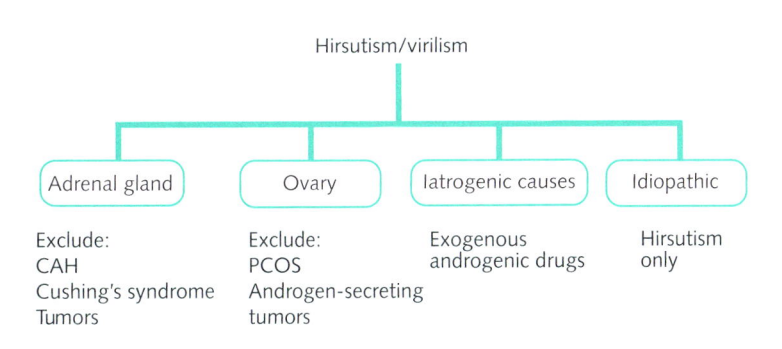

Fig. 32.5 Algorithm for hirsutism and virilism.

- What are the main causes of precocious puberty?
- Name three treatment options for women with PCOS.
- Does a normal ultrasound scan exclude PCOS?
- Is it possible for CAH to present in adult life and how?

Further reading

Hillard PA, et al. (2002) *Novak's Gynecology*, 13th ed. (Lippincott Williams & Wilkins, Philadelphia).

Speroff L, et al. (2005) *Clinical Gynecologic Endocrinology and Infertility*, 7th ed. (Lippincott Williams & Wilkins, Phildelphia).

33. Prenatal Diagnosis

Diagnosis of an ever-expanding number of conditions can now be made prior to birth. This allows for optimal preparation for the birth of an affected baby, including the place and mode of delivery (a tertiary care center rather than a community hospital might be appropriate) and the involvement of neonatal or pediatric surgical teams, if necessary. The parents can be psychologically prepared for any intervention and can be put in touch with appropriate support groups. In some cases, once fully counseled, the parents might decide to terminate the pregnancy.

Prenatal diagnosis is not just about invasive procedures, which are detailed below. Ultrasound alone is used to diagnose many structural abnormalities, such as spina bifida and heart defects. Once structural anomalies have been diagnosed, the suspicion that the fetus might have an underlying chromosomal abnormality could arise and the parents would then be offered genetic testing.

Who is offered prenatal diagnosis?

- Women who have a family history of a disorder.
- Women who have had a previous pregnancy/baby affected by a disorder.
- Women whose babies are at increased risk of chromosomal disorders, as suggested by the maternal age alone, the result of serum screening ("triple" or "quad" test), or nuchal translucency scanning.
- Women who have a "routine" ultrasound scan that reveals an abnormality.
- Women who have acquired an infection in pregnancy and there is any doubt as to whether the fetus is also infected.

Some of the most common conditions suitable for prenatal diagnosis are listed in Fig. 33.1.

Techniques for prenatal diagnosis

Ultrasound

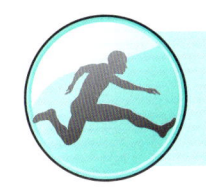

> Every ultrasound should be considered to be an opportunity for prenatal diagnosis.

Most centers advocate performing scans to examine the fetal anatomy in detail between 18 and 22 weeks. However, many women now have routine scans much earlier in pregnancy: dating scans take place at 7–12 weeks' gestation and those for nuchal translucency at 10–14 weeks (Fig. 33.2); basic anatomy can be checked at this stage, and some abnormalities will be apparent.

Amniocentesis

> Amniocentesis has a 0.5% risk of miscarriage. Careful counseling prior to diagnostic procedures is vital; the risk of the baby being affected should always be weighed against the risk of miscarriage caused by the procedure.

Transabdominal aspiration of amniotic fluid from around the fetus under continuous ultrasound guidance allows fetal cells (amniocytes) to be separated from the amniotic fluid and cultured to determine their genetic makeup (Fig. 33.3). Amniocytes can also be analyzed for the absence of certain enzymes to diagnose the presence of fetal

Prenatal Diagnosis

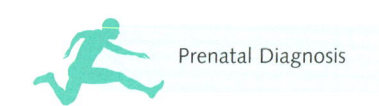

	Conditions suitable for prenatal diagnosis
Type of disorder/abnormality	Description
Chromosomal disorders	Trisomies, e.g. Down syndrome (trisomy 21), Edwards' syndrome (trisomy 18) and Patau's syndrome (trisomy 13)
	Triploidies
	Sex chromosome anomalies, e.g. Turner's syndrome (XO), Klinefelter's syndrome (XYY) X-linked disorders, e.g. Duchenne muscular dystrophy, hemophilia, fragile X
	Autosomal disorders, e.g. Huntington's disease, cystic fibrosis, thalassemia, sickle-cell disease, Tay–Sachs disease, spinal muscular atrophy
Structural abnormalities	Neural tube defects, e.g. spina bifida or anencephaly
	Congenital heart defects
	Renal tract anomalies
	Skeletal dysplasias
Metabolic	CAH
Fetal infection	Toxoplasmosis
	Rubella
	Parvovirus
	Listeria
Fetal anemia	Fetal parvovirus infection
	Rhesus hemolytic disease

Fig. 33.1 Conditions suitable for prenatal diagnosis.

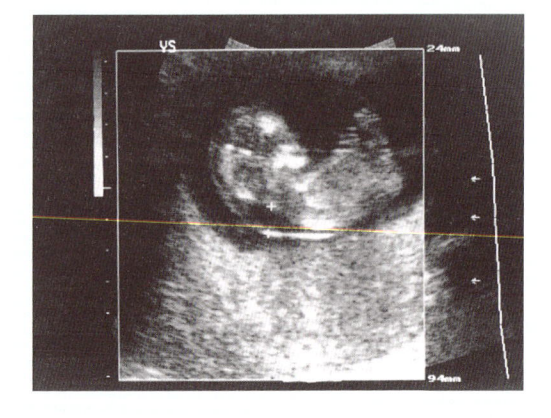

Fig. 33.2 Ultrasound scan showing increased nuchal thickness. Reproduced with kind permission from *High Risk Pregnancy* (2nd ed.), published by WB Saunders.

inborn errors of metabolism or can be examined to diagnose infection, such as toxoplasmosis.

Amniocentesis is performed after 15 weeks, ideally at around 16 weeks. Prior to this there are insufficient viable amniocytes within the fluid. Results of cell culture to determine karyotype or to look for specific gene anomalies can take around 2 weeks. With more expensive equipment the culture time can be reduced to 6 days, but the national average is around 11 days. In around 1% of cases the cells will fail to culture.

Faster results (within 24–72 h) can be obtained by using fluorescent in situ hybridization (FISH) or polymerase chain reaction (PCR). These techniques give patients a "preliminary" result, which is confirmed by culture, although many patients now make decisions regarding the future of the pregnancy on the basis of the preliminary result.

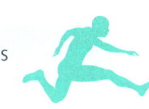

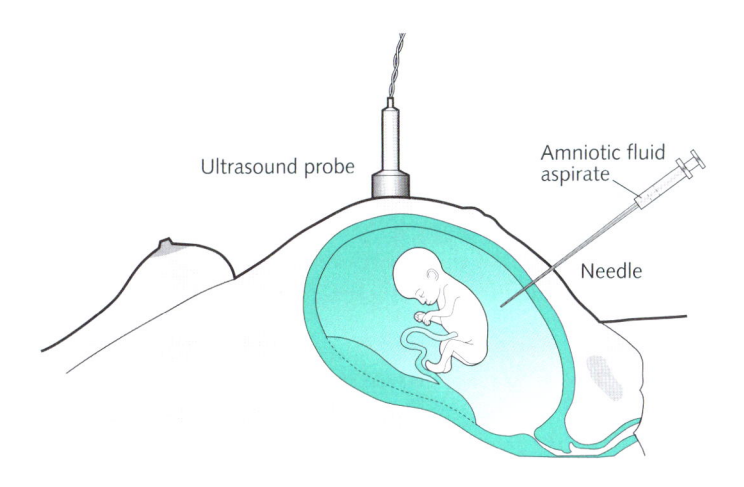

Fig. 33.3 Amniocentesis.

Because amniocentesis causes trauma to the uterus, with a risk of fetomaternal hemorrhage, anti-D is given to rhesus-negative women.

Chorionic villus sampling

> CVS can be performed earlier in pregnancy than amniocentesis, so it gives the parents the option of earlier termination. However, it carries a higher risk of miscarriage of 1%.

CVS allows biopsy of chorionic villi under continuous ultrasound guidance to obtain a sample of cells that is examined to determine genetic makeup. It is performed from 11 to 14 weeks and has a 1% risk of miscarriage. It can be performed transabdominally or transcervically (Fig. 33.4), depending on the preference of the operator. Some operators will always use the transcervical route with low-lying placenta. Like amniocentesis, it causes trauma to the uterus, so anti-D is given to rhesus negative women.

Results can be obtained more quickly from CVS samples, without resorting to FISH or PCR, because the mass of DNA obtained is greater than that from amniocentesis. "Direct" CVS results (in which a karyotype is determined without waiting for cell culture) are available within 3 days, although a complete result from culture is still considered the gold standard. However, FISH and PCR can still be used to reduce the result time to a minimum.

CVS has a false-positive rate of 1%, which is higher than amniocentesis, due to the mosaicism of chorionic villi, which might show an abnormal karyotype when the fetus is normal. It also has a false-negative rate of 0.1%, related to contamination with maternal cells.

Fetal blood sampling

This is carried out by transabdominal needle aspiration of blood from the fetal hepatic vein or the umbilical cord (when the procedure is known as cordocentesis) under continuous ultrasound guidance. Conditions that can be diagnosed include:
- Chromosomal anomalies: if abnormalities are suspected later in pregnancy (because of ultrasound findings or early onset growth retardation) then this method might be preferable to amniocentesis or CVS.
- Fetal anemia.
- Fetal thrombocytopenia, e.g. where the mother has autoimmune thrombocytopenia.
- Fetal infection, using fetal IgM as a measure of immune response.

Prenatal Diagnosis

Fetal blood sampling can also be used for treatment of fetal conditions, e.g. to give transfusions, but this application is not considered in this chapter.

The complications include bleeding from the needling site (which can be fatal for the fetus), fetal bradycardia as a reaction to vasospasm of the umbilical artery, chorioamnionitis, and rupture of the membranes.

Like the procedures above, it causes trauma to the uterus, so rhesus-negative women are given anti-D.

Pre-implantation genetic diagnosis

Pre-implantation genetic diagnosis (PGD), which is only available at a few centers at present, is performed on eight-cell embryos created by IVF. One or two cells are removed and subjected to FISH or PCR to obtain a genetic diagnosis. Normal embryos are replaced into the uterus and develop normally, despite the "insult" of having had cells removed at an early stage. Abnormal embryos are discarded.

This process is used by couples who have a high (25–50%) chance of conceiving a baby who will be affected by a genetic abnormality that would lead to the parents opting to terminate the pregnancy. It allows the parents to avoid having to choose to terminate a viable pregnancy, because only unaffected embryos are replaced.

As it can only be performed on IVF embryos, PGD carries all the risks and uncertainties associated with IVF pregnancies, i.e. the side effects of the drugs, the medical intervention, and the fact that only about 25% of embryos that are replaced into the uterus will implant.

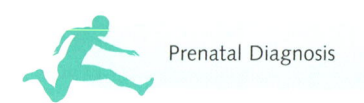

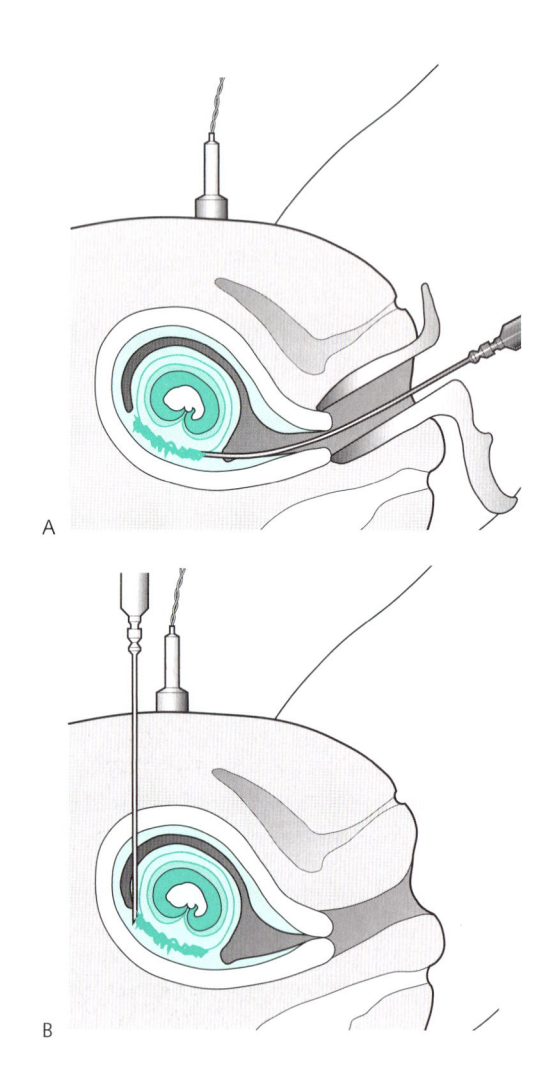

Fig. 33.4 CVS. (A) Trans-cervical. (B) Transabdominal.

- What are the three main advantages of prenatal diagnosis?
- At what gestation is nuchal translucency scanning performed?
- What are the main differences between amniocentesis and CVS?
- Which technique is used to quantify fetal platelet levels?
- Why is anti-D given after the invasive procedures described?

Further reading

Gabbe SG, et al. (2002) Obstetrics: *Normal and Problem Pregnancies*, 4th ed. (Churchill Livingstone, New York).

34. Multiple Pregnancy

A multiple pregnancy is one in which two or more fetuses are present, that is, it is not a singleton pregnancy.

Multiple pregnancies are important to the obstetrician because they represent a high-risk pregnancy. The risk of all pregnancy complications is greater than in a singleton pregnancy, including preterm labor and IUGR. Perinatal mortality for a multiple pregnancy is about five times greater than that of a singleton.

- A multiple pegnancy is a high-risk pregnancy.
- Perinatal mortality rate is increased four to five times compared with a single fetus, mainly due to the risk of preterm labor.

Incidence of multiple pregnancy

The most common type of multiple pregnancy is a twin pregnancy, with an incidence of 1 in 80 pregnancies. The incidence of spontaneous triplets is 1 in 100,000. The incidence of any multiple pregnancy increases with increasing maternal age. There has also been a rise over the last 2 decades, especially in Western countries, due to the increasing use of assisted conception techniques.

There is an ethnic variation in the frequency of multiple pregnancy (Fig. 34.1).

Diagnosis of multiple pregnancy

Nowadays, multiple pregnancies are normally diagnosed by routine dating ultrasound scan at 12–14 weeks' gestation. The diagnosis should be excluded in a patient who presents with hyperemesis gravidarum. Clinical examination of the patient will reveal a large-for-dates uterus or the clinician will be able to palpate multiple fetal parts in later pregnancy (Fig. 34.2).

Etiology of multiple pregnancy

Twins
The majority of twins (75%) are dizygotic, i.e. they arise from the fertilization (by two sperm) of two ova; monozygotic twins (25%) arise following the fertilization of a single ovum that then completely divides, so that each twin has the same genetic makeup.

However, rather than knowing the zygosity of a multiple pregnancy, the clinically important issue is the chorionicity of the pregnancy. This relates to the placentation of the pregnancy. If the placentas are separate, with separate amnions and chorions (dichorionic diamniotic twins), then the blood supply to each fetus during the pregnancy is independent.

Conversely, if there are blood vessel anastomoses between the placentas (monochorionic diamniotic twins or monochorionic monoamniotic twins), then there is a risk of uneven distribution of blood. This results in discordant growth, with one twin showing signs of growth restriction and the other getting larger (see the section "Twin-to-twin transfusion syndrome"). Thus, diagnosing chorionicity determines the level of surveillance necessary in that particular pregnancy.

Dizygotic twins
Two ova from the same or different ovaries are released simultaneously and fertilized by two separate spermatozoa. Therefore, each fetus has its own chorion, amnion and placenta—dichorionic diamniotic placentation. If implantation occurs close together, then the placentas can become fused. Subsequently, the twins can be of the same or different sexes and have different genetic constitutions, i.e. they have no more similarities than any other brother and sister.

The incidence of dizygotic twins varies widely between different populations, probably for

Ethnic variation in the frequency of twin pregnancies			
Country	Monozygotic	Dizygotic	Total
Nigeria	5.0	50	55
England and Wales	3.5	9.0	12.5
Japan	3.0	1.5	4.5
US	3.0	31.1	34

Fig. 34.1 Ethnic variation in the frequency of twin pregnancies shown as twinning rates per 1000 pregnancies. An increase in the rate of dizygotic twins in the US is due to both increased maternal age at birth and increased use of fertility drugs and assisted reproductive technologies.

Presentation of twin pregnancies at term	
Presentation	Percentage of pregnancies
Twin 1 cephalic/twin 2 cephalic	45
Twin 1 cephalic/twin 2 breech	37
Twin 1 breech/twin 2 breech	10
Other presentations including transverse	8

Fig. 34.2 Presentation of twin pregnancies at term.

multifactorial reasons, such as genetic and nutritional factors. It also increases with increasing maternal age and increasing parity.

Monozygotic twins

A single ovum is fertilized by a single sperm and subsequently the zygote divides into two at various stages of embryonic development. This gives rise to different structural arrangements of the membranes (Fig. 34.3).

About two-thirds of monozygotic twins have monochorionic diamniotic placentation, i.e. a single blastocyst implants, developing a single chorion; the inner cell mass divides into two, so that each embryo has its own amnion.

A third of monozygotic twins establish at an earlier stage than this, at the eight-cell stage, so that two separate blastocysts form and implant; such twins will thus have dichorionic diamniotic placentation.

The least common origin of monozygotic twins occurs by later splitting of the inner cell mass, before the appearance of the primitive streak, to produce a single amniotic cavity—monochorionic monoamniotic twins. Splitting even later than this causes conjoint twins to develop.

The incidence of monozygotic twins is constant around the world, at about 4 per 1000 births.

Triplets

Pregnancies of higher order multiples (i.e. three or more fetuses) are less commonly formed by separate ova. In the case of a triplet pregnancy, there are usually two ova, one of which splits as described above for monochorionic twins.

In such a pregnancy, and especially one of higher order, it is appropriate to counsel the parents about selective fetal reduction. The chorionicity of the pregnancy must be known to select the appropriate fetus. The procedure cannot be performed on a monochorionic twin because it shares placental circulation with its co-twin and, therefore, the drugs would affect both fetuses.

Diagnosis of chorionicity
Antenatally

Ultrasound assessment of the membrane dividing the amniotic sacs diagnoses the chorionicity; this is done before 16 weeks' gestation. Figure 34.4 shows the thicker insertion of the membrane, known as the lambda sign, that is found in a dichorionic pregnancy and the thinner T sign of a monochorionic pregnancy. If there is no dividing membrane between the fetuses, then they share the placental blood flow and are monochorionic monoamniotic twins.

Fetal sex can also be assessed by ultrasound. If they are different, then the pregnancy must be dichorionic. Localization of the placental sites is also important. If the placentas can be seen completely separately, then, again, the pregnancy must be dichorionic.

Postnatally
At this stage, chorionicity can be determined by:
- Macroscopic and microscopic examination of membranes.
- Analysis of red-blood-cell markers.
- DNA probes.

Etiology of multiple pregnancy

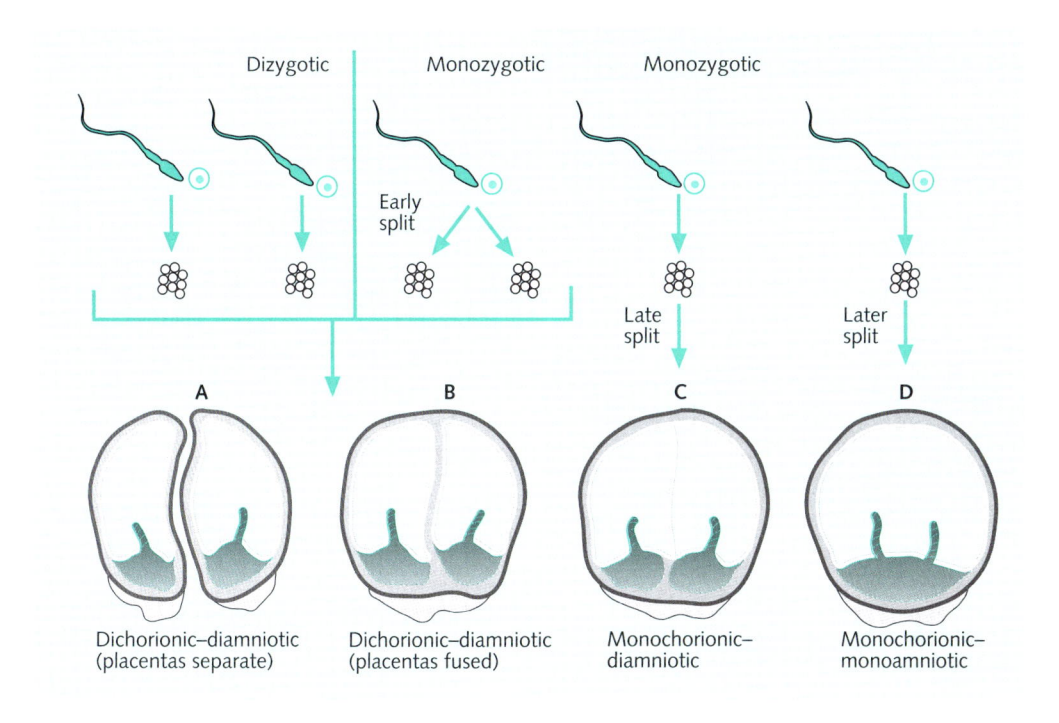

Fig. 34.3 Dizygotic and monozygotic twinning.

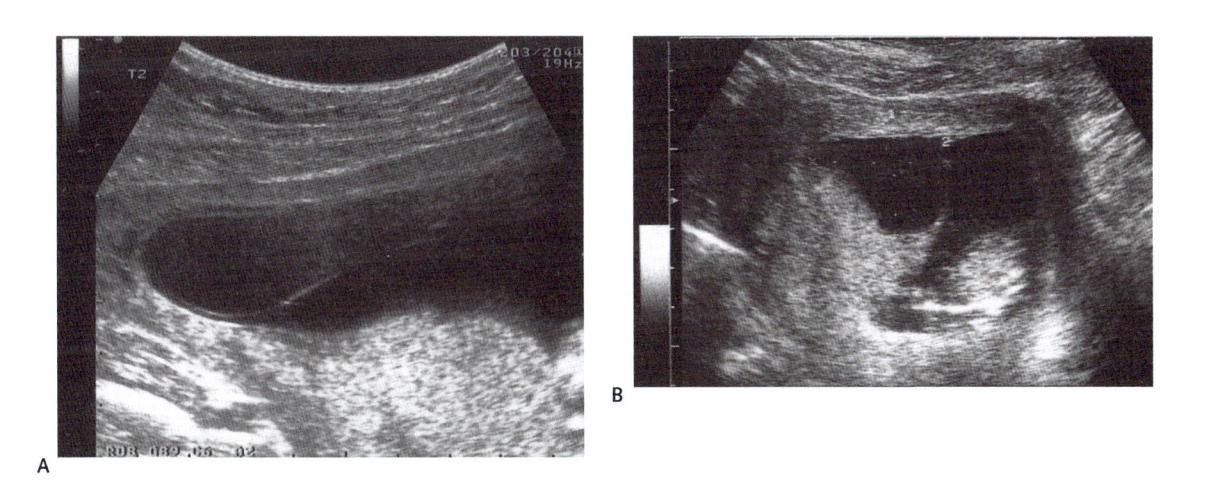

Fig. 34.4 Diagnosis of chorionicity. (A) The T sign is indicative of monochorionic diamniotic pregnancy. (B) The lambda sign is indicative of dichorionic diamniotic pregnancy.

185

Complications of multiple pregnancy

A multiple pregnancy must be treated as a high-risk pregnancy. The majority of pregnancy-related complications are more common in multiple pregnancies; there are also certain problems that are specific to multiple pregnancies.

> The mother is at risk of any complication associated with a singleton pregnancy, but the risks are increased.

> The psychologic sequelae of a multiple pregnancy on the mother and her family, including existing children, should not be underestimated.

Fetal malformations
The frequency of fetal malformations is thought to be almost double in a twin pregnancy compared with a singleton pregnancy, especially for monochorionic twins. In terms of screening for chromosomal anomalies (see Chapter 33), parents must be counseled about the possibility of a greater risk of pregnancy loss than in a singleton pregnancy with an invasive procedure. Separate sampling must be performed with dichorionic twins. There is also the potential dilemma of finding an abnormality in only one fetus; selective fetocide can result in the loss of the apparently normal fetus as well as the abnormal one.

Antenatal assessment of fetal well-being and growth
In a high-risk pregnancy, antenatal care should be more frequent, managed by a perinatologist in a unit with facilities for regular ultrasound scans to check fetal growth and neonatal care facilities in case of preterm labor and delivery.

In a multiple pregnancy, serial ultrasounds every 2 to 4 weeks are necessary to exclude IUGR. This is especially important in pregnancies with monochorionic placentation, which are at greater risk of discordant growth between the two fetuses and TTTS (see below).

Preterm labor
Spontaneous preterm labor occurs in 30% of twin pregnancies (Fig. 34.5). The use of tocolytics (see Chapter 38) might be considered to allow in utero transfer to a hospital with neonatal intensive care facilities and to allow time for steroids administered to the mother to improve lung maturation.

Pregnancy-induced hypertension
Hypertension is about three times more common in multiple pregnancies than in singleton pregnancies because of the larger size of the placental bed (see Chapter 35). It often develops earlier and is more severe.

Antepartum hemorrhage
The incidence of placental abruption and placenta previa can be increased in multiple pregnancies. In addition, multiple pregnancies are at increased risk of PPH due to increased uterine distention and atony after delivery.

Twin-to-twin transfusion syndrome
This occurs in 5–15% of monochorionic twin pregnancies: blood is shunted across placental vascular anastomoses from twin to twin, such that the donor becomes anemic and growth restricted, with oligohydramnios, and the recipient becomes plethoric with polyhydramnios. This syndrome

Multiple pregnancies	
Number of fetuses	Mean gestation (days)
1	280
2	245
3	231
4	203

Fig. 34.5 Mean gestations for multiple pregnancies.

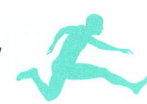

usually occurs in the second trimester and results in fetal death in up to 80% of cases.

Treatment of this condition is still under discussion. Some facilities have performed amnioreduction (i.e. taking off some of the excess fluid under ultrasound guidance to reduce the stretching of the uterus and, therefore, the risk of preterm labor). Other groups advocate laser treatment to the placental anastomoses to reduce the discordant blood flow between the fetuses.

With monochorionic placentation, fetal death of a twin in utero puts the surviving twin at risk of neurological damage and the mother at risk of developing DIC, as thromboplastins are released into the circulation. The pregnancy can usually be managed conservatively until the surviving twin reaches a gestation with improved likelihood of survival; 80% of surviving twins can be delivered vaginally.

Intrapartum management of a twin pregnancy

Figure 34.6 provides a summary of the management of a vaginal delivery in a twin pregnancy.

Delivery of twin pregnancy
Delivery of multiple pregnancies should be managed in a unit with neonatal intensive care facilities. For a twin pregnancy, the mode of delivery depends on the presentation of the first twin; if it is anything other than cephalic, cesarean section is usually the method of choice. In the case of higher order multiple pregnancies, delivery is almost always by cesarean section.

In a twin pregnancy, if the first twin presents as cephalic and there are no other complications, then a vaginal delivery is usually planned. The onset of labor can be spontaneous or induced; induction might be advised for similar reasons to a singleton pregnancy (e.g. post dates) or for an indication more specific to a twin pregnancy, such as IUGR. The woman needs intravenous access and a sample of serum saved in the blood bank because of the risk of PPH (see below). An epidural block is often recommended to allow later manipulation of twin two (see below).

Both FHRs should be monitored continuously, either both per abdomen or with a fetal scalp electrode on the first twin. If there is an abnormality in the heart rate pattern of twin one, then FBS might be appropriate (see Chapter 16). A problem with twin two should lead to immediate delivery by cesarean section. The reasons for augmentation of labor and for instrumental delivery of twin one are similar to those in a singleton pregnancy (see Chapter 41).

Once the first twin is delivered, the lie and presentation of the second twin must be determined by abdominal palpation and ultrasound. External cephalic version (ECV) can be used to establish a longitudinal lie. Intravenous oxytocin might be necessary to maintain uterine contractions, and the delivery of the second twin occurs either as a cephalic presentation or by breech extraction; again, the reasons for instrumental delivery or cesarean section are similar to those of a singleton pregnancy.

Complications
Postpartum hemorrhage
PPH (see Chapter 42) is more likely with a multiple pregnancy than a singleton because of the larger placental site. Uterine atony due to the increased volume of the uterine contents (two fetuses, two placentas, etc.) is a contributing factor. Active management of the third stage of labor is therefore appropriate; further treatment might include routine use of a postpartum oxytocin infusion.

The intrapartum management of twin pregnancy

- Neonatal intensive care unit facilities
- Allow vaginal delivery if normal pregnancy and twin one cephalic presentation
- Intravenous access/CBC/T&S
- Continuous FHR monitoring and/or fetal scalp electrode to twin one
- Intravenous oxytocin infusion to start after delivery of twin one to maintain contractions
- Intravenous oxytocin infusion for third stage to reduce risk of PPH

Fig. 34.6 The intrapartum management of twin pregnancy.

Locked twins
This is a very rare complication of vaginal deliveries. The delivery proceeds with the first twin presenting as a breech but the aftercoming head of the first twin is prevented from entering the pelvis by the head of the cephalic-presenting second twin. If this is diagnosed in the first stage of labor, then a cesarean section should be performed; during the second stage, general anesthesia is necessary to allow manipulation.

Higher order multiple pregnancies

In comparison with twin pregnancies, higher order multiples are associated with a higher perinatal mortality rate and an increased incidence of the antenatal complications mentioned above. Fertility treatments have increased the numbers of high-order pregnancies and, in the case of IVF, guidelines in the US now advise that a maximum of two to three embryos should be replaced (see Chapter 28).

Selective fetocide (fetal reduction)
Selective fetocide is a technique in which intracardial or pericardial potassium chloride is given to one or more fetuses in a high-order multiple pregnancy to improve the outcome of the remaining fetuses. Despite the procedure-related risk of miscarriage, the incidence of complications is low and improvements are seen in terms of reduction in rates of miscarriage and preterm labor. However, ethical dilemmas arise with respect to abortion in general, as well as possible miscarriage of the entire pregnancy.

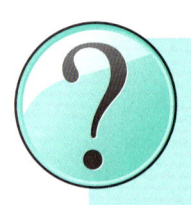

- How is chorionicity diagnosed?
- Why is chorionicity important in the management of a twin pregnancy?
- What are the potential complications of a twin pregnancy?
- Discuss the intrapartum management of a twin pregnancy.
- What are the potential advantages and disadvantages of selective fetal reduction?

Further reading
Creasy RK, et al. (2003) *Maternal-Fetal Medicine: Principles and Practice*, 5th ed. (WB Saunders, Philadelphia).

Gabbe SG, et al. (2002) *Obstetrics: Normal and Problem Pregnancies*, 4th ed. (Churchill Livingstone, New York).

35. Hypertension in Pregnancy

Hypertension can predate the pregnancy or might have been induced by the pregnancy. In some cases, hypertension is part of the syndrome of pre-eclampsia. Hypertensive disorders of pregnancy affect around 1 in 10 pregnancies.

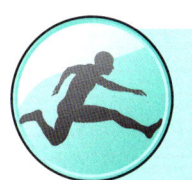

> Owing to the physiological changes seen in pregnancy, blood pressure falls in the first and second trimesters, reaching its lowest at around 23 weeks. From then on the blood pressure rises again until it has reached prepregnancy levels at term.

Nonproteinuric hypertension in pregnancy

Hypertension diagnosed prior to or early in pregnancy

This group includes known hypertensives and those whose hypertension is diagnosed in the first trimester, when the high blood pressure cannot be thought to be due to the pregnancy and was almost certainly present prior to pregnancy, but never measured. The risk factors for pre-existing hypertension are:
- Increasing maternal age.
- A family history.
- Medical disorders (e.g. diabetes, renal disease).
- Certain ethnic groups, including those of Asian, African–American, and South Pacific island origin.
- Obesity

Hypertension in a young woman not known to have any medical problems should be investigated to exclude the more unusual causes of hypertension: coarctation of the aorta, renal artery stenosis, Conn's syndrome, Cushing's syndrome, and pheochromocytoma.

Pregnancy-induced hypertension

Nonproteinuric hypertension that occurs in the second half of pregnancy can be thought of as a separate entity to essential hypertension and pre-eclampsia, but it is closely linked with both. Typically, it resolves within 6 weeks of delivery. The clinical sequelae are the same as those seen with essential hypertension and the management has the same aims.

Effects of nonproteinuric hypertension in pregnancy

The risks are threefold:
- Maternal health: above MAP levels of 125 mmHg there is a risk of cerebral hemorrhage.
- Fetal health: pregnancies affected by essential hypertension are more susceptible to IUGR
- High risk of developing pre-eclampsia.

Management of essential hypertension and pregnancy-induced hypertension

Women known to be hypertensive prior to pregnancy should ideally receive preconception counseling, with advice about diet, weight, and exercise to maximize control. If necessary, her antihypertensive medication can be changed to drugs that are considered safe in the first trimester. If hypertension is first diagnosed in early pregnancy, then an underlying cause should be sought (see Chapter 13).

As the risk of developing pre-eclampsia will be higher than for a normotensive woman, it is important that the patient knows the symptoms and signs to look out for, and to report them to her midwife or doctor. Some studies have shown value in Doppler scanning at 26 weeks' gestation to look for changes in vessels that are said to predict pre-eclampsia. However, as there is no treatment to prevent the development of pre-eclampsia, predicting it might not be helpful.

Low-dose aspirin can reduce the risk of an "at-risk" woman from developing severe pre-eclampsia early in pregnancy (before 32 weeks), but it must be started at around 12 weeks' gestation. Drug treatment that lowers blood pressure (see below) cannot prevent the development of pre-eclampsia, but it can reduce the risk of cerebral hemorrhage. Mother and fetus are closely observed with blood pressure and urinalysis checks and regular scans to monitor fetal growth.

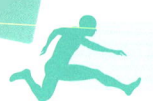

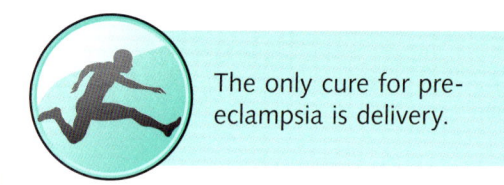

> The only cure for pre-eclampsia is delivery.

Pre-eclampsia

The risk factors for developing pre-eclampsia are:
- Primiparous.
- Age >35 or <18.
- Essential hypertension.
- Multiple pregnancy.
- Previous pregnancy affected by pre-eclampsia.
- Family history (e.g. patient's mother or sister, with the strongest link being if the patient's sister had pre-eclampsia).

> The recurrence rate of pre-eclampsia is around 10%, but is higher if there is another medical problem contributing to the hypertension or if the next pregnancy is with a new partner.

Pathology

Pre-eclampsia is a multisystem disorder affecting different organs throughout the body. The underlying pathology relates to blood vessels and the chemicals that control them; women with pre-eclampsia have abnormal vessel responses to pregnancy. In normal pregnancy the peripheral resistance falls; in pre-eclampsia the drop in peripheral resistance is not as marked. Compared with a normal pregnancy, the woman has increased sensitivity to pressor agents, reduced prostacyclin (a vasodilator) levels, and increased thromboxane (a vasoconstrictor) levels. There is relative hemoconcentration due to less of the normal expansion in blood volume. The end-organ effects are shown in Fig. 35.1.

The symptoms and investigation of high blood pressure are detailed in Chapter 13.

Management of pre-eclampsia

Treating high blood pressure in pre-eclampsia is important for the same reasons as with essential hypertension, i.e. to prevent intracerebral bleeds and to protect fetal health. However, treatment will not alter the course of the disease; the only treatment for pre-eclampsia is to end the pregnancy, i.e. to deliver the baby. If the pregnancy has reached term and the cervix is favorable, then induction of labor is sensible. If the cervix is not ripe and the pre-eclampsia is not severe, then it would be necessary to ripen the cervix with a ripening agent such as prostaglandin or misoprostil. Magnesium sulfate is also usually started to prevent the progression to eclampsia (discussed further in this chapter).

In labor, continuous monitoring is wise because the fetus will be more prone to distress and because treatment for high blood pressure can cause sudden hypotension, resulting in abruption and fetal compromise. Fluid restriction should be exercised if the mother has severe pre-eclampsia. Blood pressure can be controlled with intravenous hydralazine or labetalol, or intermittent doses of nifedipine.

When pre-eclampsia occurs preterm (before 37 weeks' gestation), decisions about induction and delivery are more difficult. Bearing in mind the problems encountered by premature babies, it might be prudent to wait, monitor the condition of mother and baby, and try to achieve fetal maturity. In severe pre-eclampsia, however, the benefit of remaining in utero will not be great, as compromised placental perfusion will result in little, if any, fetal growth.

Pre-eclampsia can be described as "fulminating", i.e. severe and of rapid onset. In these cases, delivery is more likely to be by cesarean section, unless the woman is already in labor and is progressing rapidly. The classification of severity of pre-eclampsia depends on a combination of signs and symptoms (Fig. 35.2).

Eclampsia

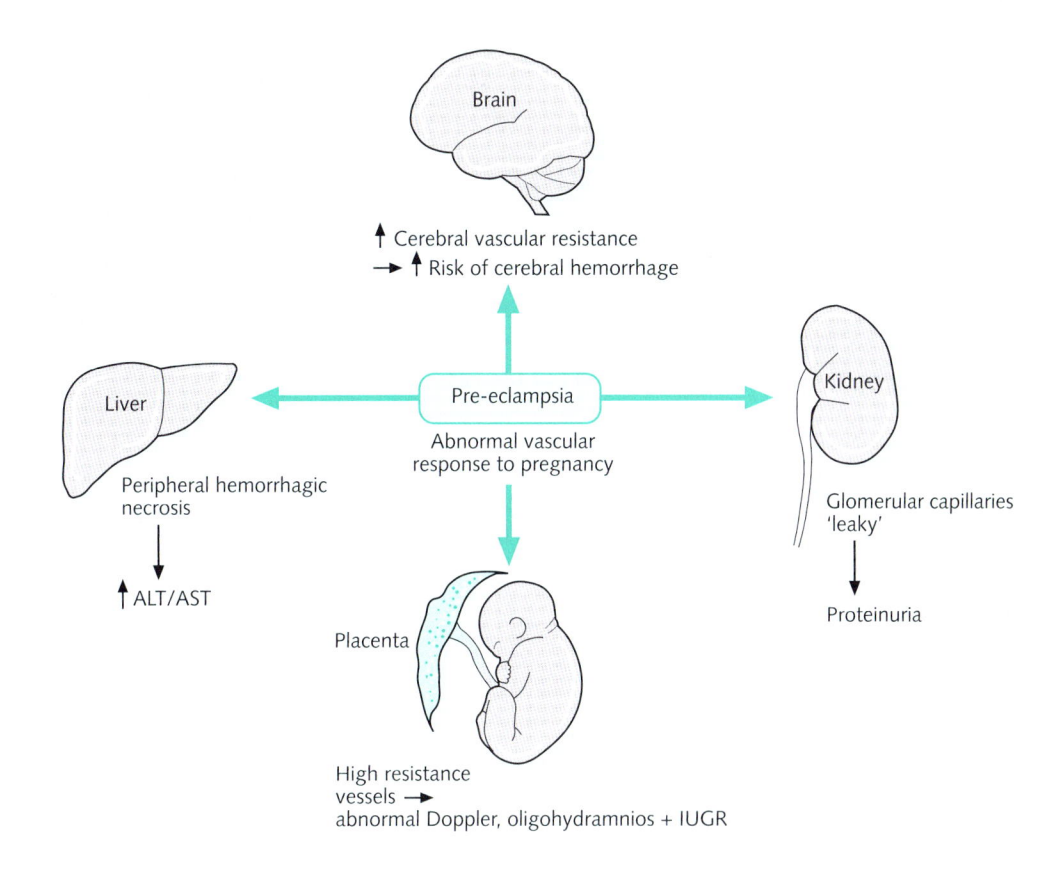

Fig. 35.1 End-organ effects of pre-eclampsia.

The criteria needed to diagnose severe pre-eclampsia

- BP ≥ 160/110 mmHg on two readings 6 h apart and proteinuria 3+ or more.
- BP > 140/90 mmHg and proteinuria 1+ and at least one of the following:
  - Oliguria: urine output <400–500 mL in 24 h
  - Visual disturbance/headache/right upper quadrant pain
  - Platelets <100, ALT >50 (i.e. evidence of HELLP syndrome)
  - Uteroplacental insufficiency/IUGR

Fig. 35.2 The criteria needed to diagnose severe pre-eclampsia.

Complications of pre-eclampsia

The fetal and maternal effects of pre-eclampsia are reduced by careful control of the blood pressure and good fluid management, but these measures will not necessarily prevent complications. These are:
- Eclampsia.
- Renal failure.
- Hepatic rupture.
- HELLP.
- Cerebral hemorrhage.
- DIC.
- Pulmonary edema.
- Increased perinatal mortality and morbidity due to increased preterm delivery, uteroplacental insufficiency and abruption (particularly in HELLP and severe pre-eclampsia).

Eclampsia

Eclampsia is defined as seizures secondary to pre-eclampsia. The appearance is the same as a grand mal epileptic seizure. It can occur in women who have previously been completely well through pregnancy, in whom there has been no suspicion of pre-eclampsia. Eclampsia affects 1 in 1600 pregnancies. Around 40% of eclamptic seizures happen postnatally, but usually within 48 h of delivery. The mortality rate is between 0.5 and 5.5%. The differential diagnosis includes epilepsy, meningitis, cerebral thrombosis, and intracerebral bleed.

Complications of eclampsia

As in severe pre-eclampsia, these are both fetal and maternal:
- Abruption (which can lead to fetal death and DIC).
- Pulmonary edema.
- Cerebral hemorrhage.
- Liver rupture.
- Retinal detachment.
- Death.

Management of eclampsia

- The first priority is to assess the ABCs of resuscitation. The airway should be secured and ventilation provided if necessary.
- Next, the convulsions must be addressed. Magnesium sulfate is given as an intravenous bolus followed by an infusion to reduce the risk of further seizures. If the initial seizure continues, then intravenous diazepam is used.
- The blood pressure can be controlled using an intravenous hydralazine infusion.
- If this occurs in the antenatal period, then delivery is achieved once the mother is stable.
- Close observation is needed for 24 h after the seizure, including regular assessment of reflexes while on magnesium (see below) and strict fluid restriction of 125 mL/h.

Drug therapy for hypertensive disorders of pregnancy

- Methyldopa has been used for a long time with no risks to the fetus. Side effects for the mother include lethargy and diarrhea. Postnatally, if antihypertensives are still required, methyldopa is no longer the drug of choice because depression is a possible side effect.
- Beta-blockers such as labetalol are also used in tablet form and as an infusion (for rapid control of severe hypertension), although in one small study it was shown that they might cause fetal growth retardation. They are contraindicated in asthmatics.
- Calcium antagonists (e.g. nifedipine) are added if a single therapy has failed to control the blood pressure. The side effects are headaches and flushing.
- Angiotensin-converting enzyme inhibitors are contraindicated in pregnancy, as they can cause fetal renal failure.
- Hydralazine is used as an intravenous infusion to control severe blood pressure. It causes vasodilation and can, therefore, cause headaches and flushing.
- Magnesium sulfate is used as an intravenous infusion for the prevention of further seizures after an eclamptic seizure. It has been suggested, but not proven, that it is useful for prophylaxis in women with severe pre-eclampsia who seem at high risk of eclampsia. Magnesium toxicity can cause neuromuscular blockade, resulting in cardiopulmonary arrest, so careful monitoring of respiratory rate, tendon reflexes, and symptoms of double vision/slurred speech is important.

It is often necessary to continue antihypertensive medication postnatally. All the drugs listed above are safe in breast-feeding. If the woman is a known hypertensive on treatment then she can return to her prepregnancy medication.

Eclampsia

- How common is hypertension in pregnancy?
- At what level of blood pressure does the risk of cerebral hemorrhage become much higher?
- Why is ultrasound monitoring of the fetus important in pregnancies affected by hypertension?
- Which family of antihypertensive drugs are contraindicated in pregnancy?
- Can any measures be taken to reduce the risk of pre-eclampsia in subsequent pregnancies?

Further reading

Creasy RK, et al. (2003) *Maternal-Fetal Medicine: Principles and Practice*, 5th ed. (WB Saunders, Philadelphia).

Gabbe SG, et al. (2002) *Obstetrics: Normal and Problem Pregnancies*, 4th ed. (Churchill Livingston, New York).

36. Medical Disorders in Pregnancy

Anemia

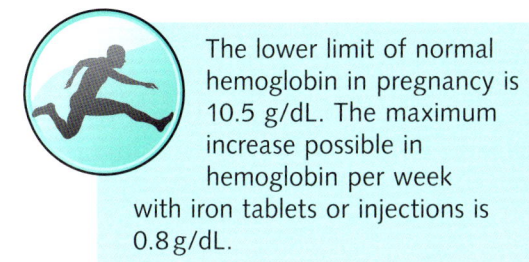

> The lower limit of normal hemoglobin in pregnancy is 10.5 g/dL. The maximum increase possible in hemoglobin per week with iron tablets or injections is 0.8 g/dL.

Plasma expansion in pregnancy results in a physiological reduction in hemoglobin concentration. The body's handling of iron and folate changes (Fig. 36.1). However, owing to the demands of the developing fetus, and in some cases aggravated by pre-existing anemia, women can become anemic in pregnancy.

The symptoms of anemia, i.e. fatigue, dizziness, fainting, are also common symptoms of pregnancy. Anemia is proven by a CBC looking at hemoglobin concentration and red cell indices.

It should not be assumed that anemia is due to lack of iron. Renal clearance of folate doubles in pregnancy, making women prone to deficiency. Measuring serum iron, ferritin, folate, and red cell folate will help to determine whether the anemia is due to deficiency of iron, folate, or both (Fig. 36. 2).

Many doctors believe that prevention is better than cure and that the disadvantages of the side effects of iron and folate tablets are outweighed by the advantages that can be conferred by taking supplements routinely in pregnancy, thus avoiding the symptoms of anemia and need for transfusions.

> Iron absorption is aided by vitamin C (so taking the tablets with orange juice helps) but impaired by caffeine (so tablets should not be taken with tea, coffee, or cola).

Asthma

This affects at least 3% of women of childbearing age and can improve, deteriorate, or stay the same during pregnancy. Peak flow and FEV_1 are unaffected by pregnancy, so remain the mainstay of monitoring asthma.

The main problem arises from women being worried to use their inhalers or to take oral steroids for fear of the possible harmful effect on the fetus. They can be entirely reassured, as the doses of drugs and the types of drug used are completely safe. The main danger to the fetus is if the woman suffers repeated severe attacks, so she should be encouraged to manage her asthma well.

Attacks in labor are very rare, but the woman should bring her inhalers with her to labor and delivery. If she has been on high doses of oral or intravenous steroids, she should be covered with stress dose steroids during labor.

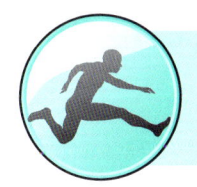

> Asthma attacks in labor are rare.

Breastfeeding while using inhalers or oral steroids is safe and might reduce the risk of the baby developing asthma in later life.

Diabetes

This section covers women with pre-existing diabetes, those with gestational diabetes, and the effect of these conditions on the fetus.

In normal pregnancy the woman becomes more resistant to her own body's insulin, partly due to the "anti-insulin" hormones (human placental lactogen, glucagons, and cortisol) secreted by the placenta. At the same time, glucose handling changes and the body loses its ability to regulate glucose levels smoothly, leading to lower fasting levels and higher postprandial levels than when not pregnant. These effects increase through the second and third trimesters.

The renal threshold for glucose also changes, so that most women will have glycosuria on urinalysis at some time in pregnancy. To cope with these changes, a pregnant woman will have doubled her insulin production by the end of pregnancy.

Pre-existing diabetes

The normal state explains some of the ways that pregnancy affects women with diabetes. The main points are that they:

- Need increased doses of insulin.
- Are more likely to experience hypoglycemic attacks.
- Might experience acceleration of the complications of diabetes (e.g. nephropathy, retinopathy).
- Can develop diabetic ketoacidosis if another factor is present (e.g. hyperemesis, infection, administration of corticosteroids; see below).

Figure 36.3 shows the complications that can occur in pregnancy when there is pre-existing diabetes.

Management

Most of the complications listed above can be reduced by good control. Preconception and early pregnancy control can be assessed by measuring the HbA1c level. The management of women with diabetes in pregnancy consists of:

- Joint care with nurses, obstetricians, and endocrinologists.
- Informing the woman: explaining to the woman why good control is so vital.

"Anti-anemic" changes	"Pro-anemic" changes
↑ Production of red blood cells	↑ Plasma volumes i.e. hemodilution
↑ Iron absorption in gut	↓ Serum iron
↑ transferrin, so ↑ total iron-binding capacity	↓ Serum ferritin
	↑ Renal clearance of folate

Fig. 36.1 Anemia in pregnancy.

	Iron deficiency	Folate deficiency
Lab results	Low hemoglobin	Low hemoglobin
	Low mean cell volume	High mean cell volume
	Low serum iron	Low serum folate
	Low serum ferritin	Low red cell folate
Risk factors	Menorrhagia	Anticonvulsant therapy
	Multiple pregnancy	Thalassemia
	Recent pregnancy	
	Recent or current breast-feeding	
	Iron-deficient diet	
Treatment	Iron tablets, solution or injections (blood transfusion)	Folate tablets
Side effects of treatment	Constipation	Few
	Indigestion	
	Green/black stools	
Food sources	Liver	Soy beans
	Red meat	Walnuts
	Kidneys beans, fresh vegetables	Kidney beans, broccoli
	Fortified cereals	Fortified cereals

Fig. 36.2 Iron- vs. folate-deficiency anemia.

Diabetes

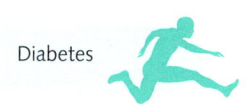

Pre-existing diabetes—complications of pregnancy	
Complication	Comment
Miscarriage	When control is poor
Intrauterine death, stillbirth	
Fetal congenital abnormality	Related to control at the time of conception: can be as low as 5% or as high as 25%
Proteinuric hypertension	Especially if there is pre-existing hypertension or nephropathy
Macrosomia (baby > 4.5 kg)	Due to fetal exposure to high levels of insulin, which is a growth-promoting hormone
Shoulder dystocia	Due to macrosomia
Polyhydramnios	Due to fetal polyuria
Candida and urinary tract infections	Due to glycosuria

Fig. 36.3 Pre-existing diabetes: complications of pregnancy.

- Dietary advice: a low-sugar, low-fat, high-fiber diet will make it easier to keep glucose levels more stable; she is likely to need to snack between meals to protect against hypoglycemia (but these can be healthy snacks!).
- Home blood-glucose monitoring and clinic HbA1c monitoring.
- Increasing insulin doses as necessary, and converting women with noninsulin-dependent diabetes to insulin.
- Fundoscopy at regular intervals to assess for retinopathy.
- Anomaly screening, in the form of a detailed anomaly scan plus fetal echocardiography.
- Scans for growth and AFI.

It is particularly important to pay attention to sugar control at times when an additional stress has been placed on the body, e.g. at times of illness, infection, or in labor, when a sliding scale or insulin drip is used for accurate control.

Corticosteroids, which might be given to the mother for the benefit of the baby when premature delivery is expected, are naturally diabetogenic and can cause high readings for a few days.

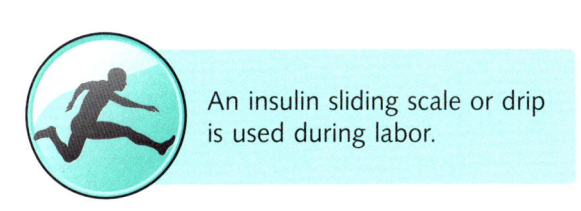

An insulin sliding scale or drip is used during labor.

Although women with diabetes are more likely to have a cesarean section, this is because of the complications listed above rather than a recommended mode of delivery. The timing of delivery relates to the control of the diabetes: if control has been good then the woman might be allowed to continue in pregnancy and to labor spontaneously, but if control has been poor, then induction of labor might be suggested to reduce the risk of intrauterine death and stillbirth after 37–38 weeks.

Postnatal considerations
The neonate is at risk of:
- Hypoglycemia.
- Respiratory distress.
- Jaundice.

It is essential to work closely with neonatology because the baby is likely to need some special care. Ongoing monitoring of the mother's glucose levels will be necessary, especially if she is breastfeeding, as her insulin requirements will take longer to return to prepregnancy levels.

Gestational diabetes
The incidence of this condition varies depending on the criteria used to diagnose it, but it is known to be far more prevalent in women of South East Asian, Mediterranean, Hispanic, and African–American origin. Other risk factors include:
- Past history of gestational diabetes.
- Previous macrosomic baby.
- Family history of diabetes.

It usually develops in the second or early third trimester; if diabetes is diagnosed earlier than this in pregnancy then the suspicion should be raised that it was present but undiagnosed prior to pregnancy, and the management plans above should be applied.

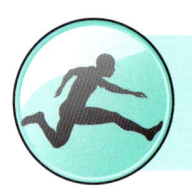

> Diabetes is diagnosed by an abnormal 3 h GTT.

Diagnosis of gestational diabetes can be made:
- On screening: screening is typically done around 24–28 weeks gestation with a 1 h glucose tolerance test (GTT). If this is abnormal, then a 3 h GTT is performed.
- As a result of maternal symptoms or signs: if the woman has recurrent infections, persistent glycosuria, or feels "large-for-dates" with macrosomia or polyhydramnios seen on scan.
- In retrospect, when HbA1c testing is done to investigate an intrauterine death/stillbirth or an unexpectedly macrosomic baby who was hypoglycemic following delivery.

These pregnancies are not at increased risk of congenital abnormality, but the risks of perinatal death and morbidity are higher than in nondiabetic pregnancies. The woman is also at increased risk of developing proteinuric hypertension.

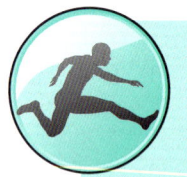

> All diabetic pregnancies are more at risk of stillbirth and neonatal morbidity and mortality, but pre-existing diabetics also have a higher risk of fetal abnormality, which gestational diabetics do not.

Management

The mainstay of management is dietary advice combined with home blood-glucose monitoring. Insulin is needed if diet fails to control glucose levels. Fetal growth and amniotic fluid volume are monitored with regular scans and a joint approach should be taken to care, ideally involving a team of endocrinologists, obstetricians, and nurses.

If on insulin, the woman is likely to need a sliding scale in labor, but this can be stopped when the third stage is complete. The neonate will be at risk of hypoglycemia, so the pediatrician should be involved.

Women who develop gestational diabetes should be made aware that they are at high risk of developing noninsulin-dependent diabetes in the future and that their attitudes and actions regarding lifestyle, weight, and diet can significantly affect this risk.

Epilepsy

Epilepsy affects 1 in 200 women of childbearing age. Pregnancy can exacerbate epilepsy, but, equally, the frequency of seizures can decline. Seizures are particularly likely around the time of labor, due to hyperventilation, dehydration, and exhaustion. Seizures do not in themselves harm the baby, but status epilepticus is dangerous for mother and fetus.

Complications

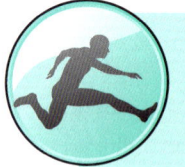

> Women who have epilepsy should take higher than normal doses of folic acid before and throughout pregnancy: preconceptually and for the first 12 weeks of pregnancy to reduce the risk of neural tube defects and facial clefts, and later to counteract the antifolate effects of anticonvulsants that make women with epilepsy more prone to folate-deficiency anemia.

The main concern for pregnant women who are epileptic is that all drugs used to treat epilepsy are teratogenic; possible effects are shown in Fig. 36.4. The rate of abnormality is around 6% for women who are being treated for their epilepsy and 4% for women not receiving treatment, compared with 3% for nonepileptic women.

Fetal and neonatal complications of anticonvulsant therapy

- Cleft lip and palate
- Neural tube defects
- Congenital heart defects
- Hemorrhagic disease of the newborn

Fig. 36.4 Fetal and neonatal complications of anticonvulsant therapy.

The discrepancy is accounted for by the inherent link between facial clefts and epilepsy that is independent of drug therapy. The teratogenic effect of the drugs used is cumulative (i.e. the risk of abnormality if the mother is on two drugs is >12%), so monotherapy is the aim.

New anticonvulsants (e.g. lamotrigine and gabapentin) have shown encouragingly low levels of teratogenesis in animal studies, but they cannot be recommended for use in human pregnancy yet because there are no data as to their safety. Although no one anticonvulsant is particularly better than another, new patients are usually started on carbamazepine in pregnancy.

The woman should not have her usual drug changed unless it is one of the new drugs or phenobarbital, which can lead to neonatal seizures and withdrawal. Control of seizures in pregnancy can deteriorate because drug levels change as a result of the difference in drug handling by the body. If seizures become frequent, then drug levels should be monitored regularly, but the question of compliance should also be addressed—the patient might need further reassurance that it is safer for her baby that she takes her medication than that she run the risk of poor control.

Anticonvulsants affect hepatic handling of vitamin K, increasing the risk of hemorrhagic disease in the newborn, so women taking medication should receive vitamin K supplements from 36 weeks, and the baby should have vitamin K at birth.

Breastfeeding when on anticonvulsants is generally considered safe. Occasionally, if the feeding coincides with a peak in drug levels, the infant might become drowsy. All that is necessary is to change the time of feeding in relation to taking the medication.

Human immunodeficiency virus

Issues to be considered include the effect of pregnancy on the course of HIV infection, the risks of maternal HIV for the fetus, and the screening of the antenatal population for HIV.

HIV is a disease of immunosuppression, and as pregnancy is a naturally immunosuppressed state it might be assumed to cause a deterioration in the condition of the woman affected. However, studies have not proven this to be the case. Women with HIV who become pregnant require specialized care, and this is not just physical, but also psychological and social.

Complications

Women with HIV seem to have higher rates of miscarriage, premature labor, and in utero growth restriction, but some of these might be accounted for by confounding variables, such as smoking, poor nutritional status, and general ill health. The main risk is of vertical transmission, i.e. of the baby becoming HIV positive, as neonatal and infant HIV infection carries a very poor prognosis. Transmission of the virus can occur antenatally or during labor (rates of around 30% without retroviral treatment and with vaginal delivery) or postnatally, through breastfeeding, which doubles the risk of transmission. Factors that increase the risk of vertical transmission are shown in Fig. 36.5.

Management

Women continuing in pregnancy should be monitored as usual, with regular blood tests for viral load and CD4 counts, but the physiological reduction in CD4 count must be taken into account. Treatment may be altered given the limited data available for the safety for the fetus of some of the newer combination regimens of antiretroviral and protease inhibitor drugs. Women at high risk of opportunistic infection, such as pneumocystis and toxoplasma, should be given prophylaxis.

The procedures that are known to increase the risk of vertical transmission are avoided if at all possible and women are offered elective cesarean section at 38 weeks. Additional protection against vertical transmission may be gained by treating the mother with zidovudine (AZT), orally for the

Medical Disorders in Pregnancy

Factors increasing the risk of vertical transmission of human immunodeficiency virus

- Advanced maternal disease, high viral load, low CD4 counts
- Procedures that risk fetal and maternal blood mixing:
  - amniocentesis / chorionic villus sampling
  - fetal blood sampling / fetal scalp electrodes in labor
  - episiotomy
- Normal or instrumental vaginal delivery
- Breast-feeding

Fig. 36.5 Factors increasing the risk of vertical transmission of HIV.

duration of the pregnancy and intravenously around the time of delivery. The baby is given AZT syrup for the first 6 weeks of life.

> Vertical transmission is reduced by giving antiretroviral therapy: orally to the mother in pregnancy, intravenously during delivery, then orally to the neonate.

Women in the developed world are advised not to breastfeed. In the developing world the risks of nonsterile bottle-feeding and the loss of the protection against common infant ailments afforded by breast-feeding might mean that breast is still best.

Screening
In the US, the Institute of Medicine has recommended that antenatal testing for HIV be part of routine care, offered to all women at their initial prenatal visit. The identification of HIV infection has considerable implications for the management of the pregnancy.

Most facilities that have adopted the offer of testing to all women have had good testing rates, and it is known that in some inner-city areas the incidence of HIV is as high as 0.5% in the population (although some of those women will already be aware of their diagnosis).

Liver disorders

Acute fatty liver
This is an extremely rare but potentially lethal liver condition of unknown etiology. The incidence is approximately 1 in 10,000 pregnancies, and it carries mortality rates of 20–30% for the fetus and 10–20% for the mother. It is associated with obesity and with multiple pregnancy.

The woman presents with nausea, malaise, and loss of appetite. She then develops severe vomiting and abdominal pain, jaundice, and ascites. Fulminant liver failure can ensue, leading to renal failure, encephalopathy (with drowsiness and confusion), and clotting anomalies, culminating in DIC.

Pathology specimens show fatty infiltration of hepatocytes, and the gold standard for diagnosis is liver biopsy, although this might be inadvisable given clotting problems. Ultrasound and MRI have been used as alternatives to visualize the fatty infiltration of the liver. Blood tests show hypoglycemia, extremely high transaminase (ALT and AST) levels, alkaline phosphatase raised to a lesser degree, and a very high uric acid.

Management is to correct hypoglycemia and clotting as far as possible and then to deliver the baby. Rapid reversal of the problem follows delivery.

> The unique symptom of cholestasis of pregnancy is itchy palms of the hands and soles of the feet.

Cholestasis of pregnancy
This disorder is of unknown etiology, but there is a strong family history and it is postulated that there is autosomal dominant inheritance. Women present in the third trimester with severe pruritus that is worst on the palms of the hands and soles of the feet; on examination there is no rash. Direct questioning might reveal pale, fatty stools, dark urine, and loss of appetite.

Investigation
LFTs show raised serum bile acids, raised transaminases (ALT and AST), mildly raised bilirubin, and alkaline phosphatase raised even higher than is usually seen in pregnancy. Other causes for liver dysfunction should be investigated, including ultrasound scanning for gallstones and serology for hepatitis. The complications are shown in Fig. 36.6.

Management
Management consists of:
- Reducing the itching: cholestyramine acts to reduce bile acids and can relieve itching, but it often causes vomiting and diarrhea. Antihistamines work for some women, but have unwelcome sedative effects. Ursodeoxycholic acid (ursodiol) lowers bile acids and reduces itching, but it is not licensed for use in pregnancy, so is prescribed with caution.

> Ursodiol lowers serum bile acids and reduces symptoms of itching, but it does not reduce the perinatal morbidity and mortality.

- Reducing the risk of fetal and maternal hemorrhage: women are prescribed daily vitamin K tablets.
- Monitoring fetal well-being: unfortunately, the drugs listed above, which reduce bile acids, have not been shown to reduce the fetal risks of cholestasis. Regular NSTs and growth scans are performed, but they probably do not make a difference in terms of preventing intrauterine death. The mother is warned to be aware of and to report any change or reduction in fetal movements.
- Delivery: once the fetus is considered sufficiently mature, i.e. around 37 weeks, cholestasis of pregnancy in itself is not an indication for elective cesarean section, but because of the increased risk of fetal distress in labor there is a higher than average chance of the woman needing operative delivery.
- Counseling: regarding the risks to this pregnancy and to future pregnancies (there is a high recurrence rate). Women should also be warned to avoid the combined OCP because it can provoke similar liver dysfunction.

Multiple sclerosis

The typical female MS sufferer is of childbearing age, but new presentation during pregnancy is unusual. The usual picture is of a relapsing and remitting course, often better in the third trimester but worse in the 6 months following delivery. The disease itself has no effect on the fetus or on pregnancy; but, if mobility is limited, then the risk of thrombosis should be considered and appropriate precautions introduced (e.g. TED stockings); if there are pre-existing bladder problems, then the risk of UTI will be higher.

Psychiatric disorders

Depression
Recognition of postpartum depression has received widespread attention in the media and in the medical literature. The subject of antenatal depression is less popular, and yet, on closer questioning, many of the women suffering from postpartum depression admit to symptoms of depression before the birth of their baby.

Society's view of pregnancy as something to be happy about and to be enjoyed can make it even harder for women to admit to depression or to ask for help. Women who suffered from depression prior to pregnancy might assume that drug treatments are contraindicated in pregnancy and that there is no point in them mentioning it to their caregivers.

Complications of cholestasis of pregnancy

Complications	Comments
PPH	Due to malabsorption of vitamin K
Intrauterine death	2–4%, with risk increasing with gestation
Premature labor	40% will deliver before 37 weeks
Fetal distress in labor	Meconium-stained amniotic fluid likely
Fetal and neonatal intracranial hemorrhage	Due to maternal absorption of vitamin K

Fig. 36.6 Complications of cholestasis of pregnancy.

Known risk factors for antenatal and postpartum depression include those common to all patients suffering from depression, and some that are specific to pregnancy (Fig. 36.7). The symptoms of depression are:
- Persistently low mood.
- Anhedonia.
- Loss of appetite.
- Insomnia or hypersomnia.
- Psychomotor agitation or retardation.
- Thoughts of self-harm.
- Anxiety (during the postpartum period, this might relate particularly to the baby, with worries of not being able to care for the baby or to love it enough).

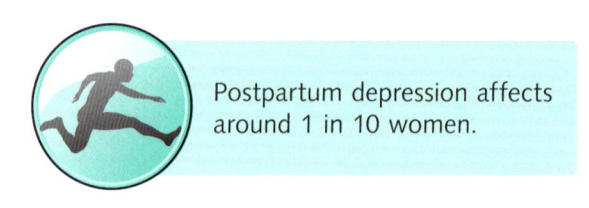

> Postpartum depression affects around 1 in 10 women.

True postpartum depression, where symptoms are present for more than 2 weeks, affects around 1 in 10 women and should be distinguished from the "baby blues," which lasts for a few days and is experienced by up to 70% of women. Once recognized, treatment should be started without delay, as most antidepressants will not have an effect for 6 weeks. Good support is vital and hospitalization is sometimes necessary. In severe cases, electroconvulsive therapy (ECT) might be used.

Drug therapy
The older tricyclic antidepressants can cause drowsiness and antimuscarinic side effects, such as dry mouth and constipation, but they have been used for years with no problems being seen for the fetus or, when breast-feeding, for the baby. However, depression outside pregnancy is often treated with selective serotonin reuptake inhibitors (SSRIs), such as sertraline (Zoloft®), fluoxetine (Prozac®), and paroxetine (Paxil®), so women will seek advice as to whether they should change their medication in pregnancy.

Sertraline has been shown to be potentially harmful to the fetus in animal studies, but it seems to be safe in breast-feeding. The other SSRIs show no evidence of teratogenicity in animal studies, but the manufacturers advise that they are avoided in pregnancy unless the benefit of their use outweighs the risk. Fluoxetine (Prozac) shows high amounts in breast milk, so should be avoided, and the manufacturers of paroxetine (Paxil) advise that it is avoided unless the benefit outweighs the risk.

In conclusion, the choice of antidepressant treatment in pregnancy and during breast-feeding should be made on a case-by-case basis, actively involving the patient in the process and discussing the risks and benefits.

Postpartum psychosis
This disorder is seen most often in women who have a history of psychiatric illness (40% of women with bipolar disorder will develop a postpartum psychosis), but this is not always the case. It usually develops between 2 days and 3 weeks after the birth. The woman exhibits symptoms of mania, with accompanying delusional thoughts and visual or auditory hallucinations. The delusions and hallucinations might pertain to the baby and sometimes manifest as a desire to harm the baby, so a careful risk assessment must be made.

Admission to hospital is necessary, if possible to a specialized mother and baby unit. Treatment consists of antipsychotic medications. Breast-feeding should be avoided if at all possible while the mother is taking these, because animal studies suggest possible adverse effects on the baby's developing nervous system. The risk of recurrence in future pregnancies is up to 50%.

Risk factors for depression during and after pregnancy

- History of postpartum depression
- History of depression unrelated to pregnancy
- IVF pregnancy
- History of abuse
- Multiple pregnancy
- Drug misuse
- Poor social support
- Low socioeconomic status
- Low educational achievement
- Poor pregnancy outcome, e.g. illness in pregnancy, premature or difficult delivery, neonatal illness or death, diagnosis of congenital anomaly antenatally or neonatally

Fig. 36.7 Risk factors for depression during and after pregnancy.

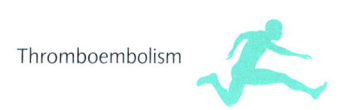

Bipolar disorder

The main problem with this condition is that the drugs used as maintenance therapy (carbamazepine and lithium) are teratogenic. The risks associated with carbamazepine can be reduced to an extent by taking 4 mg of folic acid before conception and for the first 12 weeks of pregnancy, but detailed anomaly scanning is important. Lithium has a narrow therapeutic-to-toxic ratio and close monitoring of lithium levels is needed during pregnancy as dose requirements increase in the second and third trimesters, but they then come rapidly back to normal. High maternal levels at the time of delivery lead to the danger of toxicity in the neonate.

The most likely time for acute episodes of mania to occur is not during the pregnancy but in the puerperium. Close communication between psychiatric and obstetric care providers will be very important. Breast-feeding while taking carbamazepine is safe, but lithium is present in breast milk and can lead to toxicity in the infant. Acute episodes are treated with antipsychotics (see below for their use in pregnancy and with breast-feeding).

Schizophrenia

Women who conceive when on the older antipsychotic drugs can be reassured that the risks to the baby from the medication are not high, although extrapyramidal side effects are sometimes seen in the neonate. The manufacturers of other newer drugs advise their use only if the benefit outweighs the risk in pregnancy; others are to be avoided entirely if possible.

It is known that women with schizophrenia are more prone to preterm labor and that their babies have a higher than average risk of IUGR. All of these factors should be discussed carefully with the woman, and careful communication with her psychiatrist is vital.

During the puerperium the woman is particularly vulnerable to exacerbations, so close support and observation are necessary during this time. Breast-feeding while on antipsychotic medication is not advisable.

Drug and alcohol dependence

The misuse of drugs and alcohol is linked with poor obstetric outcome in many different ways. The essence of obstetric care is to try to establish a relationship with the woman so that she will keep prenatal appointments, but the involvement of counselors, pediatricians, and social services may also be necessary.

Careful explanation of the risks for the fetus is necessary (see Chapter 45), and plans for a withdrawal program should be drawn up if the woman agrees. Intravenous drug use should prompt discussion of screening for HIV and hepatitis B and C. Many facilities have social workers with expertise in this area who will be a link between the hospital, care providers, and the mother.

Thromboembolism

PE is a leading cause of pregnancy-related deaths in the US, so thromboembolism is to be taken extremely seriously in pregnancy. The underlying problem is that pregnancy is a hypercoaguable state, with increased levels of clotting factors and fibrinogen, decreased fibrinolysis, and decreased levels of antithrombin; this state continues for at least 6 weeks postpartum. The added effects of venous pooling and increased abdominal pressure mean that pregnancy increases a woman's risk of a thromboembolic event by six times. Delivery by cesarean section raises the risk still further, by 10 to 20 times, giving the risk of developing deep vein thrombosis (DVT) after an emergency cesarean section of 1–2%. The risk factors are summarized in Fig. 36.8.

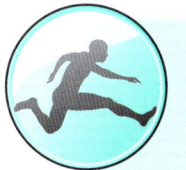

> The increased risk of thromboembolism related to pregnancy continues for 6 weeks postpartum.

The diagnosis of thromboembolism on the basis of history and examination alone is more difficult in pregnancy. Signs and symptoms are less reliable. Leg edema (which can be due to DVT) and shortness of breath (which might be due to PE) are both common symptoms in pregnancy. The best advice is to have a high index of suspicion and to employ the studies described below.

Medical Disorders in Pregnancy

Factors increasing risk of thromboembolic disease related to pregnancy

- Obesity > 80 kg
- Age > 35
- Grand multiparity
- Past medical history of TED
- Prolonged bed rest
- Varicose veins, if severe
- Thrombophilia, e.g. protein C or S deficiency, antithrombin III deficiency, activated protein C resistance (the factor V Leiden mutation), antiphospholipid antibody syndrome

Fig. 36.8 Factors increasing risk of TED related to pregnancy.

Cerebral vein thrombosis is very uncommon, but is associated with high mortality; it usually occurs in the puerperium. Once again, it can be difficult to make the diagnosis on clinical grounds; the picture is confusing, with the woman suffering from seizures (raising the suspicion of eclampsia), fever, vomiting, and photophobia (suggesting meningitis).

Work-up

The diagnosis of DVT is best made using Doppler ultrasound, unless the clot is above the inguinal ligament, in which case venography is the investigation of choice. The investigation of PE should include arterial blood gases, which show hypoxemia and hypocapnia, ECG and chest X-ray.

The chest X-ray might be normal or might show an area of infarction or effusion. In nonpregnant patients a V/Q scan, showing ventilation and perfusion, or a spiral CT scan is performed to confirm the diagnosis. Although the dose of radiation is not contraindicated in pregnancy, it might be possible to reduce exposure by making the diagnosis on the basis of a perfusion scan alone. If, however, the original chest X-ray was abnormal, then a ventilation scan will be necessary. The diagnosis of cerebral thrombosis is best made with MRI scanning.

Management

Pending the confirmation of the diagnosis of PE or DVT, the safest course of action is to anticoagulate. There is an ongoing discussion of the advantages of intravenous heparin infusion compared with intermittent low molecular weight heparin (LMWH). LMWH is used extensively by physicians for treating DVT and PE, but it is still unproven for treatment in pregnancy. It is known that larger doses of intravenous heparin are needed in pregnancy to achieve the target of prolonging the activated partial thromboplastin time by 1.5–2 times the control.

Treatment is continued for the duration of the pregnancy. Subcutaneous heparin or LMWH is used; warfarin is avoided because of its teratogenicity and the risk of maternal retroplacental bleeding and fetal intracerebral bleeds. Anticoagulation must be continued through labor and for 6 weeks postpartum.

Warfarin and heparin are both safe in breast-feeding, so some women might opt to switch to warfarin; the disadvantage is the frequent blood testing at first, but chronic treatment with heparin is not without its side effects (see below).

Prophylaxis against thromboembolism in pregnancy

As is stated above, pregnancy itself is a major risk factor for thromboembolism. Some women have added risk factors and need the protection of prophylaxis. Women with a history of thromboembolism or a strong family history should be screened before pregnancy or in the first trimester. The duration and type of prophylaxis depend on the degree of the risk (Fig. 36.9).

Treatment with heparin for long periods of time results in bone demineralization, which can lead to vertebral fractures. As pregnancy and breast-

Antithromboembolism prophylaxis in pregnancy

Risk factor	Prophylaxis
Prosthetic heart valve	Heparin through pregnancy and puerperium
Multiple DVT/PE in the past	Heparin through pregnancy and puerperium
Thrombophilia (proven or probable)	Heparin through pregnancy and puerperium
One previous DVT or PE	Aspirin through pregnancy, then heparin through labor and puerperium

Fig. 36.9 Antithromboembolism prophylaxis in pregnancy.

feeding also cause demineralization, the rate of symptomatic osteoporosis in women on long-term therapy could be as high as 2%, although bone density does improve once therapy is stopped.

A rarer, but dangerous side effect of heparin is heparin-induced thrombocytopenia. The risks of these side effects are thought to be lower with LMWH. Women on maintenance heparin have monthly platelet counts and clotting screens and, if therapy is for longer than 10 weeks in total, a dual-energy X-ray absorptiometry scan should be performed postnatally to assess bone loss. Low-dose aspirin is safe in pregnancy.

As operative delivery increases the risk of thromboembolism dramatically, prophylaxis is also given after cesarean section to some women, in the form of heparin and/or TED stockings.

Thyroid disorders

Hyperthyroidism

Hyperthyroidism affects 1 in 500 pregnant women. Most of them are hyperthyroid because they have Graves' disease, an autoimmune condition. Affected women often have a family history. Some of the symptoms and signs are similar to those of pregnancy, but the first three listed in Fig. 36.10 should raise the suspicion of thyroid disease. Blood tests reveal raised free T4 and low levels of TSH in comparison with the normal range for that stage of pregnancy.

Like other autoimmune conditions, thyrotoxicosis often improves in pregnancy, but the deterioration in the puerperium might, therefore, be more marked. If untreated in pregnancy, thyrotoxicosis can predispose to miscarriage, IUGR, premature labor and increased perinatal morbidity, and the danger of thyroid storm. In 1–2% of women, thyroid antibodies cross the placenta and cause fetal and neonatal thyrotoxicosis. This is more likely to happen if control is poor in the third trimester, and carries a risk of 15% neonatal mortality if untreated.

Management

Treatment is with methimazole or propylthiouracil. Both drugs cross the placenta and in high doses can result in fetal hypothyroidism. Efficacy of treatment is monitored with free T4 levels every other month. Women with Graves' disease should have serial ultrasound scanning looking for evidence of fetal thyrotoxicosis in the form of IUGR, goiter, or fetal tachycardia. If the condition is diagnosed, then increased doses of antithyroid drugs are administered to the mother. All neonates born to mothers with Graves' disease should have cord blood sent for thyroid function tests.

Antithyroid drugs are secreted in breast milk in small amounts, so the thyroid function of all breast-fed babies should be monitored.

Hypothyroidism

Hypothyroidism is seen in about 1% of pregnant patients. New diagnosis in pregnancy is made more difficult by the fact that many of the symptoms are similar to those of normal pregnancy; the first three features shown in Fig. 36.11 are the most useful when trying to discriminate.

Fortunately, new diagnosis in pregnancy is unusual, and the management of hypothyroidism mainly consists of the care of women who are already on replacement therapy.

Most cases are due to autoimmune destruction of the thyroid—in this process the thyroid gland can atrophy or enlarge, forming a goiter. When a goiter is present the condition is known as Hashimoto's thyroiditis. Other cases are related to

Signs and symptoms of hyperthyroidism	
• Lid lag	• Heat intolerance
• Tremor	• Palpitations
• Weight loss	• Vomiting
• Exophthalmos	• Goiter

Fig. 36.10 Signs and symptoms of hyperthyroidism.

Signs and symptoms of hypothyroidism
• Cold intolerance
• Decreased heart rate
• Delayed relaxation of deep tendon reflexes
• Weight gain
• Lethargy
• Hair loss
• Dry skin
• Constipation
• Carpal tunnel syndrome
• Goiter

Fig. 36.11 Signs and symptoms of hypothyroidism.

drug use (e.g. lithium, amiodarone) or to previous thyroidectomy. The diagnosis is confirmed by a low T4 level (normal ranges for different stages of pregnancy are used). TSH will be raised. A test for thyroid autoantibodies might be sent.

Untreated hypothyroidism leads to a higher risk of:
- Miscarriage.
- Fetal loss.
- Pre-eclampsia.
- IUGR.

It might also be related to lower intelligence in the child.

Well-controlled hypothyroidism does not affect maternal or fetal outcome, except the rare cases of fetal and neonatal hypothyroidism, where TSH-receptor-blocking antibodies cross the placenta resulting in impaired neurological development.

Thyroxine replacement does not affect fetal thyroid function, and seldom needs adjustment during pregnancy if the dose was correct prior to pregnancy. Pregnant women receiving thyroxine replacement should have thyroid function checked once in each trimester, and, if the dose is altered, 4 weeks after any alteration.

Postpartum thyroiditis

It is estimated that this condition affects 5–11% of postpartum women. Those with a family history of hypothyroidism are particularly at risk. It is caused by an autoimmune thyroiditis, which results in an imbalance of thyroid hormones; the state resulting can be hypothyroid, hyperthyroid, or a biphasic pattern of first hyperthyroidism and then hypothyroidism. Symptoms are often vague (e.g. fatigue, palpitations, lethargy, depression) and can be attributed (by the woman and her GP) to her recovery from childbirth and the demands of a new baby. It usually occurs around 12 weeks postpartum. Investigation is first with blood tests, to confirm thyroid dysfunction. A radioactive iodine scan can be done to distinguish postpartum thyroiditis from Graves' disease.

Treatment is not always necessary; the condition is usually self-limiting and treatment will not speed recovery, although it will relieve troublesome symptoms. Overactive symptoms can be treated with β-blockers, and underactive symptoms can be treated with thyroxine replacement. However, 3–4% of women will remain permanently hypothyroid, requiring replacement therapy, and around one-third will be euthyroid for a few years but then develop permanent hypothyroidism. Recurrence in future pregnancies is common.

Thyroid nodules

These are present in about 1% of women of childbearing age and are noteworthy because up to 30% might be malignant, so nodules must be investigated with fine-needle aspiration or biopsy.

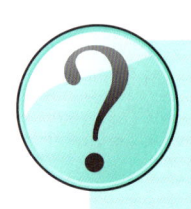

- What are the three common fetal structural abnormalities associated with anticonvulsant therapy?
- What is the main fetal concern in cholestasis of pregnancy?
- What should be done to reduce the thromboembolic risk of a woman with a thrombophilia in pregnancy?
- Why is good control of blood sugars so important for an insulin-dependent diabetic woman who is trying to conceive?
- What three steps can be taken to reduce the risk of vertical transmission of HIV?
- When is a patient with bipolar affective disorder most likely to need psychiatric care related to pregnancy?
- If a woman is hypothyroid prior to pregnancy but is well controlled on treatment, what levels should be checked during pregnancy, and how often?

Further reading

Creasy RK, et al. (2003) *Maternal-Fetal Medicine: Principles and Practice*, 5th ed. (WB Saunders, Philadelphia).

Gabbe SG, et al. (2002) Obstetrics: *Normal and Problem Pregnancies*, 4th ed. (Churchill Livingstone, New York).

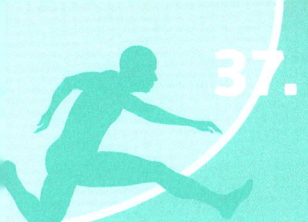

37. Antepartum Hemorrhage

Definition

An APH is defined as any vaginal bleeding that occurs after 20 weeks' gestation and before the birth of the infant.

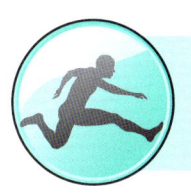

> APH is an important cause of maternal and perinatal morbidity and mortality.

Incidence

The incidence of APH is 3%.

Etiology

A summary is shown in Fig. 37.1. Placenta previa combined with placental abruption accounts for about 50% of the causes of an APH. In both cases, the bleeding comes from maternal vessels that are exposed as the placenta separates from the decidua, i.e. it is not fetal blood, although fetal hypoxia can occur as a secondary process.

Placenta previa

Definition

The placenta is wholly or partially overlying the cervix. The degree of attachment has traditionally been divided into four grades (Fig. 37.2), but, more recently, placenta previa has been classified into three degrees, either complete, partial, or marginal.

Incidence

Placenta previa occurs in 0.4–0.8% of pregnancies; this figure has altered with routine use of ultrasound scanning. The incidence is increased with:

- Increasing maternal age.
- Increasing parity.
- Multiple pregnancy.
- Previous cesarean section.
- Presence of a succenturiate placental lobe.
- Smoking.

It is associated with a maternal mortality rate of about 0.03% in the developed world. The maternal and fetal morbidity is substantially higher in developing countries because of the complications of hemorrhage and prematurity.

History
Painless vaginal bleeding

Bleeding from a placenta previa is usually unprovoked and occurs in the third trimester and in the absence of labor.

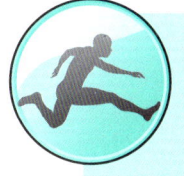

> The presence of abdominal pain is the distinguishing clinical factor between placenta previa and placental abruption.

Examination

General observations should always be performed, including maternal pulse and blood pressure. On abdominal palpation, the uterus is soft and nontender. Because the placenta is low lying, it displaces the presenting part from the pelvis so that a cephalic presentation is not engaged, or there might be a malpresentation (see Chapter 46).

With a minor degree of bleeding, a speculum can be passed to exclude a lower genital tract cause for the APH. A digital examination is contraindicated because it might provoke massive bleeding.

Diagnosis

As part of the routine 20-week ultrasound scan, the placental site is localized. If a low-lying placenta is noted, then a follow-up scan in the third trimester is usually performed to make the

Antepartum Hemorrhage

Etiology of APH

Source of hemorrhage	Type of hemorrhage
Uterine source	Placenta previa
	Placental abruption
	Vasa previa
	Circumvallate placenta
Lower genital tract source	Cervical ectropion
	Cervical polyp
	Cervical carcinoma
	Cervicitis
	Vaginitis
	Vulvar varicosities
Unknown origin (about 50%)	

Fig. 37.1 Etiology of APH.

Ultrasound scan grading of placenta previa

Grade	Description	Degree of placenta previa
I	Encroaches the lower segment	Low lying
II	Reaches the internal os	Marginal
III	Overlies the internal os in part	Partial
IV	Centrally placed in the lower segment	Complete

Fig. 37.2 Grading of placenta previa determined by ultrasound scan.

diagnosis of placenta previa. In the majority of patients, as the lower segment begins to form and the upper segment enlarges upwards, the placenta appears to move up, away from the cervical os. A transvaginal scan is the diagnostic technique of choice owing to its improved accuracy over the transabdominal mode.

Investigations
As well as an ultrasound scan, blood should be sent for hemoglobin count and T&S. Anti-D is indicated if the patient is rhesus negative. If the bleeding is heavy, cross-matching units for transfusion is indicated and a baseline clotting screen should be ordered. Renal function tests might be necessary if the urine output is poor. An NST should be done to check fetal well-being.

Management
Management depends first on assessing the severity of the bleeding and resuscitation of the patient if necessary (see Chapter 18). Immediate delivery by cesarean section might be appropriate if there is either maternal or fetal compromise.

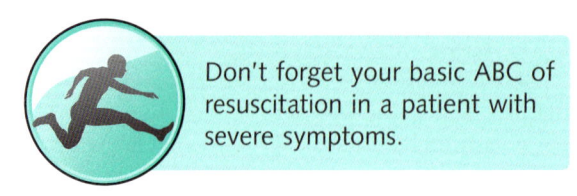

Don't forget your basic ABC of resuscitation in a patient with severe symptoms.

Expectant management depends on the gestation of the pregnancy and the placental site. If the placenta remains at or over the cervical os, then massive bleeding is likely to occur if the patient goes into labor and the cervix starts to dilate. Therefore, inpatient management is appropriate in the third trimester. Delivery by cesarean section is advised if the placenta is encroaching within 2 cm of the internal cervical os.

Complications
Placenta previa is associated with an increased risk of PPH (see Chapters 18 and 42). The lower uterine segment is less efficient at retraction following delivery of the placenta, and thus less effective occlusion of the venous sinuses results in heavier blood loss.

Placenta accreta (see Chapter 42) is also a potential complication in up to 15% of patients with placenta previa, especially those who have had a previous cesarean section. Whether this has been diagnosed preoperatively on ultrasound scan or not, preparations should be in place for potential PPH, e.g. by consulting a perinatologist and anesthesiologist.

Future pregnancy
Placenta previa has a recurrence rate of 4–8%.

Placental abruption

Definition
The placental attachment to the uterus is disrupted by hemorrhage as blood dissects under the

placenta, possibly extending into the amniotic sac or the uterine muscle.

Incidence
Placental abruption occurs in about 1% of pregnancies in the US. In the majority of cases the cause is unknown, but it is thought to be associated with:
- Maternal hypertension or pre-eclampsia.
- Abdominal trauma (e.g. assault, motor vehicle accident).
- Cigarette smoking.
- Lower socioeconomic group.
- ECV.

History
Vaginal bleeding associated with abdominal pain
The patient can present at any stage of pregnancy with a history of bleeding and constant abdominal pain, which is usually unprovoked. This might be associated with uterine contractions.

As maternal blood escapes from the placental sinuses, it tracks down between the membranes and the uterus and escapes via the cervix; this is known as a revealed hemorrhage. Sometimes, the blood remains sealed within the uterine cavity such that the degree of shock is out of proportion to the vaginal loss; this is known as a concealed hemorrhage (Fig. 37.3).

Depending on the patient's previous antenatal history, she should be asked about symptoms of pre-eclampsia, including headache, blurred vision, nausea, and epigastric pain (see Chapter 35).

Examination
The general maternal condition, including pulse and blood pressure, should be assessed. On abdominal palpation the uterus is typically tender. As bleeding extends into the uterine muscle, a tonic contraction can occur, making the uterus feel hard. Fetal parts are difficult to palpate. If the placental site is known (i.e. if placenta previa has been excluded), then a digital examination might be appropriate to diagnose the onset of labor.

Maternal hypertension and proteinuria must be excluded due to the association between abruption and pre-eclampsia. If present, liver tenderness, hyperreflexia, and clonus should be excluded (see Chapter 35).

Work-up
Blood should be sent for hemoglobin count and T&S. Anti-D is indicated if the patient is rhesus negative. If the bleeding is heavy or if the patient is in shock, then cross-matching units for transfusion is indicated and a baseline clotting screen should be ordered.

Renal function tests might be necessary if the urine output is poor or in conjunction with LFTs if pre-eclampsia is suspected. Urinalysis should be

Revealed hemorrhage   Concealed hemorrhage

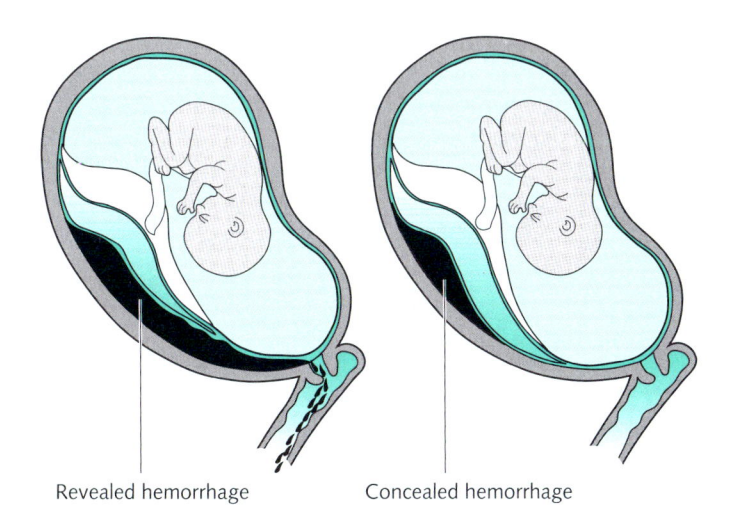

Fig. 37.3 Types of placental abruption.

done to exclude proteinuria; if present, a 24-h urine protein level may be helpful to determine the degree of renal involvement more accurately (see Chapter 35).

An NST should be done to check fetal well-being and also to monitor uterine activity. There might be palpable uterine contractions or the uterus might simply be irritable with irregular activity.

An ultrasound scan is of limited value, since only a large retroplacental hemorrhage will be seen. The diagnosis of abruption is made on clinical grounds (Fig. 37.4).

Management
As for placenta previa, management of a placental abruption must start with assessment of the severity of the symptoms. In a situation where the patient is clinically well and the fetus is not compromised, expectant management might allow the symptoms to resolve. However, in a more serious situation, active resuscitation of the patient could be necessary (see Chapter 18) with immediate delivery of the fetus as a life-saving procedure for the mother and fetus, regardless of gestation.

Complications
- Accurate assessment of blood loss is necessary to assess the risks of developing DIC and renal failure (see Chapter 18).
- PPH occurs in 25% of cases.
- Sheehan's syndrome as a result of PPH (pituitary necrosis secondary to hypovolemic shock).

Management of a patient with an APH

- Hemoglobin
- T&S/cross-match
- Rhesus status
- Renal function tests
- LFTs
- Continuous fetal monitoring
- Ultrasound scan

Fig. 37.4 Management of a patient with an APH.

Future pregnancy
The risk of recurrence is about 6%.

Vasa previa

This is a rare cause of APH. There is a velamentous insertion of the cord and the vessels lie on the membranes that cover the internal cervical os, in front of the presenting part. When the membranes rupture, the vessels can be torn and vaginal bleeding occurs. Unlike placenta previa and placental abruption, this blood is fetal blood and the fetus must be delivered urgently before it exsanguinates.

If the condition is suspected, a Kleihauer test can be performed on the per vagina loss to test for the presence of fetal red blood cells.

Circumvallate placenta

This type of placenta develops secondary to outward proliferation of the chorionic villi into the decidua, beneath the ring of attachment of the amnion and chorion. This does not interfere with placental function, but it is associated with APH and intrapartum hemorrhage.

Unexplained antepartum hemorrhage

No specific cause is found in up to 50% of cases of APH. The cervix should be visualized with a speculum examination and the date of the patient's last Pap smear checked. However, perinatal mortality with any type of APH is double that of a normal pregnancy, suggesting that placental function might be compromised. Therefore, it might be appropriate to consider delivery at term, by inducing labor.

- What are the main causes of APH?
- How is the differential diagnosis made between placenta previa and placental abruption?
- What laboratory studies are appropriate for the patient who presents with an APH?
- What is the management of placental abruption?
- What are the main complications of placenta previa?

Further reading
Gabbe SG, et al. (2002) Obstetrics: *Normal and Problem Pregnancies*, 4th ed. (Churchill Livingstone, New York).

38. Premature Labor

Premature labor is defined as labor occurring after 20 weeks' gestation and before 37 weeks' gestation, so diagnosis depends upon the calculation of the estimated date of delivery. It is important to establish whether a labor is preterm for several reasons:
- Preterm labor is less predictable, and has more complications, than labor at term.
- There is an increased risk of fetal distress in labor.
- Neonatal problems are likely, so the pediatric team must be involved.

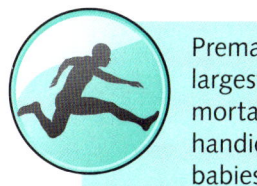

> Prematurity is the single largest cause of neonatal mortality and long-term handicap in otherwise normal babies: premature babies have a 100-fold increased risk of dying than term babies.

- In most circumstances an effort can be made to stop the labor to administer corticosteroids to the mother, which will boost fetal lung surfactant production and, therefore, reduce neonatal respiratory distress.

> Corticosteroids (e.g. betamethasone or dexamethasone) are given to the mother as two intramuscular injections 24 h apart. They have been shown to significantly reduce neonatal respiratory distress by stimulating fetal surfactant production and are recommended for any woman in threatened preterm labor between 24 and 34 weeks' gestation. It is not known whether more than one course of steroids is beneficial, but the effect is thought to decline over time.

Incidence

The incidence of preterm labor is currently around 6% in the US, but this varies in different populations and the incidence is increasing. Risk factors for premature labor are shown in Fig. 38.1, with the most significant association being a history of a previous preterm labor.

The main causes of preterm delivery are shown in Fig. 38.2. Infection is thought to play a part in at least 20% of cases (see Fig. 38.3 for common pathogens implicated in preterm labor). Iatrogenic preterm delivery, accounting for one-third of preterm deliveries, occurs when obstetricians decide that delivery is necessary in the interests of fetal or maternal health, due, for example, to

Characteristics of women more at risk of preterm labor

- BMI <19
- Low social class
- Poor social support
- African–American race
- Extremes of reproductive age (under 20 and over 35)
- Domestic violence
- Smoking
- Previous preterm labor
- Bacterial vaginosis
- Chronic medical conditions

Fig. 38.1 Characteristics of women more at risk of preterm labor.

Causes of preterm delivery

- Infection (e.g. chorioamnionitis, maternal pyelonephritis/appendicitis)
- Uteroplacental ischemia (e.g. abruption)
- Uterine overdistention (e.g. polyhydramnios, multiple pregnancy)
- Cervical incompetence
- Fetal abnormality
- Iatrogenic

Fig. 38.2 Causes of preterm delivery.

Premature Labor

Pathogens implicated in preterm labor

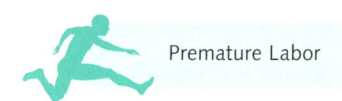

- Sexually transmitted: *Chlamydia, Trichomonas,* syphilis, gonorrhea
- Enteric organisms: *Escherichia coli, Streptococcus faecalis*
- Bacterial vaginosis: *Gardnerella, Mycoplasma* and anaerobes
- Group B streptococcus (if a very heavy growth)

Fig. 38.3 Pathogens implicated in preterm labor.

Management checklist for patient presenting in threatened preterm labor

- Assess for signs of a precipitant of preterm labor, e.g. sepsis, polyhydramnios, abruption, severe pre-eclampsia, cholestasis of pregnancy. Take blood tests as appropriate. Perform urinalysis and send clean catch urine for culture
- Determine frequency and regularity of contractions. Monitor the fetal heart
- Perform a sterile speculum examination to examine the cervix. Perform wet mount and endocervical swabs. Start continuous electronic fetal monitoring if there is cervical dilatation.
- Ascertain fetal presentation (cephalic or breech)
- Give corticosteroids
- Give antibiotics if ruptured membranes or if obvious signs of sepsis
- Consider tocolysis
- Contact pediatrician and arrange transfer out if necessary and appropriate
- Discuss mode of delivery

Fig. 38.4 Management checklist for patient presenting in threatened preterm labor.

severe pre-eclampsia, or when ultrasounds have shown severe IUGR of the fetus.

Clinical evaluation and investigation of women in preterm labor

As preterm labor is often rapid and is almost always unexpected, some women will arrive in an advanced state of labor; in this case the mother should be assessed to make sure that she is stable (and not, for instance, in shock due to a large abruption), examined vaginally to check the dilatation of the cervix, and fetal monitoring commenced. The pediatricians must be informed. As abnormal lie and presentation are far more common in preterm pregnancy, an ultrasound scan should be performed.

If the presentation is less acute, then a history should be taken and examination performed with the aim of finding out what the underlying cause of the threatened preterm labor is, and laboratory work and/or studies arranged as appropriate. Any woman admitted with abdominal pain or discharge should have a speculum examination to allow inspection of the cervix (Fig. 38.4). Premature labor does not always present with obvious contractions, and the cervix can undergo so-called "silent" dilatation.

Cervical dilatation confirms labor, but if the cervix is closed in the presence of uterine contractions the diagnosis of "threatened" preterm labor is made. Around half of women presenting with symptoms of threatened preterm labor are either not in labor or stop laboring spontaneously. If membranes have ruptured, delivery is far more likely.

The clinical picture alone does not allow us to predict accurately which women will stop contracting spontaneously, so the management plan is formulated on the assumption that delivery will occur. Transvaginal scans to examine the length of the cervix have been used, where cervical shortening is a predictor of preterm delivery (Fig. 38.5). Evidence of fetal fibronectin in the mother's cervical secretions can be used; its absence has proved to be a reassurance that delivery is very unlikely, but it is not a very sensitive test.

Communication with the pediatric team is vital. Some hospitals do not have facilities for treating babies born under certain gestations, and in these cases transfer to the nearest tertiary care center is made, preferably in utero, i.e. transfer of the mother before she has delivered. If the mother is seriously unwell or if delivery is imminent, then transfer of the baby can be arranged after delivery. Unless the mother is in advanced labor on arrival, there will be an opportunity for her and her partner to meet one of the pediatricians to find out what is likely to happen if her baby is born at an early gestation. They can be given a realistic outlook and warned about some of the problems that premature babies encounter. A tour of the neonatal intensive care unit could be arranged.

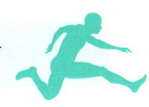

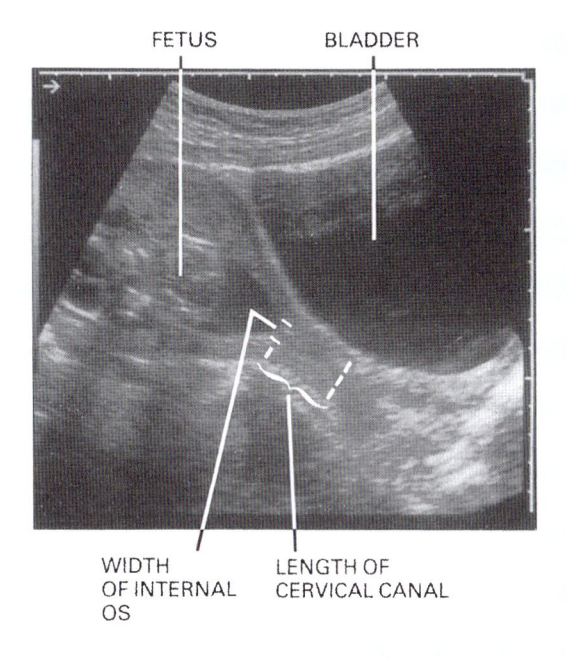

Fig. 38.5 Transvaginal scan of cervical canal. Reproduced with kind permission from *Obstetric Ultrasound: How, Why and When*, published by Churchill Livingstone.

The main problems encountered by children surviving premature delivery are cerebral palsy, chronic lung disease, visual and hearing deficits, and learning difficulties.

Treatment of women presenting in preterm labor

Although the mortality and morbidity of preterm infants has been reducing over the last decade, this cannot be ascribed to improved obstetric management, other than the increased administration of corticosteroids to the mother. Sadly, our attempts to stop preterm labor are unsatisfactory, being often ineffective and exposing women and their babies to drugs with significant side effects. Part of the problem is our lack of knowledge about what triggers preterm labor.

Tocolysis

The different drugs used to try to stop contractions are shown in Fig. 38.6. Ethanol infusion is not included, but it was used routinely until the 1970s. The common factor of all the drugs is that none has been shown to result in improved neonatal morbidity or mortality. Most have been shown to delay delivery for some time (24–48 h), which gives the obstetricians the opportunity to administer corticosteroids and, if necessary, transfer to another hospital able to offer neonatal care. With all drugs, the side effects on mother and fetus must be balanced against the benefit of prolonging the pregnancy. Tocolysis should not be used for all cases of preterm labor; instances when it might be inadvisable include:

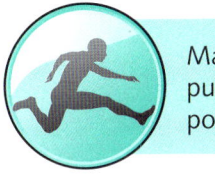

Magnesium sulfate can cause pulmonary edema, a potentially fatal side effect.

- Maternal illness that would be helped by delivery, e.g. pre-eclampsia.
- Evidence of fetal distress.
- In the presence of chorioamnionitis.
- When there has been significant vaginal bleeding.
- Once the membranes have ruptured.

Antibiotic therapy

Antibiotics are given prophylactically if the membranes have ruptured before term (around a third of cases) to protect the fetus from ascending infection. If the membranes are intact, then the mother is screened for infection (vaginal and cervical swabs, blood cultures if feverish) and started on prophylactic antibiotics until culture results are available.

Cervical cerclage

When there is cervical incompetence resulting in cervical dilatation but the patient is not actively laboring, a suture can be placed in the cervix to attempt to reduce the prolapse of membranes that

215

Premature Labor

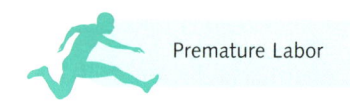

Drugs used to treat preterm labor

Beta agonists (e.g. ritodrine, salbutamol, terbutaline)
Administered as intravenous infusion or subcutaneous injection. Act on β receptors in myocardium to cause relaxation. Common side effects, occurring in up to 80% of mothers, include tachycardia, headache, tremor, nausea and vomiting, hyperglycemia, and hypokalemia. Similar effects are seen on the fetus. The potentially fatal side effects of pulmonary edema and myocardial ischemia occur in around 5% of women.

Calcium channel blockers (e.g. nifedipine)
Block calcium channels in the myometrium, interrupting contraction. Their effectiveness has been questioned, and they have the potential to alter uteroplacental blood flow, causing fetal compromise. Maternal side effects are less common than with β agonists, but include headache, flushing, and tremor.

Oxytocin receptor antagonists (e.g. atosiban)
This newly developed family of drugs has been proved to delay delivery, but not to influence neonatal outcome. Atosiban seems to be well tolerated, with fewer side effects than other drugs, but it is expensive. Given as an intravenous infusion. Side effects occur in around 8% of mothers, who experience flashing and headache.

NSAIDs (e.g. indomethacin)
NSAIDs are effective tocolytics, acting on the cyclo-oxygenase enzyme that catalyzes production of prostaglandin, which is vital for labor. They are cheap and easy to administer orally. Side effects in the mother are mild, consisting of GI upset (nausea, heartburn) and headache. However, they have potentially serious fetal side effects, causing premature closure of the ductus arteriosus (which can result in pulmonary hypertension, tricuspid regurgitation, and heart failure) and reducing renal function, leading to oligohydramnios. The neonatal complications necrotizing enterocolitis and intracerebral hemorrhage are also more common. The fetal effects are temporary, and the neonatal effects are more common with prolonged administration of the drug, but the fetal morbidity that has been seen in the past has dissuaded clinicians from using NSAIDs. The use of indomethacin is relatively contraindicated after 32 weeks for this reason.

Magnesium sulfate
This competes at calcium channels in the myometrium. Given as intravenous infusion. Maternal side effects are uncommon but potentially serious, occurring in around 5% and consisting of blurred vision, loss of tendon reflexes, pulmonary edema, and arrhythmias. Fetal and neonatal side effects include reduced FHR variability, hypotonia, and respiratory depression. Magnesium sulfate has also been linked to increased maternal and perinatal mortality, so it is used with caution.

Nitric oxide donors (e.g. glyceryl trinitrate patches)
Nitric oxide donors act on myometrium in vitro to cause relaxation. They have few side effects for mother or fetus, but their effectiveness in vivo has not been proved.

Fig. 38.6 Drugs used to treat preterm labor.

will otherwise ensue. Once the membranes prolapse into the vagina they weaken and their rupture is likely, followed by delivery or the development of infection. The MacDonald suture, which is inserted vaginally as high in the cervix as possible, is used most commonly (Fig. 38.7). Other options are the Shirodkar suture, which is inserted vaginally but involves the dissection of the bladder off the cervix, and an abdominal cerclage, which is a suture inserted into the cervix at laparotomy, which can be placed higher.

However, insertion of a suture can introduce infection or result in rupture of the membranes during the procedure.

Mode of delivery

The cesarean section rate might be presumed to be higher because of a higher incidence of low-lying placenta, fetal distress, and abnormal lie in prematurity, but there is also a trend to deliver all preterm babies by cesarean section, although there is no firm evidence to show that this is safer for the baby than vaginal delivery, especially when the presentation is cephalic. Cesarean section might have higher morbidity for the mother when performed at very early gestations because the lower segment is less well formed.

Management of future paregnancier

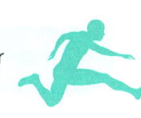

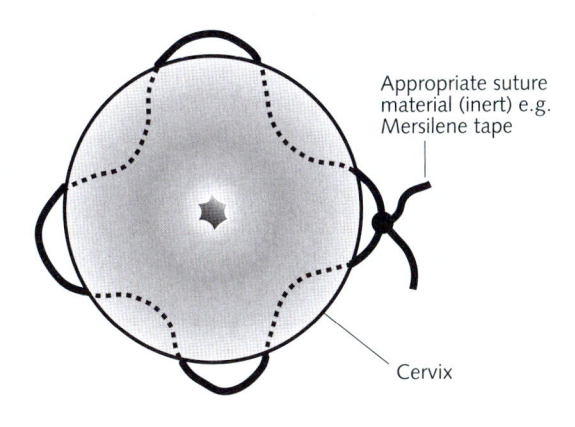

Fig. 38.7 The MacDonald suture.

Management of future pregnancies

Any woman who has labored prematurely is more at risk of doing so again in her next pregnancy. In many cases there will be nothing that can be done to prevent this. Exceptions are when:
- Labor has been due to treatable, persistent infection, e.g. bacterial vaginosis.
- There is cervical incompetence.

Where infection has been proven it should be treated and the mother screened regularly for recurrence during subsequent pregnancies and treated as necessary.

Cervical incompetence can be treated by insertion of a cervical suture, either electively in early pregnancy (usually around 13–14 weeks after the high risk of early miscarriage has passed), or, if the cervix is monitored regularly in pregnancy with transvaginal scanning, when ultrasound shows that the cervix is shortening.

The prescription of prophylactic tocolytics to women at increased risk of recurrent preterm labor is not helpful, but some clinicians prescribe prophylactic corticosteroids at a point in the pregnancy before the last baby delivered.

- Between which weeks of pregnancy can labor be said to be premature?
- What is the greatest risk factor for premature labor?
- What is the purpose of antenatal steroid administration, and how are they given?
- What is the fibronectin test?
- What proportion of women presenting with symptoms of preterm labor will deliver at that time?

Further reading
Gabbe SG, et al. (2002) *Obstetrics: Normal and Problem Pregnancies*, 4th ed. (Churchill Livingstone, New York).

39. Malpresentation and Malpositions of the Occiput

Malpresentation

Any presentation other than a vertex presentation is a malpresentation. The vertex is the area between the parietal eminences and the anterior and posterior fontanelles. The most common malpresentation is the breech presentation, but others include shoulder, brow, and face presentations.

Malpresentation can occur by chance, but it can also be caused by fetal or maternal conditions that prevent the vertex from presenting to the pelvis (Fig. 39.1). In all cases, management must include exclusion of important conditions such as fetal abnormality, pelvic masses, and placenta previa.

Breech presentation

Apart from the general causes of malpresentation, breech presentation is particularly associated with prematurity. The incidence of breech presentation increases with decreasing gestation:
- Term: 3%.
- 32 weeks: 15%.
- 28 weeks: 25%.

Classification of breech presentation
There are three types of breech presentation:
- Extended or frank breech.
- Flexed or complete breech.
- Footling breech.

Just over half of breech presentations are extended, and the remainder are divided roughly equally between flexed and footling. With an extended breech, the hips are flexed and the knees extended with the feet situated adjacent to the fetal head. Flexed and footling breeches are flexed at both the hips and knees, but in the latter the feet present to the maternal pelvis, not the breech (Fig. 39.2).

Diagnosis
The head can be felt as a hard lump at the uterine fundus by the examiner and the patient. Auscultation of the fetal heart at a higher level than is usual with a cephalic presentation might suggest a breech presentation, although this is not a reliable sign. Vaginal examination can confirm the diagnosis, although if there is any doubt ultrasound examination is indicated, which will also determine the type of breech presentation.

Complications
There is an increased perinatal mortality and morbidity associated with vaginal breech delivery when compared with cephalic presentation of comparable birth weight and gestation. This is usually associated with difficulty in delivering the aftercoming head. The fetal trunk is softer than the head and can pass through a borderline pelvis, resulting in entrapment of the aftercoming head. Moulding of the fetal head as it passes through the pelvis can only occur after the body has delivered and in a relatively short period of time. Rapid compression and decompression of the head during delivery can produce intracranial injury. The presence of nuchal arms, i.e. when the fetal arms are extended posteriorly behind the head and sometimes crossed behind the head in the hollow of the neck, reduces the available space for delivering the aftercoming head. Unfortunately, no method of antenatal assessment (clinical, radiologic, or ultrasonic) will guarantee easy delivery of the aftercoming head.

Perinatal mortality
Four major causes account for the increased perinatal mortality associated with vaginal breech delivery. The relative importance of these depends on the gestational age of the fetus:
- Prematurity.
- Cord prolapse.
- Birth trauma.
- Congenital anomaly.

> There has been a recent move towards more elective cesarean sections in breech presentation because of proven lower perinatal risks.

Cord prolapse can occur if the cervix is poorly applied to the presenting part and is most likely to occur with a footling breech (Fig. 39.3). Birth trauma is associated with difficulty in delivery of the aftercoming head or soft-tissue injury due to excessive traction to the fetus. The causes of death associated with birth trauma following vaginal breech delivery include:
- Intracranial hemorrhage/tentorial tear.
- Spinal cord injury.
- Soft-tissue injury.
- Liver rupture.
- Adrenal hemorrhage.

Perinatal morbidity
Morbidity is also usually associated with difficulty in delivering the aftercoming head. Although the morbidity is distressing for all concerned with the delivery, the neonate usually makes a complete recovery. Typical injuries associated with vaginal breech delivery include nerve palsies, fractures, and soft-tissue injuries (Fig. 39.4).

Management
There are three management options for a breech presentation:
- ECV.
- Planned vaginal breech delivery.
- Elective cesarean section.

Following the publication of a large, randomized, prospective trial in the *Lancet*, the tendency is now to deliver most breech presentation babies by cesarean section. This trial indicated a significantly lower incidence of complications in term breech babies born by cesarean section than by the vaginal route.

External cephalic version
The fetus is turned to a cephalic presentation by manual manipulation through the maternal anterior abdominal wall. This is now usually performed at around 37 weeks' gestation, by which time most

Causes of malpresentation	
Type of cause	Description
Maternal	Contraction of the pelvis
	Pelvic tumor
	Müllerian abnormality
	Multiparity
Fetoplacental	Placenta previa
	Polyhydramnios
	Multiple pregnancy
	Fetal anomaly • hydrocephalus • extension of the fetal head by neck tumor • anencephaly • decreased fetal tone

Fig. 39.1 Causes of malpresentation.

Frank breech   Footling breech   Complete breech

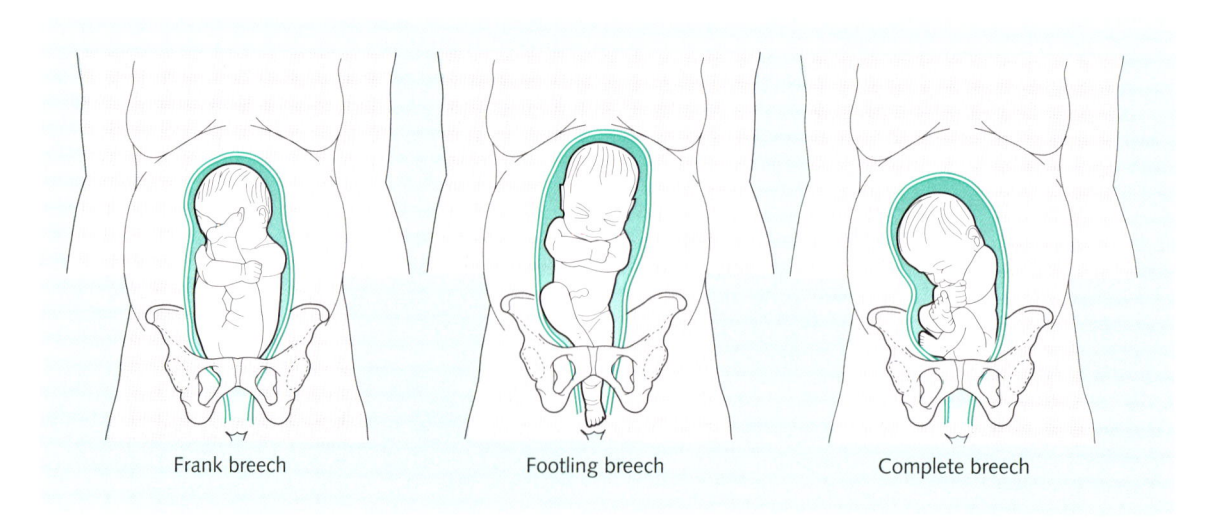

Fig. 39.2 Classification of breech presentation.

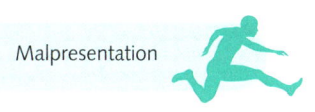

Malpresentation

Incidence of cord prolapse associated with fetal presentation	
Fetal presentation	Incidence (%)
Cephalic	0.5
Extended breech	1.0
Flexed breech	4.0
Footling breech	18.0

Fig. 39.3 Incidence of cord prolapse associated with fetal presentation.

Fetal injuries associated with vaginal breech delivery	
Type of injury	Description
Nerve palsies	Brachial plexus palsy
	Facial nerve palsy
Fractures	Clavicle
	Upper limb
Soft-tissue injury	

Fig. 39.4 Fetal injuries associated with vaginal breech delivery.

breeches will have spontaneously turned. Contraindications to ECV include:
- Pelvic mass.
- APH.
- Placenta previa.
- Previous cesarean section or hysterotomy.
- Multiple pregnancy.
- Ruptured membranes.

ECV can be performed with the aid of tocolytics, to reduce uterine activity, and under ultrasound control. It should be performed on labor and delivery because of the small risk of fetal distress requiring immediate cesarean section (<1%). The fetus can be rolled forwards or backwards and version is successful in about half the cases. Extended breeches are more difficult to turn because the legs 'splint' the fetus. Rhesus-negative women should be given anti-D Ig following attempted version because of the possibility of fetomaternal hemorrhage.

Antenatal assessment for vaginal breech delivery

Antenatal assessment for vaginal breech delivery includes assessment of:
- Fetal size.
- The maternal pelvis.

It is important to exclude a macrosomic fetus prior to vaginal breech delivery and this is best done by ultrasound estimated fetal weight (EFW). A fetus with an EFW of greater than 3.8 kg is probably best delivered by cesarean section. Ultrasound EFW at term is associated with an error of at least 10%. Measurement of the pelvic inlet and outlet is rarely performed now, because of the inaccuracies and poor predictive value, unless there is a significant past history of pelvic injury or rickets.

Management of labor with a breech presentation
(Figs 39.5–39.14)

Delivery should be in an obstetric unit with an attendant neonatologist because vaginal breech delivery should be regarded as high risk. Management of the first stage of labor should be as for a vertex presentation, although some obstetricians do not advocate the use of oxytocin in the presence of secondary arrest preferring to perform a cesarean section. Continuous FHR monitoring is recommended. Exclusion of cord prolapse is mandatory when the membranes rupture or if the FHR pattern becomes abnormal. Epidural anesthesia is recommended because of the increased level of manipulation during delivery. In only half of planned vaginal breech deliveries will vaginal delivery be successful, because of the lower threshold to perform cesarean section.

During the second stage, the breech should be allowed to descend onto the pelvic floor before active pushing is commenced. If descent does not occur this could indicate disproportion or an unexpectedly large fetus, and cesarean section is indicated. Delivery in the lithotomy position allows access for the attendant to perform any necessary manipulation to the fetus. Routine episiotomy is recommended to further increase access and prevent delay due to the soft tissues. Two procedures are particularly valuable in the delivery of a breech presentation:
- Lovset's maneuver.
- The Mauriceau–Smellie–Veit maneuver.

Lovset's maneuver

Lovset's maneuver is used when the arms are extended. Grasping the fetal pelvis and upper

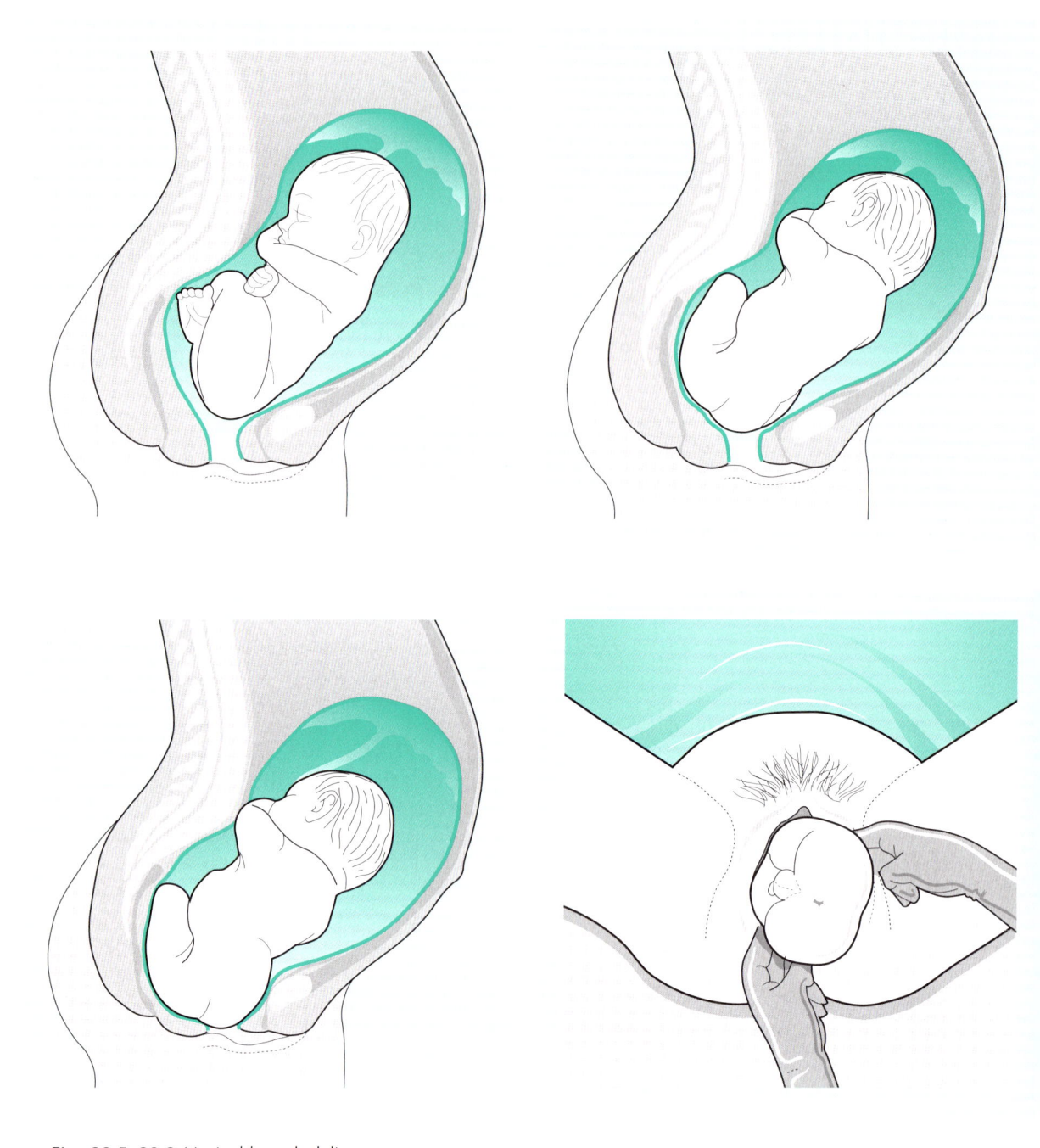

Figs 39.5–39.8 Vaginal breech delivery.

thighs, gentle downwards traction is applied until the anterior shoulder lies behind the symphysis pubis and the inferior border of the scapula is visible. This allows the posterior shoulder to descend into the pelvic cavity. With the back uppermost, the fetal trunk is rotated through 180° to bring the posterior shoulder to an anterior position under the pubic arch. If the arm does not deliver spontaneously it is easily delivered using a finger. The posterior shoulder will now be situated in the sacral curve and, again with the back uppermost, the fetal trunk is rotated 180° in the

Malpresentation

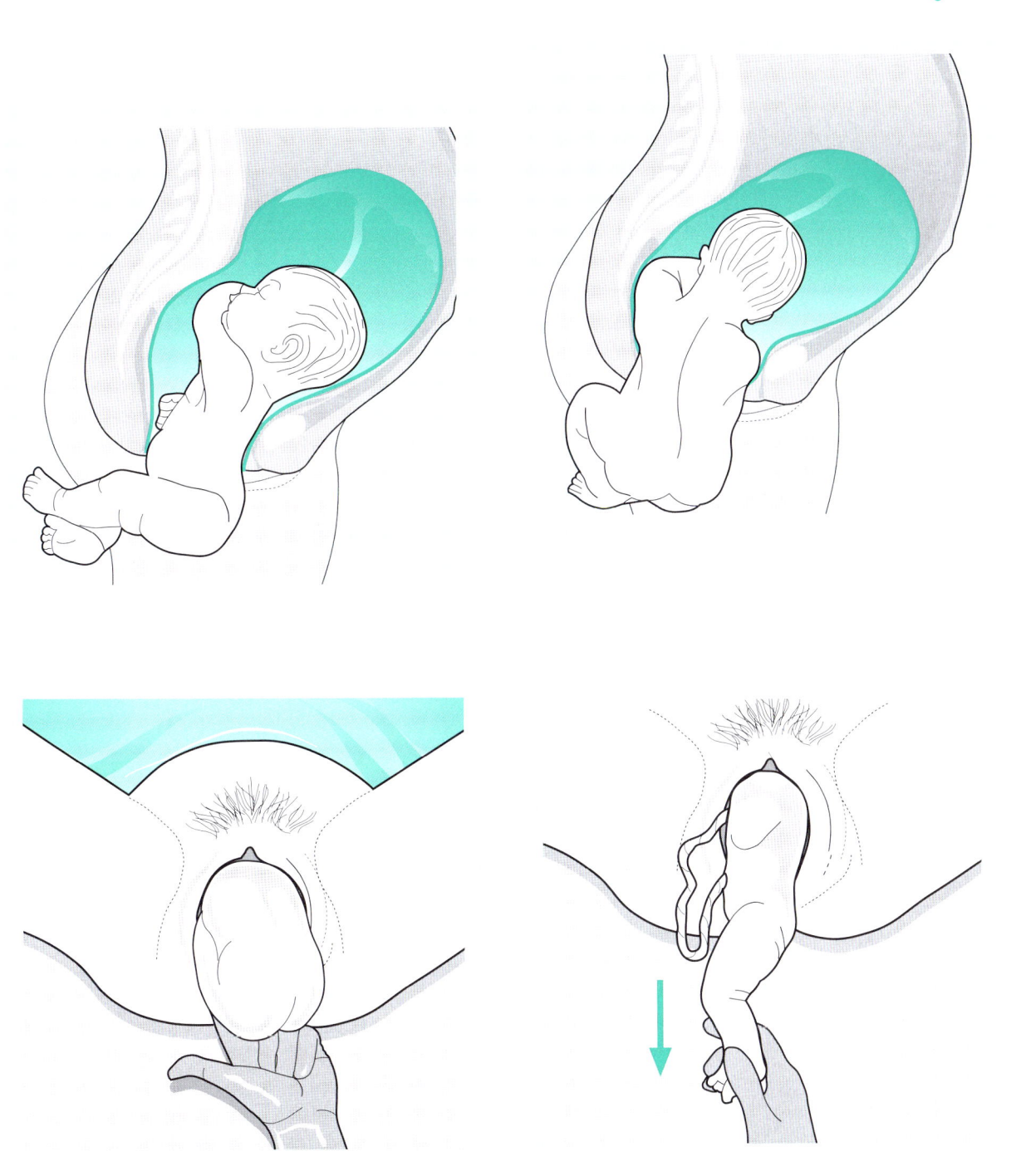

Figs 39.9–39.12 Vaginal breech delivery (continued).

223

Malpresentation and Malpositions of the Occiput

A B

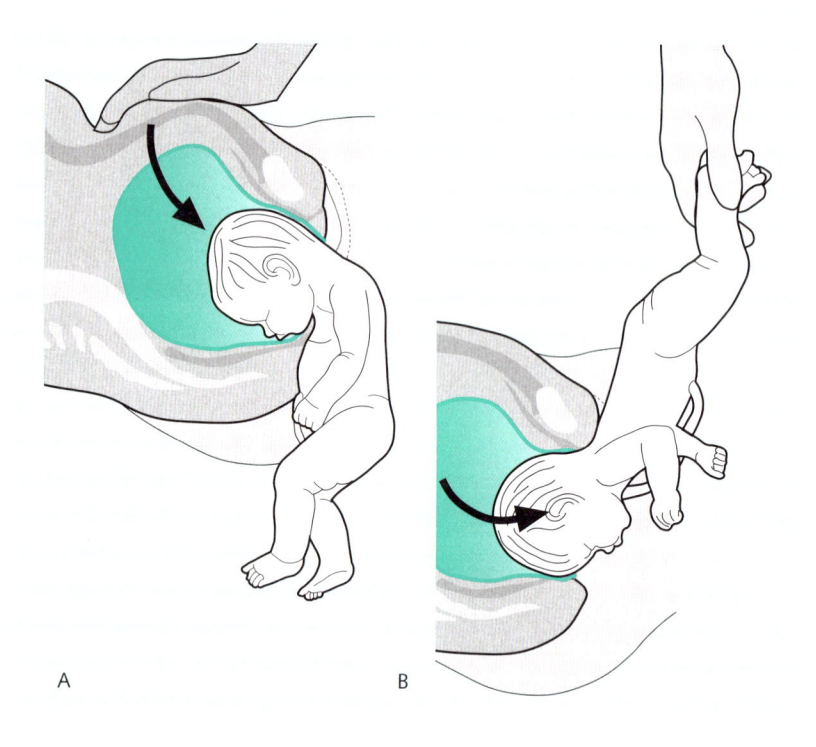

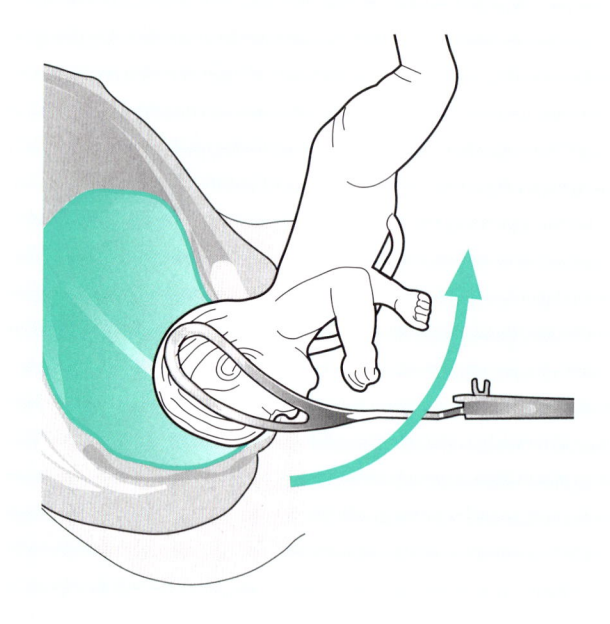

Figs 39.13–39.14 Vaginal breech delivery (continued).

opposite direction to bring the posterior shoulder anteriorly to lie under the pubic arch. The second arm will then deliver easily.

As soon as the trunk has been delivered, the fetal circulation will be compromised because the head will be compressing the cord at the level of the pelvic brim. Therefore, delivery of the head is necessary in a matter of minutes to avoid asphyxia. The body of the fetus should be allowed to hang downwards while the head descends into the pelvis. The head usually enters the pelvis transversely and, during descent, undergoes rotation until the occiput lies beneath the pubic arch. If the head does not rotate and descend then the Mauriceau–Smellie–Veit maneuver can be used (often remembered as the "smelly feet" maneuver by students!).

The Mauriceau–Smellie–Veit maneuver

This maneuver maintains flexion of the head as downwards traction is applied. With the body of the fetus lying on the attendant's lower arm, and with the fingers of this arm in the vagina, the middle finger is used to apply pressure on the fetal jaw or gently inserted in the mouth to flex the fetal head. The index and middle finger of the other hand are placed over the fetal shoulders and used to apply downwards traction until the occiput lies under the pubic arch. The fetal legs are then grasped and elevated, extending the back and, by further gentle pressure on the fetal jaw, continuing flexion of the head allows delivery. Forceps can also be used to deliver the aftercoming head.

Elective cesarean section for breech presentation

The vast majority of breeches are now delivered by cesarean section, either emergency or elective. Some of the indications for elective cesarean section include:
- Footling breech.
- Maternal request.
- Ultrasound EFW > 3.8 kg.
- Suboptimal pelvimetry.
- Failed ECV.
- Twins, where the first twin presents by the breech.
- Breech plus another complication (e.g. PIH, previous cesarean section, diabetes mellitus).

As more and more breeches are delivered abdominally, gaining the required skills and experience needed for vaginal breech delivery is more difficult, and it is likely that in the future we will see even fewer breeches delivered vaginally. Some would argue that this is not necessarily a retrograde step, particularly in light of the recent data.

Transverse lie and unstable lie

A transverse lie occurs when the long axis of the fetus lies transverse or oblique to the long axis of the uterus, usually with the shoulder presenting (Fig. 39.15). When the fetal lie is different at each palpation, the lie is said to be unstable.

The incidence of transverse lie diagnosed in labor with a single fetus is approximately 1 in 500 women, but many more will have been identified and managed appropriately antenatally.

The causes of transverse lie include the general causes of malpresentation shown in Fig. 39.1, but there is particular association with:
- Multiparity, where the tone of the uterus and anterior abdominal wall is poor.
- Premature labor.
- The second twin.
- Uterine anomalies/fibroids.

The diagnosis of a transverse lie is usually made antenatally and the findings on abdominal palpation include the:
- Fetal head palpable laterally in the maternal abdomen.
- Fundal height being lower, and the uterus wider, than expected.

Vaginal examination, which should be avoided until placenta previa has been excluded, will reveal an empty pelvis.

The most serious complication of a transverse lie is cord prolapse, and this is associated with spontaneous rupture of membranes, which can occur antenatally or in labor. As the shoulder usually presents, the arm can prolapse and, in an unsupervised situation, obstructed labor, infection, and uterine rupture can occur. Treatment depends on the situation at the time of diagnosis and is aimed at:
- Correcting the malpresentation.
- Avoiding serious complications.

If the diagnosis is made antenatally, then exclusion of causes of malpresentation is important. Elective abdominal delivery at or approaching term is indicated in the presence of pelvic contraction,

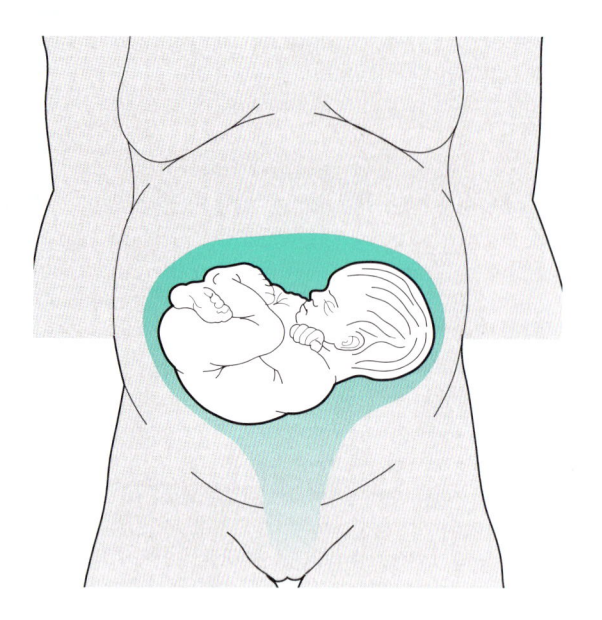

Fig. 39.15 Transverse lie.

placenta previa or a pelvic mass. In their absence, ECV can be attempted. At term, an unstable lie can be managed expectantly because spontaneous version to a cephalic presentation often occurs due to the increase in uterine activity. Transverse lie can be corrected by ECV followed by induction of labor. If the lie remains unstable then cesarean section is indicated.

If a transverse lie is diagnosed in early labor, then ECV should be attempted only if the membranes are intact. If successful, artificial rupture of membrane (AROM) with the head in the pelvis can stabilize the lie by inducing uterine contractions. If version is not successful or the membranes have ruptured, then cesarean section is indicated.

Following delivery of the first twin, if the second twin lies transversely the membranes must not be ruptured until external version to a longitudinal lie has been performed. When the presenting part has descended into the pelvis, AROM can be performed and vaginal delivery expected.

Face presentation

The incidence of face presentation is 1 in 300 labors and occurs when the head is fully extended (Fig. 39.16).

The causes of extension of the fetal head include congenital tumors of the neck, but these are rare. Face presentation is more likely to occur when a normal fetus holds its head in an extended position. Historically, anencephaly is associated with face presentation, but this is now rare due to increased prenatal diagnosis and termination of pregnancy.

Diagnosis is usually made during vaginal examination in labor when the supraorbital ridges, the bridge of the nose, and the alveolar margins in the mouth are palpable (Fig. 39.17). During labor, the face becomes edematous and might be mistaken for a breech presentation.

Mechanism of labor

The chin (mentum) is the denominator and in 75% of cases the position is mentum anterior. The submentobregmatic diameter is 9.5 cm, so vaginal delivery is possible. Vaginal delivery occurs by flexion of the head, which is possible only in the mentum anterior position (Fig. 39.18).

> Face presentation will deliver vaginally if it is mentum anterior, but not if it is mentum posterior.

Malpresentation

Fig. 39.16 Face presentation.

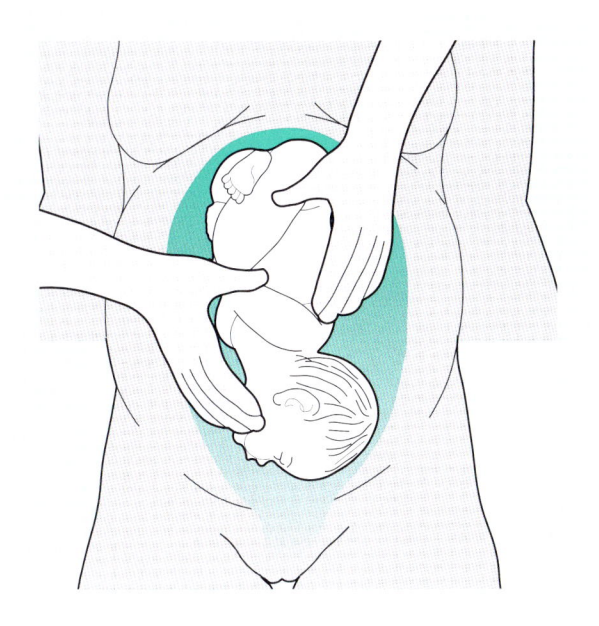

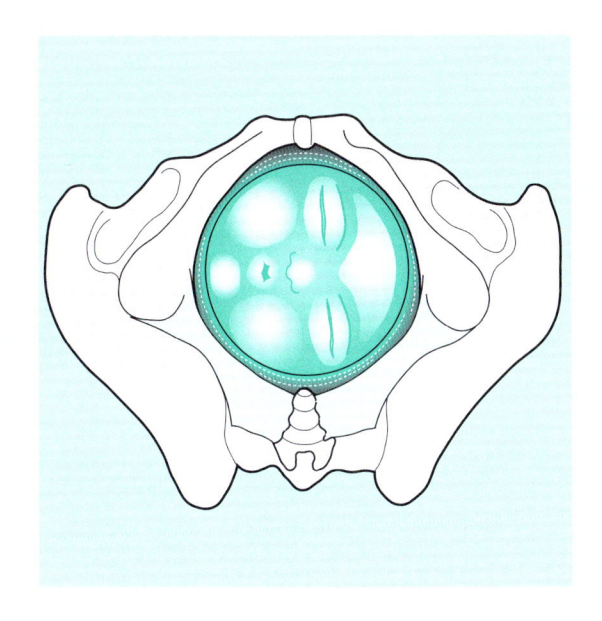

Fig. 39.17 Vaginal examination findings in face presentation.

Management of a face presentation in labor is essentially the same as for a vertex presentation. Vaginal examination should be performed when the membranes rupture to exclude a cord prolapse. Mentum posterior positions rotate spontaneously to mentum anterior in 50% of cases, usually in the second stage of labor, and in those that do not a cesarean section is indicated. Cesarean section should also be performed when the FHR pattern is abnormal, because a fetal blood sample for pH measurement should not be taken from the face. Traction forceps can be applied to a mentum

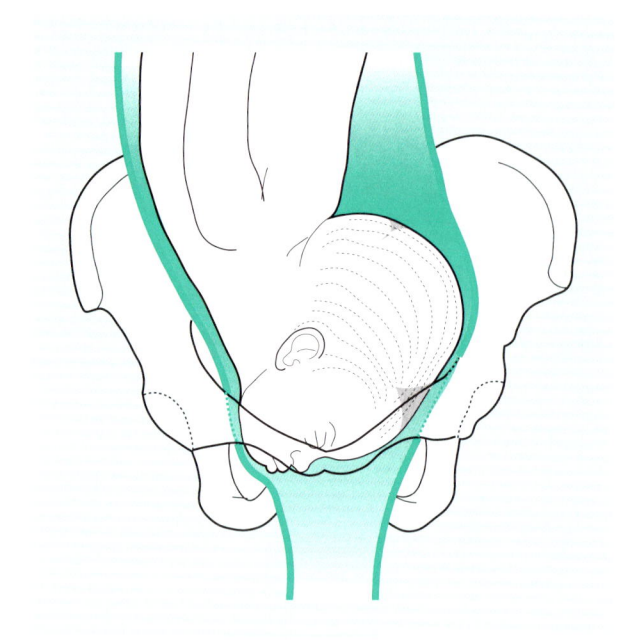

Fig. 39.18 Vaginal delivery of face presentation.

anterior position to correct delay in the second stage.

The face is nearly always swollen and bruised following a face presentation, and the parents should be warned about this. Care must be taken during vaginal examination, because the fetal eyes can be damaged by trauma or antiseptic lotions.

Brow presentation
The incidence of brow presentation is approximately 1 in 500 labors and the causes are the same as for a face presentation.

Brow presentation should be suspected on abdominal palpation when there is prominence of the head on the side of the back in the presence of an unengaged head. Vaginal examination reveals a high presenting part, a palpable forehead with orbital ridges in front and the anterior fontanelle behind.

Mechanism of labor
The membranes tend to rupture early in labor and there is an increased risk of cord prolapse. With a brow presentation, the mentovertical diameter—one of the longest diameters of the fetal head (13 cm)—presents. An average-sized fetus will not engage with a normal-sized pelvis and obstructed labor results. When the fetal head is small in relation to the maternal pelvis descent might occur, allowing flexion of the head as it hits the pelvic floor.

In the absence of disproportion, labor should be allowed to continue. Further extension might occur to a face presentation or flexion to a vertex position.

Malposition

The fetal head normally engages in an occipitotransverse position. With descent, the head rotates to an occipitoanterior position, presenting the narrowest diameter for delivery through the outlet. Any position that does not follow this pattern is regarded as a malposition; the two most important are:
- Occiput posterior (OP) position.
- Deep transverse arrest.

Theoretically, brow and face presentations could be regarded as malpositions, but they are more commonly regarded as malpresentations.

Occiput posterior position
In approximately 20% of women, in early labor the fetus will present with an OP position.

Anthropoid and android pelvises, which have an anteroposterior diameter equal to or greater than the transverse diameter, predispose to an OP position. An anterior placenta is said to be associated with OP position.

An OP position is the most common cause of an unengaged head at term in a primigravida. Abdominal palpation reveals:
- A prominent fundus.
- A lower abdomen that is flattened or concave.
- A fetal back that can be palpated posteriorly.
- Fetal limbs that can be palpated anteriorly.

In labor, vaginal examination will ascertain the position by identifying the sutures and fontanelles. If the anterior fontanelle is at all palpable vaginally, then the head is deflexed. If only the posterior fontanelle can be palpated, then the head is well flexed. The degree of flexion of the head is important in the mechanism of labor.

Mechanism of labor

If the occipitofrontal diameter (11.5 cm) presents to a borderline pelvis then engagement will not occur, resulting in an obstructed labor requiring cesarean section. If the pelvis is adequate and the fetus not macrosomic, then the mechanism of labor with an OP position depends on the degree of flexion of the fetal head. When the head is well flexed, rotation to an anterior position usually occurs as the occiput hits the pelvic floor first and rotates forward. When the head is deflexed, a persistent OP position is usual, although delivery in an OP position is possible if the pelvis is large enough.

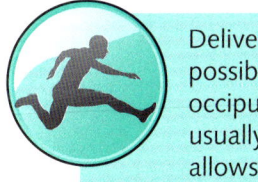

> Delivery of an OP position is possible, but rotation and occiput anterior delivery is usually preferable because this allows better flexion of the head and, therefore, less perineal trauma.

The first stage of labor should be managed in the normal way. During the second stage, if the head rotates anteriorly then normal delivery can be anticipated. An episiotomy is recommended if the fetus is delivered OP because a wider diameter presents and increases the risk of severe perineal trauma. If rotation fails to occur spontaneously, then this can be achieved using the following techniques:
- Manual rotation.
- Rotational forceps.
- Vacuum extraction with spontaneous rotation.

Excluding those women who require cesarean section for CPD, the outcome for an OP position in labor is as follows:
- 70% rotate and spontaneously deliver occipitoanterior.
- 10% fail to rotate and deliver OP.
- 20% need assistance with rotation.

Deep transverse arrest

Deep transverse arrest is said to have occurred when a poorly flexed head arrests in the transverse position at the level of the ischial spines.

Deep transverse arrest usually occurs when a transverse position fails to rotate to an anterior position. The head is neither flexed enough for the occiput nor extended enough for the brow to influence rotation. An android pelvis, where the side walls are convergent, can prevent descent of the head to the pelvic floor, where rotation normally occurs.

Diagnosis is by vaginal examination in the presence of failure to progress in the second stage of labor. The head is at the level of the ischial spines, the sagittal suture is in the transverse position, and both anterior and posterior fontanelles are usually palpable.

Rotation is required and can be achieved either manually or by rotational forceps. The fetal head should not be rotated in the presence of fetal acidosis, because intraventricular hemorrhage might be precipitated. Cesarean section is indicated in this situation.

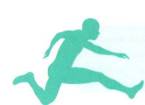

- What is the difference between a malposition and a malpresentation?
- What are the possible reasons for a malpresentation?
- What are the different types of breech presentation and what are their relative risks with regard to vaginal delivery?

Further reading

Gabbe SG, et al. (2002) *Obstetrics: Normal and Problem Pregnancies*, 4th ed. (Churchill Livingstone).

Hannah ME, et al. (2000) Planned caesarean section versus planned vaginal birth for breech presentation at term: a randomized multicentre trial. *Lancet* 356(9239):1368–9.

40. Labor

Labor is divided into three stages:
- First stage: from the onset of established labor until the cervix is fully dilated.
- Second stage: from full dilatation until the fetus is born.
- Third stage: from the birth of the fetus until delivery of the placenta and membranes.

Onset of labor

Prior to the onset of labor, painless intermittent uterine tightenings, known as Braxton Hicks contractions, become increasingly frequent. As the presenting part becomes engaged, the fundus descends, reducing upper abdominal discomfort, and pressure in the pelvis increases. The signs and symptoms that define the actual onset of labor are:
- Painful regular contractions.
- A "show" (passage of a mucoid plug from the cervix, often blood stained).
- Rupture of the membranes.
- Cervical dilatation and effacement.

Labor is diagnosed when there are regular painful contractions in the presence of an effaced cervix, which is 3 cm or more dilated, with or without a show or ruptured membranes.

The exact cause of the onset of labor is not known. To some degree it might be mechanical, because preterm labor is seen more commonly in circumstances in which the uterus is overstretched, such as multiple pregnancies and polyhydramnios. Prostaglandins might play a role; they are thought to be present in the decidua and membranes in late pregnancy and are released if the cervix is digitally stretched at term to separate the membranes ("stripping of membranes").

Progress in labor

Once the diagnosis of labor has been made, progress is assessed by monitoring:
- Uterine contractions.
- Dilatation of the cervix.
- Descent of the presenting part.

The rate of cervical dilatation is expected to be approximately 1 cm/h in a nulliparous woman and approximately 2 cm/h in a multiparous woman. A labor curve is commonly used to chart the observations made in labor (Fig. 40.1) and to highlight slow progress, particularly a delay in cervical dilatation or failure of the presenting part to descend (see Chapter 15).

Progress is determined by the three factors:
- Passages.
- Passenger.
- Powers.

Passages
Bony pelvis
The pelvis is made up of four bones, the:
- Two innominate bones.
- Sacrum.
- Coccyx.

The passage that these bones make can be divided into inlet, cavity and outlet (Fig. 40.2). The pelvic inlet is bounded by the pubic crest, the iliopectineal line, and the sacral promontory. It is oval in shape, with its longest diameter being transverse. The cavity of the pelvis is round in shape. The pelvic outlet is bounded by the lower border of the pubic symphysis, the ischial spines, and the tip of the sacrum. Again, the shape is oval, but with the larger diameter being anteroposterior (Fig. 40.3).

When a woman stands upright, the pelvis tilts forward. The inlet makes an angle of about 55° with the horizontal; this varies between individuals and different ethnic groups. The presenting part of the fetus must negotiate the axis of the birth canal, with the change of direction occurring by rotation at the pelvic floor.

Soft tissues
The soft passages consist of:
- Uterus (upper and lower segments).
- Cervix.
- Pelvic floor.
- Vagina.
- Perineum.

Labor

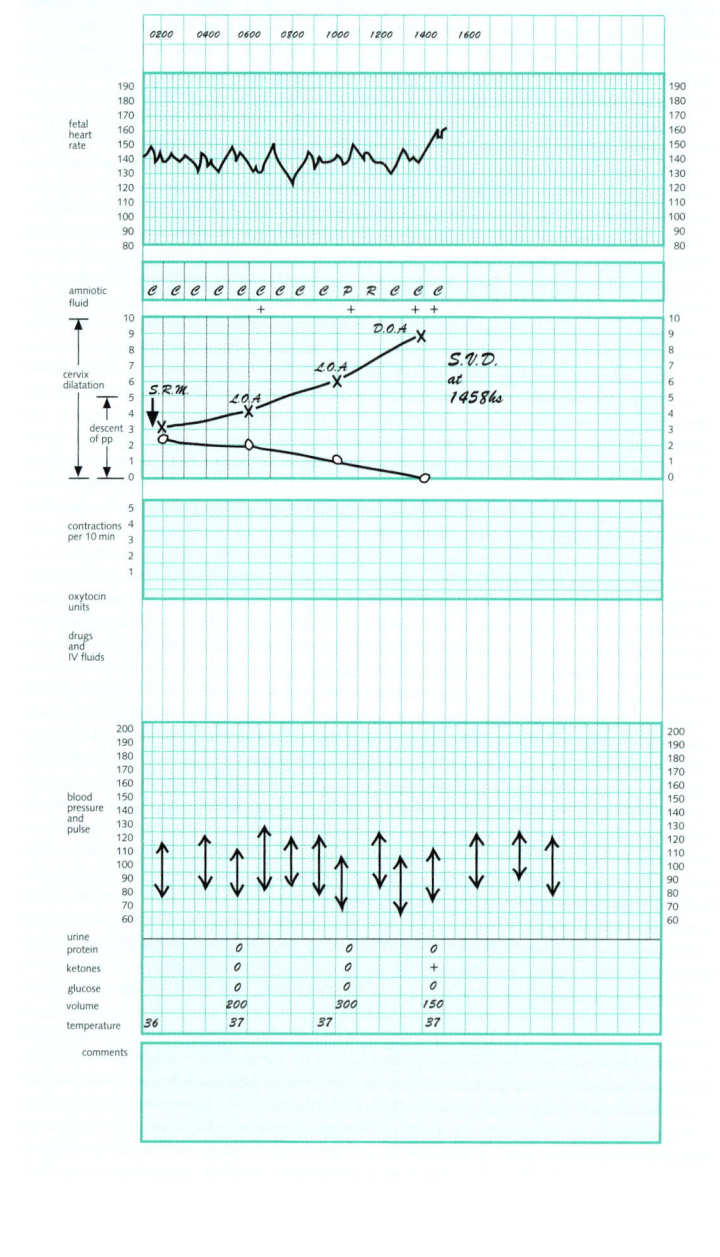

Fig. 40.1 A labor curve.

The upper uterine segment consists mainly of the fundus and is responsible for the propulsive contractions that deliver the fetus. The lower segment is the part of the uterus that lies between the uterovesical fold of the peritoneum and the cervix. It develops gradually during the third trimester, and then more rapidly during labor, incorporating the cervix, to allow the presenting part to descend.

The pelvic floor consists of the levator ani group of muscles, including pubococcygeus and iliococcygeus arising from the bony pelvis to form a muscular diaphragm along with the internal obturator muscle and piriformis muscle (see Chapter 27). As the presenting part of the fetus is pushed out of the uterus it passes into the vagina, which has become hypertrophied during pregnancy. It hits the pelvic floor, which acts like a

Progress in labor

Fig. 40.2 The bony pelvis.

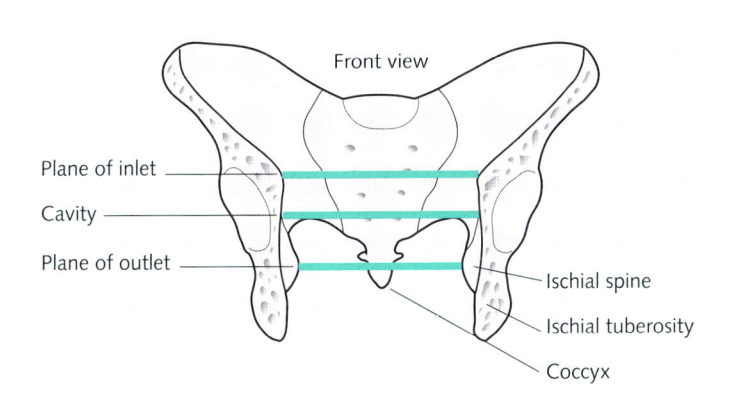

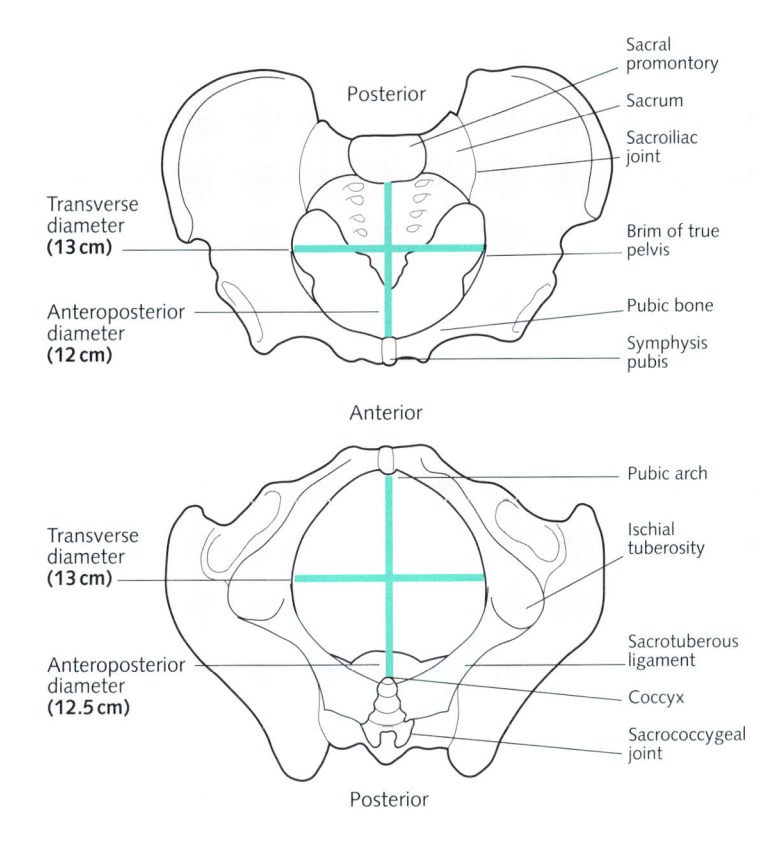

Fig. 40.3 The dimensions of the pelvic inlet and the pelvic outlet.

gutter to direct it forward and allow rotation. The perineum is distal to this and stretches as the head passes below the pubic arch and delivers.

Passenger

The fetal skull consists of the face and the cranium. The cranium is made up of two parietal bones, two frontal bones, and the occipital bone, held together by a membrane that allows movement. Up until early childhood, these bones are not fused and so can overlap to allow the head to pass through the pelvis during labor; this overlapping of the bones is known as molding.

Labor

Figure 40.4 shows the anatomy of the fetal skull, including the sutures between the bones, and the fontanelles. These are important landmarks that can be felt on vaginal examination and enable the position of the fetus to be assessed.

The size and presentation of the fetal skull determine the ease with which the fetus passes through the birth canal. Figure 40.5 shows the diameters of the fetal skull. The one that presents during labor depends on the degree of flexion of the head; thus, the suboccipitobregmatic diameter represents a flexed vertex presentation, giving the smallest diameter for delivery, along with the submentobregmatic diameter, which corresponds to a face presentation. The widest diameter is the mentovertical one, a brow presentation, which usually precludes vaginal delivery.

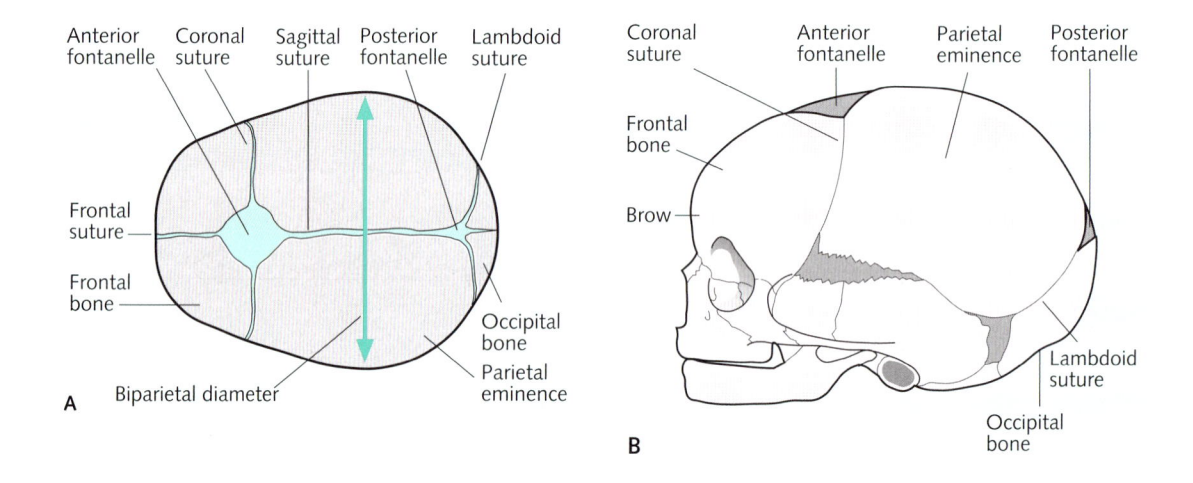

Fig. 40.4 The fetal skull from above (A) and from the side (B), showing the landmarks.

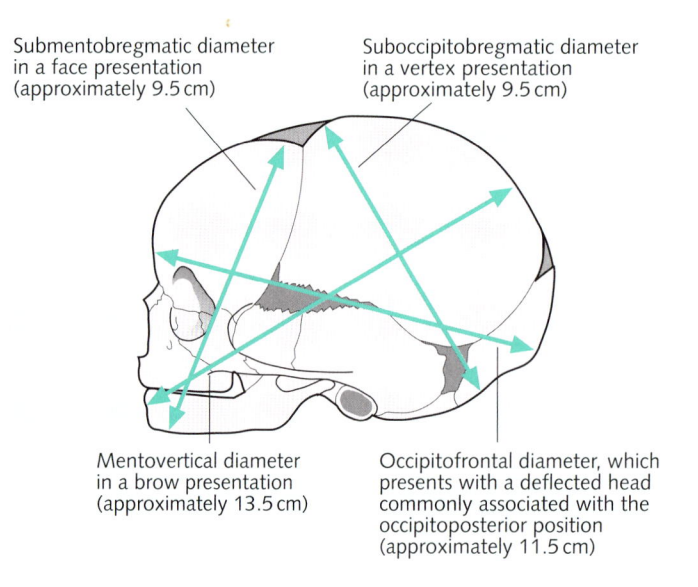

Fig. 40.5 Diameters of the fetal skull.

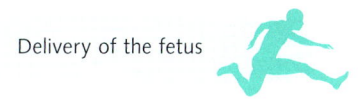

Power

The myometrial component of the uterus acts as the power to deliver the fetus. It consists of three layers:
- Thin outer longitudinal layer.
- Thin inner circular layer.
- Thick middle spiral layer.

From early pregnancy, the uterus contracts painlessly and intermittently (Braxton Hicks contractions). These contractions increase after the 36th week until the onset of labor. Each contraction starts from the junction of the fallopian tube and the uterus on one side, spreading down and across the uterus with its greatest intensity in the upper uterine segment.

During labor, the contractions are monitored for:
- Intensity.
- Frequency.
- Duration.

The resting tone of the uterus is about 6–12 mmHg; to be effective in labor this increases to an intensity of 40–60 mmHg. There should be three or four coordinated contractions every 10 min, each lasting 60–90 s.

In the second stage of labor, additional power comes from voluntary contraction of the diaphragm and the abdominal muscles as the mother pushes to assist delivery.

Mechanisms of normal delivery: action of the uterus

The myometrium acts like all muscle, i.e. it contracts and relaxes, but it also has the ability to retract so that the fibers become progressively shorter. This effect is seen in the upper segment muscle: progressive retraction causes the lower segment to stretch and thin out, resulting in effacement and dilatation of the cervix (Fig. 40.6).

Delivery of the fetus

Active contractions of the uterus of increasing strength, frequency, and duration cause passive movement of the fetus down the birth canal. At the beginning of labor, the lie, presentation, and engagement of the fetus are assessed (see Chapter 46). As labor progresses (Fig. 40.7), the neck becomes fully flexed so that the

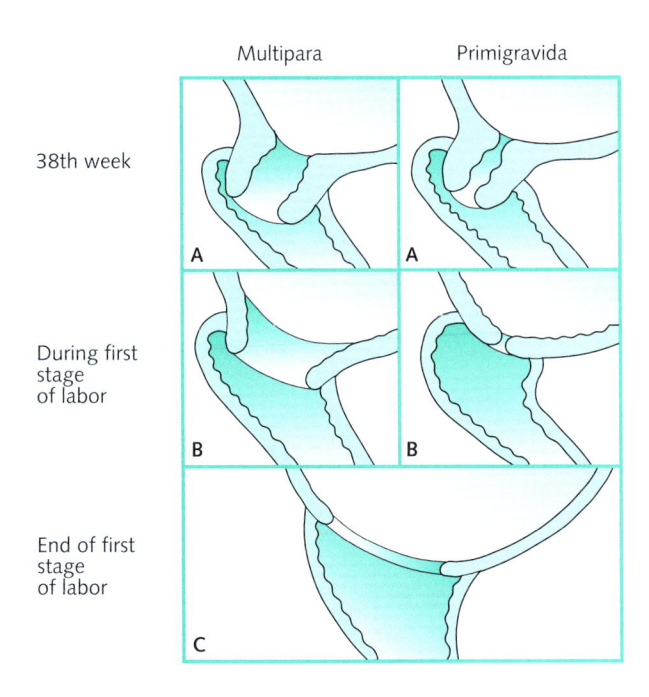

Fig. 40.6 Dilatation and effacement of the cervix in late pregnancy and labor.

Labor

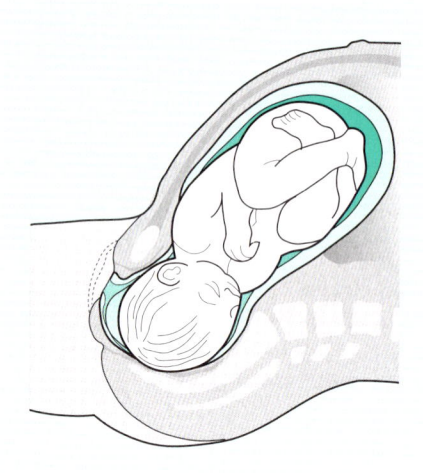

Fig. 40.7 Early labor. There has been flexion of the fetal head. The cervix is effaced but has not yet begun to dilate.

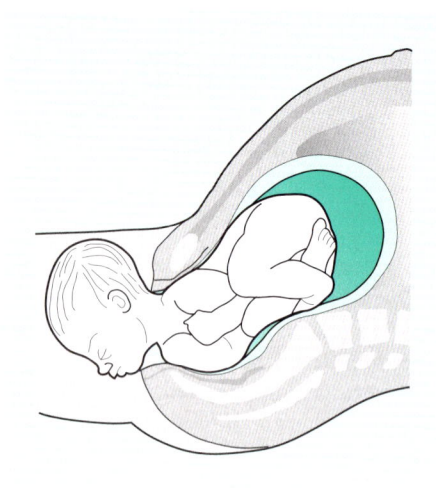

Fig. 40.9 Delivery of the head. Extension of the fetal neck occurs as the head passes under the pubic symphysis to deliver the head. The shoulders are still in the transverse diameter of the midpelvis.

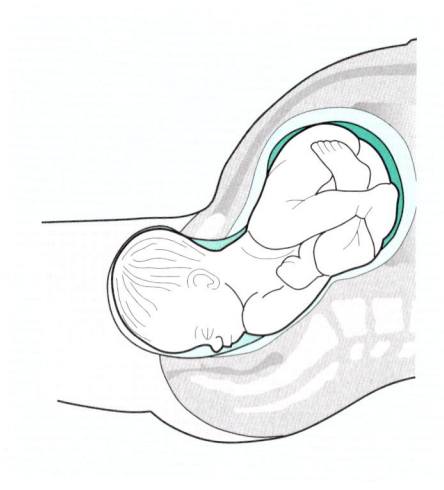

Fig. 40.8 The second stage of labor. The head has undergone internal rotation to bring the occiput into the anterior position. The cervix is fully dilated.

extension round the pubic bone delivers the face (Fig. 40.9).

Delivery of the head brings the shoulders into the pelvic cavity, with the head oblique to the line of the shoulders. Restitution occurs: the head rotates to the natural position in relation to the shoulders (Fig. 40.10). Finally, in the process of external rotation, continuing descent and rotation of the shoulders brings their widest diameter (the bisacromial diameter) into the anteroposterior diameter of the pelvic outlet. This enables the anterior shoulder to pass under the pubic symphysis. Lateral flexion of the fetus delivers the posterior shoulder and the rest of the body follows (Fig. 40.11).

suboccipitobregmatic diameter is presenting (see above).

Descent occurs when the head is engaged, followed by internal rotation to bring the occiput into the anterior position when it reaches the pelvic floor. In the second stage of labor, the occiput descends below the symphysis pubis (Fig. 40.8) and the movement of extension pushes the head forward and delivers the occiput. Increasing

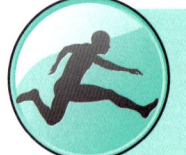

Cardinal movements of labor:
- Engagement.
- Descent.
- Flexion.
- Internal rotation.
- Extension.
- External rotation (restitution).
- Expulsion.

Management of the first stage of labor

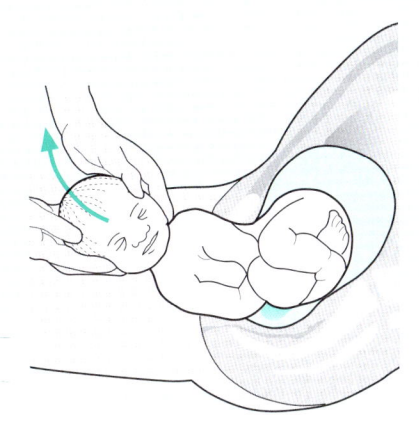

Fig. 40.11 Delivery of the shoulders. The anterior shoulder passes below the pubic symphysis, aided by downwards and backwards traction of the head from the obstetrician. The posterior shoulder delivers as the head is gently lifted upward.

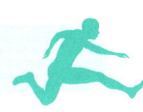

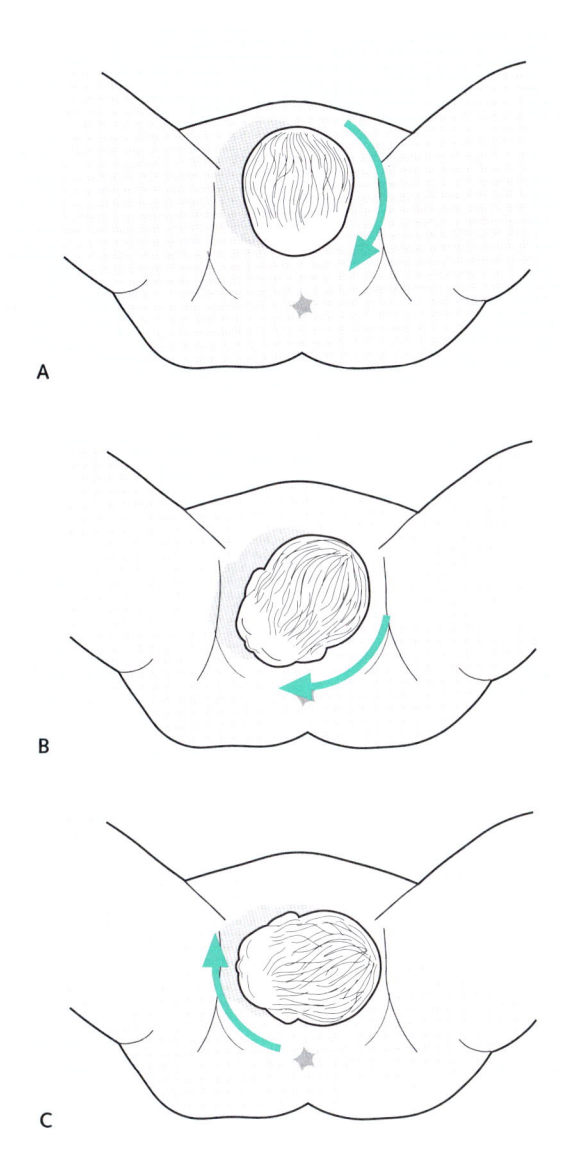

Fig. 40.10 External rotation (restitution). The head distends the perineum as it delivers in the occipitoanterior position and the external rotation occurs.

Management of the first stage of labor

When a patient presents in the first stage of labor, routine assessment includes:
- Mother: pulse, blood pressure, temperature, urinalysis, analgesia requirements.
- Fetus: presentation and engagement of the presenting part, FHR pattern (see Chapter 16).
- Contractions: frequency, duration, intensity.
- Vaginal examination: degree of cervical effacement, cervical dilatation, station of presenting part above ischial spines, position of presenting part, presence of caput or molding.
- Amniotic fluid: clear/blood stained, presence of meconium.

Maternal monitoring

The patient is encouraged to mobilize if possible and might be allowed to eat, depending on her risk of needing an operative procedure. There is delayed gastric emptying during pregnancy and labor and, therefore, a risk of inhalation of regurgitated acid stomach contents, causing aspiration pneumonia if the patient is given a general anesthetic.

The need for analgesia during labor varies markedly between different women, depending on their antenatal preparation. Nonpharmacological techniques include the use of psychoprophylaxis, hypnosis, massage, and transcutaneous electrical nerve stimulation. The pharmacologic methods are summarized in Fig. 40.12.

Fetal monitoring

Different degrees of fetal monitoring are appropriate, depending on the clinical picture. For

Labor

Pharmacologic methods of analgesia in labor

	Technique	Indication	Effectiveness	Duration of effect	Side-effects
Oxygen/nitrous oxide	Inhalation of 50:50 mixture with onset of contraction	First stage	<50% Takes 20–30s for peak effect	Time of inhalation only	Does not relieve pain
Meperidine	Intramuscular injection 25–50 mg	First stage	<50% Takes 15–20 min for peak effect	Approximately 3 h	• Nausea and vomiting—give with an antiemetic • Respiratory depression in the neonate (this is easily reversed with intramuscular naloxone)
Pudendal block	Infiltration of right and left pudendal nerves (S2, S3 and S4) with 0.5% lidocaine	Second stage for operative delivery	Within 5 min	45–90 min	—
Perineal infiltration	Infiltration of perineum with 0.5% lidocaine at posterior fourchette	Second stage prior to episiotomy Third stage for suturing of perineal lacerations	Within 5 min	45–90 min	—
Epidural anesthesia	Injection of 0.25% or 0.5% bupivicaine via a catheter into the epidural space (L3–4)	First or second stage cesarean section	Complete pain relief in approximately 95% of women	Bolus injection every 3–4 h or continuous infusion	• Transient hypotension—give intravenous fluid load • Dural tap • Risk of hemorrhage if abnormal maternal clotting • Increased length of second stage because of reduced pelvic floor tone and loss of bearing-down reflex
Spinal anesthesia	Injection of 0.5% bupivicaine into the subarachnoid space	Any operative delivery; manual removal of the placenta	Immediate effect	Single injection lasting 3–4 h	Respiratory depression

Fig. 40.12 Pharmacologic methods of analgesia in labor.

238

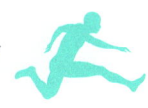

example, continuous fetal monitoring is advisable in a high-risk pregnancy, such as the presence of IUGR or if there is meconium-stained amniotic fluid (see Chapter 16). In a low-risk pregnancy, intermittent monitoring might be sufficient, approximately every 15 min during and after a contraction.

In some patients, abdominal monitoring can be difficult, e.g. if the patient is obese, and so a fetal scalp electrode can be applied directly once the membranes are ruptured. If monitoring suggests that the FHR pattern is abnormal, then it might be appropriate to measure the fetal pH by taking a blood sample from the fetal scalp (see Chapter 16).

Management of the second stage of labor

Once the cervix is fully dilated, the patient is encouraged to use voluntary effort to push with the contractions. If she has an epidural anesthetic in situ she might be unaware of an urge to push, and so a further hour can be allowed for the presenting part to descend with the contractions alone.

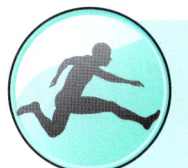

> Descent of the presenting part (fetal station) is assessed during vaginal exam in relation of the presenting part to the level of the ischial spines.
> - Zero is at the level of the ischial spines.
> - Negative 1–3 is 1–3 cm above the ischial spines.
> - Positive 1–3 is 1–3 cm below the ischial spines.

Delivery of the infant is conducted as a sterile procedure, in the left lateral or dorsal position. As the head descends, the perineum distends and the anus dilates. Then the head crowns: the BPD has passed through the pelvis and there is no recession between contractions. The attendant applies pressure on the perineum to maintain flexion of the head and, once the occiput is free, encourages extension to allow delivery. The neck is felt to exclude the presence of the cord.

After external rotation, lateral flexion of the head towards the anus dislodges the anterior shoulder with the next contraction. Lifting the head in the opposite direction delivers the posterior shoulder. Holding the shoulders, the rest of the body is delivered either onto the bed or the mother's abdomen. Finally, the cord is clamped and cut.

Management of the third stage of labor

Active management of the third stage has been shown to reduce the incidence of PPH (see Chapter 42). Management involves:
- Using an oxytocic drug.
- Clamping and cutting the cord.
- Controlled cord traction.

In most units, oxytocin (20 units in 1000 mL isotonic solution) is given with delivery of the anterior shoulder; it takes about 2–3 min to act. As the placenta detaches from the uterine wall, it descends into the lower segment and the cut cord will appear to lengthen. There is slight bleeding, and the fundus becomes hard. Suprapubic pressure along with controlled cord traction is commonly used, once the placenta has separated, to reduce the incidence of uterine inversion (Fig. 40.13). The

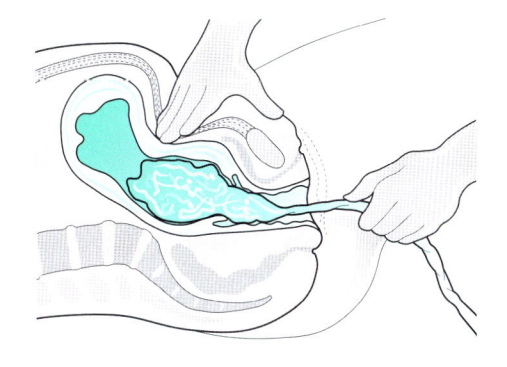

Fig. 40.13 Controlled cord traction to deliver the placenta.

239

placenta and membranes must be checked to ensure that they are complete.

Finally, the vagina, labia, and perineum are examined for lacerations. The uterine fundus is palpated to check that it is well contracted, approximately at the level of the umbilicus. The estimated blood loss should be recorded.

Induction of labor

Definition
Induction of labor is the artificial initiation of uterine contractions prior to spontaneous onset, resulting in delivery of the baby.

Indications
The rate of induction varies widely between different institutions and even within different institutions. Figure 40.14 shows possible reasons for induction of labor, maternal or fetal. In the US, the most common indication is prolonged pregnancy.

Methods
Prior to induction of labor, the favorability of the cervix should be assessed to give an indication of the likely success of the procedure. This is usually done by using the Bishop score (see Chapter 46); a higher score suggests a more favorable cervix.

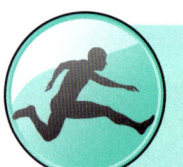

With regard to the Bishop score to assess the cervix:
- Unfavorable cervix = hard, long, closed, not effaced (low Bishop score).
- Favorable cervix = soft, beginning to dilate and efface (high Bishop score).

Prostaglandins
Local application of a prostaglandin, usually prostaglandin E2, given as a vaginal gel, has been shown to ripen the cervix as part of the induction process and reduce the incidence of operative delivery when compared with use of oxytocin alone (see below). Used locally, the GI side effects are minimized. Strict guidelines have been produced to restrict the dose of prostaglandin given, to reduce the risk of uterine hyperstimulation.

Amniotomy
Artificial rupture of the membranes is thought to cause local secretion of endogenous prostaglandins, and thus is performed using an amnihook. It might be part of the induction process, or accelerate slow progress in labor. It can also be done with an abnormal FHR strip to exclude meconium-staining of the amniotic fluid, or to apply a fetal scalp electrode.

Oxytocin
An intravenous infusion of synthetic oxytocin (pitocin) is commonly used to induce labor, to stimulate contractions after amniotomy. The dose must be carefully titrated according to the strength and frequency of the uterine contractions, and continuous fetal monitoring is necessary. Uses of oxytocin include:
- To augment labor after spontaneous rupture of the membranes without the onset of contractions.
- In primary dysfunctional labor (see below).

Complications
Figure 40.15 lists the possible complications associated with the use of amniotomy and oxytocin.

Indications for the induction of labor	
Type of indication	Description
Maternal	Severe pre-eclampsia
	Diabetes
	Social
Fetal	Prolonged pregnancy
	Intrauterine growth restriction

Fig. 40.14 Indications for the induction of labor.

Amniotomy and oxytocin associated complications	
Treatment	Complication
Amniotomy	Cord prolapse
	Infection
	Bleeding from a vasa previa
	Placental separation
	Failure to induce efficient contractions
	Amniotic fluid embolism
Oxytocin	Abnormal FHR pattern
	Hyperstimulation of the uterus
	Rupture of the uterus
	Water intoxication

Fig. 40.15 Complications associated with the use of amniotomy and oxytocin.

Causes of abnormalities of the bony pelvis	
Type of cause	Description
Congenital	Osteogenesis imperfecta
	Dislocation of the hip
Acquired	Kyphosis of the thoracic or lumbar spine
	Scoliosis of the spine
	Spondylolisthesis
	Pelvic fractures
	Rickets/osteomalacia
	Poliomyelitis in childhood

Fig. 40.16 Causes of abnormalities of the bony pelvis.

Failure to progress in labor

As described above, progress in labor is related to the passages, the passenger (i.e. the baby), and the power.

The diagnosis of labor is made in the presence of regular contractions, with the cervix effaced and at least 3 cm dilated. There might also be a show or ruptured membranes.

Failure to progress related to the bony pelvis

Abnormal bony shape
Antenatal X-ray pelvimetry and routine pelvic assessment by vaginal examination are no longer commonplace. However, certain points in a patient's history and examination can give clues to the likelihood of failure to progress in labor (Fig. 40.16).

Cephalopelvic disproportion
With CPD, the size of the pelvis is not in proportion to the fetus. It should be suspected antenatally if the head does not engage, particularly in a woman of short stature. Usually, a trial of labor is still appropriate, but in some cases an elective cesarean section is planned.

During labor, CPD is diagnosed if the head remains high on abdominal palpation. This is confirmed on vaginal examination by the relationship of the head to the ischial spines (known as the station) and the presence of caput (swelling under the fetal scalp caused by reduction in venous return) and molding.

Failure to progress related to the soft tissues of the pelvis
Uterus
A uterine malformation, such as the presence of a midline septum, might prevent the fetus from lying longitudinally, so that a malpresentation is responsible for failure to progress. This can also be caused by uterine fibroids, which often increase in size during pregnancy and might obstruct labor; a cervical fibroid might even necessitate cesarean section.

Cervix
Failure of the cervix to dilate during labor, despite adequate uterine contractions, may be secondary to

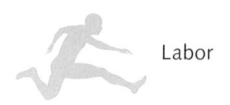

cervical scarring causing cervical stenosis. This could be the result of a LEEP or cone biopsy.

Vagina
Congenital anomalies of the vagina rarely cause problems with respect to labor and delivery, except for patients who have had reconstructive surgery. Other types of surgery, such as a colposuspension for urinary stress incontinence or repair of a vesicovaginal fistula, might indicate the need for an elective cesarean section at term, but more to prevent recurrent symptoms than because of possible slow progress in labor.

Vulva
Previous perineal tears or episiotomy should not present difficulties during delivery. More problematic is a female circumcision, which usually necessitates an elective episiotomy to prevent more severe tears and the risk of fistula formation.

Ovary
Ovarian cysts in pregnancy are usually incidental findings at routine ultrasound. They can present with abdominal pain during pregnancy, secondary to torsion or hemorrhage (see Chapter 12). Rarely, they cause slow progress in labor if they fail to rise up out of the pelvis as the uterus increases in size.

Failure to progress related to the passenger
Fetal size
The possibility of a large infant might be suggested by the patient's past medical history, e.g. insulin-dependent diabetes or from the antenatal history, with development of gestational diabetes or fetal hydrops secondary to rhesus isoimmunization or parvovirus infection (see Chapter 11).

Abdominal palpation is not particularly accurate as a method of diagnosing a large baby, although it should be suspected if the presenting part fails to engage in labor. Ultrasound is more accurate, provided that gestational age has been correctly estimated early in pregnancy. During labor, signs of CPD may indicate a large infant (see above).

Fetal abnormality
Routine ultrasound scanning is likely to diagnose abnormalities such as a congenital goiter or a lymphangioma. These extend the neck, resulting in a face presentation. Abdominal enlargement, such as in the presence of ascites or an umbilical hernia, may make delivery difficult.

Abnormalities of the fetal skull, such as anencephaly, should be suspected in labor if the head does not engage and the sutures feel widely spaced on vaginal examination.

Fetal malposition
Labor is more prolonged if the occiput is in the posterior or transverse position. This can be determined abdominally by easy palpation of fetal parts and confirmed on vaginal examination by checking the positions of the sutures and fontanelles (see Chapter 46).

Fetal malpresentation
Malpresentation of the fetus is defined as a nonvertex presentation (see Chapter 39). This can be:
- Face.
- Brow.
- Breech.
- Shoulder.

Failure to progress related to the power
Uterine palpation monitors frequency, duration, and intensity of the contractions. The tocometer checks the frequency and duration, but the recording of the intensity can be altered by position of the monitor on the abdomen and maternal obesity. In some facilities, intrauterine-pressure catheters are used to monitor contraction pressure. Inefficient uterine action can be diagnosed if labor is prolonged and the contractions are:
- Uncoordinated.
- Fewer than three or four in 10 min.
- Lasting less than 60 s.
- Less than 40 mmHg.

CPD and a malpresentation should be excluded. Then, careful use of oxytocic drugs, most commonly intravenous pitocin infusion, can improve the contractions. Caution must be taken to avoid too frequent contractions, because this can reduce the oxygen exchange in the placental bed and lead to fetal hypoxia. Continuous electronic monitoring is advisable.

Particular care is essential in a multiparous patient because the diagnosis of inefficient uterine action is much less common than in a primiparous patient. A fetal malposition, malpresentation, or fetal size should be considered as the causes of the slow progress; inappropriate use of oxytocic drugs is more commonly associated with uterine rupture in this group.

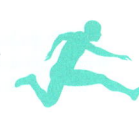

- How do you diagnose labor?
- What maternal factors affect the progress of labor?
- What fetal factors affect the progress of labor?
- What comprises active management of the third stage of labor?
- What are the interventions in induction of labor, and their complications?

Further reading
Gabbe SG, et al. (2002) *Obstetrics: Normal and Problem Pregnancies*, 4th ed. (Churchill Livingstone, New York).

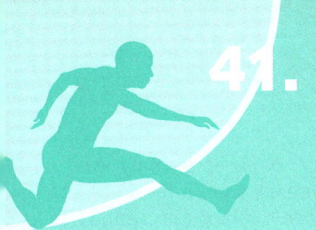

41. Operative Intervention in Obstetrics

For all interventions in obstetrics, the following general principles apply:
- Make sure all documentation includes the time and date, and a legible signature.
- Clearly record the indication for the intervention, the abdominal and vaginal examination findings as appropriate, and the operative findings, including any complications.
- Obtain informed consent from the patient, either verbal or written, depending on the procedure.

Episiotomy

The purpose of an episiotomy is to increase the diameter of the vulval outlet by making an incision in the perineal body. The indications for this procedure are shown in Fig. 41.1. Since the 1980s, the routine episiotomy rate has been reduced dramatically because studies have demonstrated its association with increased blood loss, as well as long-term morbidity such as pain and dyspareunia.

To make them easier to remember, the indications for any intervention can be divided into maternal and fetal.

Two techniques are used for episiotomy (Fig. 41.2). Both should be performed with adequate analgesia, either an epidural or perineal infiltration with local anesthetic, and should start in the midline at the posterior fourchette.

1. Midline: this technique is widely used in the US and, although it is easier to repair and likely to result in less postpartum pain, it is more likely to involve the anal sphincter if it extends.
2. Mediolateral: widely used in the UK, this type of incision is more likely to protect the anal sphincter if the incision extends during delivery.

Repair of an episiotomy should be performed by an experienced operator. There should be adequate light and appropriate analgesia. A three-layer

Indications for episiotomy

Type of indication	Description
Maternal	Female circumcision
	Consider if previous perineal reconstructive surgery
Fetal	Shoulder dystocia
	To precipitate delivery in cases of an abnormal FHR tracing when the presenting part is on the perineum
	Consider in instrumental delivery
	Consider in breech delivery

Fig. 41.1 Indications for episiotomy.

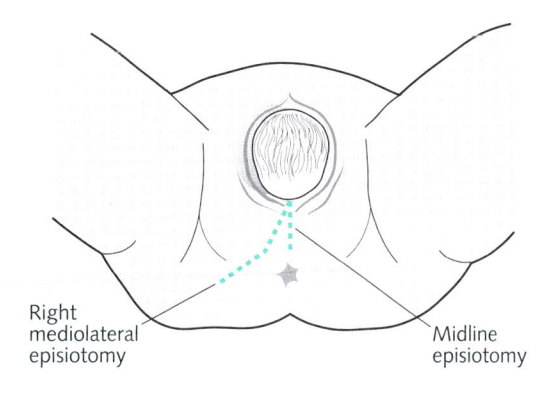

Fig. 41.2 Types of incision for episiotomy.

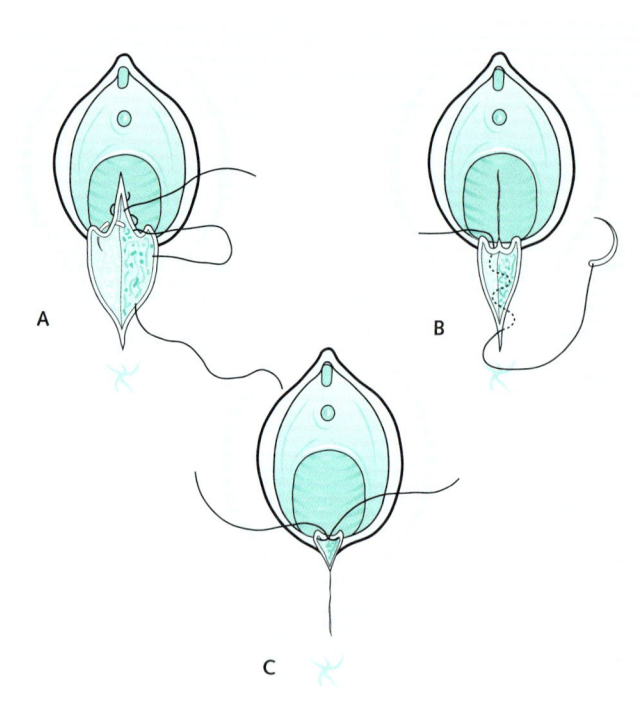

Fig. 41.3 Repair of an episiotomy. A. Suturing the vaginal wall. B. Suturing the perineal muscles. C. Tying the strands together—the knot disappears beneath the vaginal mucosa.

technique is usual with absorbable subcuticular sutures (Fig. 41.3):
- First layer, vaginal skin: identify the apex of the incision and suture in a continuous layer to the hymen to oppose the cut edges of the posterior fourchette.
- Second layer, perineal body: deep sutures to realign the muscles of the perineal body.
- Third layer, perineal skin: continuous or interrupted subcuticular sutures to close the skin.

At the end of the procedure, all needles and swabs should be checked. An examination of the vagina should be performed to ensure that the apex of the episiotomy is secure. Rectal examination should ensure that the rectal mucosa has not been broached by any deep sutures, because this can result in fistula formation.

Perineal repair

Approximately 70% of mothers who deliver vaginally will sustain some degree of perineal trauma. This can be classified as:

- first degree: involves skin only.
- second degree: involves skin and perineal muscle.
- third degree: includes partial or complete rupture of the anal sphincter.
- fourth degree: as for 3rd degree, but with the tear involving the anal mucosa.

The principles for repair are the same as for episiotomy. Some first-degree tears can be allowed to heal by secondary intention if they are not actively bleeding. It is very important to recognize and repair appropriately any damage to the anal sphincter or mucosa; failure to do so can result in long-term morbidity, such as incontinence of flatus or feces (this occurs in approximately 5% of women).

Vacuum delivery

Since the 1950s, when the vacuum extractor was invented in Sweden, it has increasingly been seen as the instrument of choice for assisted vaginal delivery. Metal cups were used initially, either anterior or posterior, and subsequently silicone

Forceps delivery

Indications for vacuum delivery

Type of indication	Description
Maternal	Delay in 2nd stage due to maternal exhaustion
Fetal	Delay in 2nd stage due to fetal malposition (occipitoposterior or occipitotransverse position)
	Abnormal FHR tracing

Fig. 41.4 Indications for vacuum delivery.

Criteria for instrumental vaginal delivery

1. Adequate analgesia: perineal infiltration/pudendal block/epidural anesthesia (see Chapter 40)
2. Abdominal examination: estimation of fetal size—suspicion of fetal macrosomia relative contraindication
3. Vaginal examination: cervix fully dilated—head below the ischial spines, known fetal position, note presence of caput or molding
4. Adequate maternal effort and regular contractions necessary for vacuum delivery
5. Empty bladder for forceps delivery

Fig. 41.5 Criteria for instrumental vaginal delivery.

rubber cups were developed; the former are more likely to be associated with vaginal trauma, but they might be more appropriate for delivery in certain situations, such as the presence of excessive caput on the fetal head. Both types are available in different diameters, depending on the gestation of the fetus. It is not an appropriate instrument at less than 34 weeks gestation.

Indications for vacuum delivery
These are shown in Fig. 41.4.

Technique for vacuum
The criteria shown in Fig. 41.5 must be fulfilled. Instrumental delivery should not be attempted if the head is above the ischial spines because of the risks to the fetus—a cesarean section is indicated.

Both types of cup rely on the same technique. The cup is applied in the midline over the occiput, avoiding the surrounding vaginal mucosa; the pressure in the connecting pump is raised to $-0.8\,kg/cm^2$.

Complications of instrumental delivery

Type of complication	Description
Maternal	Genital tract trauma (cervical/vaginal/vulvar) with risk of hemorrhage and/or infection
Fetal	Vacuum delivery is likely to cause neonatal scalp injuries or, less commonly, a cephalohematoma (subperiosteal bleed)
	Forceps can cause bruising if not appropriately applied, or possibly facial nerve palsy or depression skull fracture

Fig. 41.6 Complications of instrumental delivery.

Traction with the maternal contractions and with maternal effort should be along the pelvic curve, i.e. initially in a downwards direction and then changing the angle upwards as the head crowns. This action basically mimics the passage of the fetal head during a normal delivery, but uses the vacuum pump to increase traction and flexion.

The operator should judge whether an episiotomy is needed and the procedure should be complete within approximately 15 min of cup application. The tracing should monitor the FHR throughout and, in most facilities, it is standard practice for a neonatologist to be present. Complications are listed in Fig. 41.6.

Forceps delivery

Over the last three or four centuries, forceps have been used for delivery. There are two main types of forceps (Fig. 41.7):
- Nonrotational or traction forceps (Simpson's, Anderson's, Neville–Barnes, or Wrigley's).
- Rotational forceps (Keilland's).

Indications for forceps
These differ slightly from those for the vacuum, mainly because the vacuum requires maternal effort and adequate contractions (Fig. 41.8). Nonrotational forceps are suitable only for certain positions of the fetal head: direct occipitoanterior or direct occipitoposterior.

247

Operative Intervention in Obstetrics

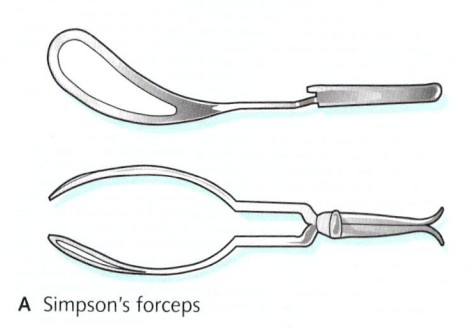

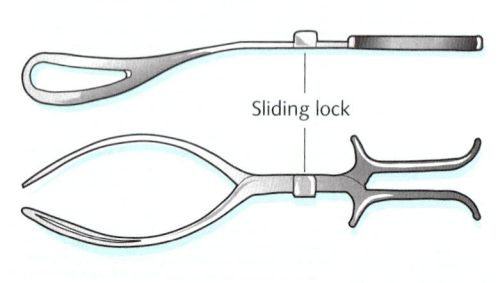

A Simpson's forceps

Sliding lock

B Keilland's forceps

Fig. 41.7 Types of forceps.

Indications for forceps rather than vacuum delivery		
Type of indication	Description
Maternal	Medical conditions complicating labor, e.g. cardiovascular disease
	Unconscious mother, i.e. conditions where the mother is unable to assist with pushing
Fetal	Gestation less than 34 weeks
	Face presentation
	Known or suspected fetal bleeding disorder
	Aftercoming head of a breech
	At cesarean section

Fig. 41.8 Indications for forceps rather than vacuum delivery.

By contrast, the mode of action of the vacuum cup allows rotation to take place during traction, and so it is suitable for a malposition (see Chapter 15). With a decline in the use of rotational forceps in some facilities due to fetal and maternal complications, it is essential to define the fetal position before attempting delivery so that the appropriate instrument is chosen.

Technique for forceps
As for the vacuum, the necessary criteria must be fulfilled (see Fig. 41.5). The blades of nonrotational forceps are applied to the head, avoiding trauma to the vaginal walls. The direction of traction is similar to that of the vacuum, with episiotomy more likely to be performed when the head crowns than with the vacuum (Fig. 41.9).

Use of the rotational forceps involves a slightly different technique: the knobs on the blades must always point towards the occiput; asynclitism can be corrected using the sliding mechanism of the handles and then rotation achieved prior to traction in the manner described above.

Cesarean section

Cesarean section was first described by the ancient Egyptians. It was used increasingly throughout the twentieth century, such that rates of 15–20% are now common in the US. The lower segment procedure, i.e. low transverse cesarean section (LTCS), was introduced in the 1920s and has largely replaced the "classical" midline uterine incision. Although the latter is sometimes indicated for preterm delivery with a poorly formed lower segment or for a preterm abnormal lie, it is associated with higher rates of hemorrhage and rupture in future pregnancies (up to 10% for midline operation vs. <1% for lower segment procedure).

Indications for low transverse cesarean section
These are shown in Fig. 41.10.

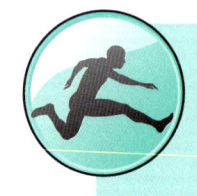

It is not appropriate to attempt an instrumental delivery if the fetal head is above the ischial spines. An LTCS should be performed.

Cesarean section

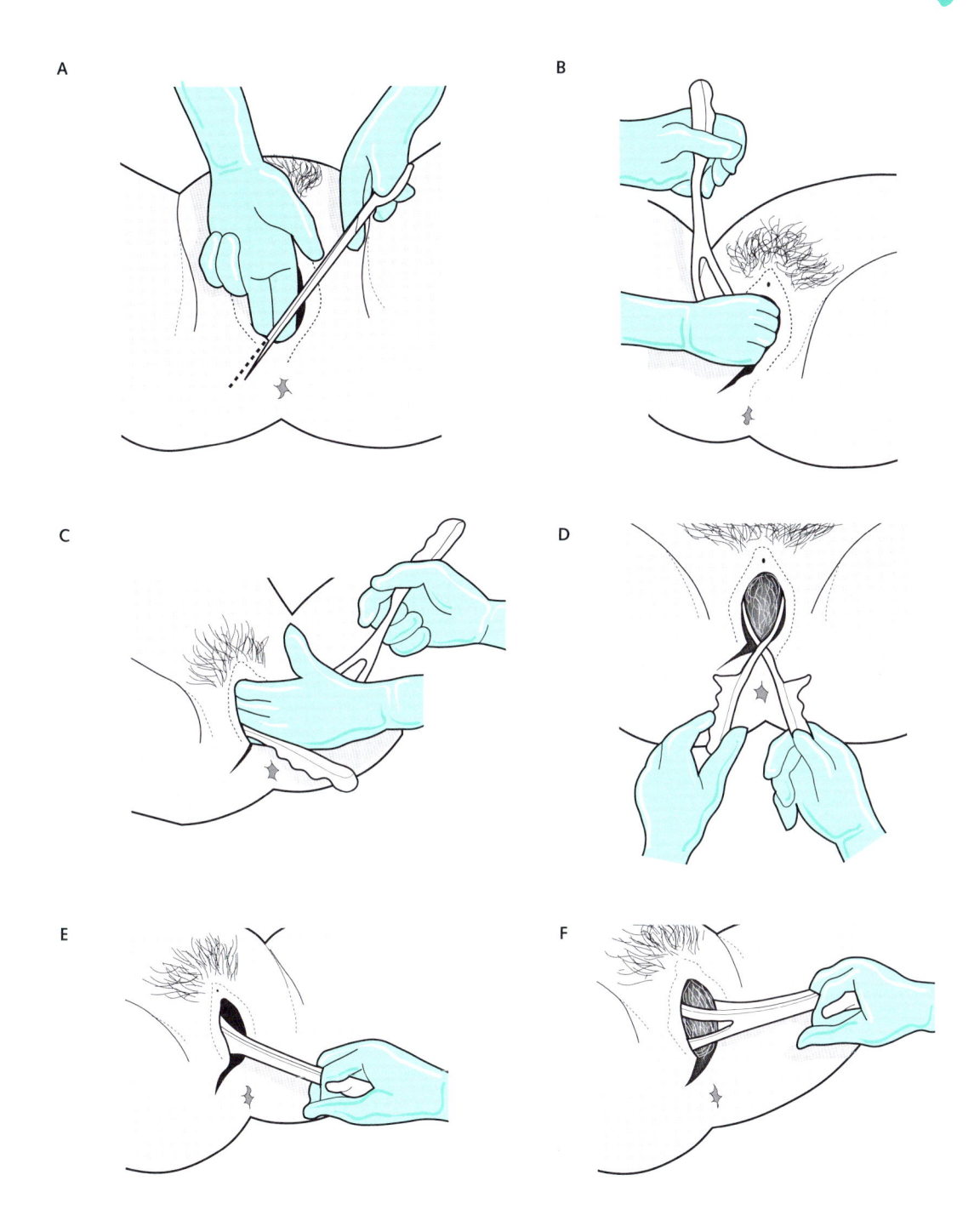

Fig. 41.9 Forceps delivery.

Technique for low transverse cesarean section

Under general or regional analgesia, depending on the indication for LTCS, a low transverse skin incision is made. The rectus sheath is divided and the uterovesical peritoneum is incised to allow the bladder to be reflected inferiorly. The lower uterine segment is

249

Operative Intervention in Obstetrics

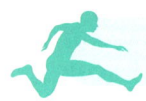

Indications for lower transverse cesarean section	
Type of indication	Description
Maternal	Two previous LTCSs
	Placenta previa
	Maternal disease, e.g. fulminating pre-eclampsia
	Maternal request with no obstetric indication
Fetal	Breech presentation
	Twin pregnancy if the presentation of first twin is not cephalic
	Abnormal FHR tracing or abnormal fetal blood pH
	Cord prolapse
	Delay in first stage of labor, e.g. due to malpresentation or malposition

Fig. 41.10 Indications for LTCS.

incised transversely and the fetus is delivered manually.

Intravenous oxytocin is given by the anesthesiologist and the placenta and membranes are removed. The angles of the uterine incision are secured to ensure hemostasis and then the uterus is closed with an absorbable suture, usually in two layers. The rectus sheath is secured to avoid incisional hernias and finally the skin is closed with either an absorbable or nonabsorbable suture.

Complications of low transverse cesarean section

Although LTCS has become an increasingly safe procedure, particularly with the introduction of regional anesthesia, there is still significant morbidity associated with it:

- Hemorrhage: it is important to cross-match blood for certain patients (e.g. those with placenta previa).
- Gastric aspiration: particularly with general anesthetic (aspiration pneumonia); this is reduced by routine use of antacids.
- Infection: reduced by routine use of prophylactic antibiotics.
- TED: consider prophylaxis in all patients.
- Future pregnancy: subject to trial of labor (see below) or repeat cesarean section with an increasing risk of complications.

Trial of labor

In patients who have had a pregnancy complicated by cesarean section, options for future deliveries should be discussed. In the case of a classical cesarean, the possibility of scar rupture is high (up to 10%) and thus repeat cesarean would be recommended.

With LTCS for a nonrepeatable cause, e.g. cord prolapse, then a trial of vaginal delivery might be appropriate, providing the patient is fully counseled. Certain measures are advisable during labor to exclude the possibility of scar rupture, which would mean immediate cesarean section:

- Intravenous cannula.
- CBC and T&S sample available in laboratory.
- Continuous FHR monitoring.
- Monitor vaginal blood loss to exclude internal bleeding.
- Monitor abdominal pain: scar rupture can present with continuous pain, as opposed to intermittent contractions.

With appropriate monitoring, vaginal delivery rates of 75% can be expected, with a scar rupture rate of <1%.

- What criteria must be fulfilled for an instrumental delivery?
- What are the differences in the indications for vacuum compared with forceps?
- What is the technique for repair of an episiotomy?
- What complications are associated with LTCS?
- What precautions are necessary in a patient undergoing a trial of labor?

Further reading

Gabbe SG, et al. (2002) *Obstetrics: Normal and Problem Pregnancies*, 4th ed. (Churchill Livingstone, New York).

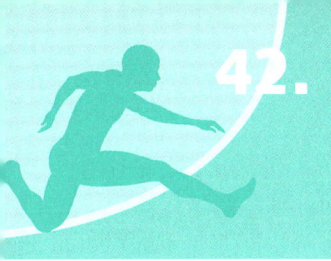

42. Complications of the Third Stage of Labor and the Puerperium

Postpartum hemorrhage

Definition
PPH is defined as vaginal bleeding of more than 500 mL after a vaginal delivery or >1000 mL after a cesarean delivery. It can be either early or late:
- Early: occurring within 24 h of delivery.
- Late: occurring after the first 24 h and within 6 weeks of delivery.

Early postpartum hemorrhage

Incidence of early postpartum hemorrhage
The incidence of early PPH in the developed world is about 5% of deliveries; this is in contrast to developing countries, where it can occur in 28% of deliveries and is still a major cause of maternal mortality.

Etiology of early postpartum hemorrhage
The main causes of early PPH are shown in Fig. 42.1.

Uterine atony
The most common cause of PPH is uterine atony, when there is a failure of contraction and retraction of the uterus after the infant has been delivered. Risk factors include:

Causes of early postpartum hemorrhage	
Cause	Frequency (%)
Uterine atony	Approximately 90%
Genital tract trauma • Retained placenta/placenta accreta • Coagulation disorders • Uterine inversion • Uterine rupture	Approximately 7%

Fig. 42.1 Causes of early PPH.

- Multiple pregnancy.
- Grand multiparity.
- Polyhydramnios.
- Fibroid uterus.
- Prolonged labor.
- Previous PPH.
- APH, especially placenta previa or abruption.

In the case of a twin pregnancy, for example, there is overdistention of the uterus, which might reduce its ability to contract effectively, as well as a larger placental site, which can bleed. Fibroids can also restrict efficient contraction of the uterus, depending on their position. APH secondary to placental abruption impairs the normal function of the uterine muscle because of damage caused by bleeding into the myometrium. The lower segment of the uterus does not contract after delivery, and so a patient with placenta previa is at risk of hemorrhage from the placental bed.

Genital tract trauma
A PPH can occur after any type of delivery, but it is more common in certain circumstances. For example, a difficult forceps delivery might cause cervical lacerations as well as needing an episiotomy for delivery. At cesarean section, delivery of a deeply engaged presenting part or a large infant might cause extension of the uterine incision and result in heavy bleeding.

Prevention
In the first instance, prevention of early PPH involves treatment of anemia during pregnancy and identifying patients who might be at risk. These women might be obvious antenatally, such as the patient with a known inherited coagulation factor deficiency or one who has had a previous PPH. Equally, PPH might be anticipated during labor, e.g. the patient who has a prolonged labor ending with a difficult instrumental delivery of a large baby.

Active management of the third stage of labor is routine in most obstetric units, with the patient's consent. It involves:

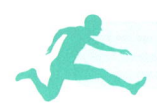

- Use of an oxytocic drug.
- Controlled cord traction to deliver the placenta (Brandt–Andrews method).
- Clamping and cutting the umbilical cord.

Prophylactic use of oxytocics in particular is known to reduce the incidence of PPH by 30–40%. Oxytocin is most commonly used in the US (20 units of oxytocin in 1000 mL of isotonic solution).

Management

History, examination and management of the patient who has a PPH is described in Chapter 17. Treatment must start with basic resuscitation (ABC), depending on the patient's condition and the extent of the bleeding. It is important to get an accurate estimation of the blood loss; it is frequently underestimated. Intravenous access must be established. Blood is sent for hemoglobin, platelets, clotting, and cross-matching. In cases of massive obstetric hemorrhage, generally classified as ≥2000 mL, a multidisciplinary approach to management is very important, involving co-management between the obstetrician, the anesthesiologist, and the hematologist.

> Multidisciplinary management is important with:
> - Hematologists in cases of massive PPH.
> - Infectious disease specialists in cases of sepsis of uncertain origin that does not respond to regular treatment.
> - Psychiatrists in cases of postpartum mental illness.
>
> All these disorders are associated with maternal mortality.

Retained or incomplete placenta

The cause of the bleeding must be identified so that appropriate management can be instigated. If the placenta is still in situ, then delivery should be attempted by controlled cord traction. Once delivered, the placenta must be examined to ensure that the cotyledons and the membranes are complete. If the placenta is still retained, manual removal is necessary under regional analgesia. This is usually performed with antibiotic prophylaxis and with further doses of uterotonics.

Examination of the patient under anesthesia allows exploration of the uterus if the placenta is thought to be incomplete. It also enables suturing of genital tract trauma, such as cervical or vaginal lacerations, once uterine atony is excluded as the cause of the PPH.

Uterine atony

With uterine atony, the uterus is palpated and contractions are induced by massaging the uterus abdominally. Further uterotonic drugs are given, commonly intravenous oxytocin, initially as a single dose, then proceeding to an intravenous infusion. Prostaglandin may be beneficial. This is commonly given in the form of carboprost (PGF$_{2\alpha}$) injected intramuscularly or intramyometrially (also known as Hemabate).

In severe cases, surgery is necessary and even life saving. This includes bilateral uterine artery ligation or bilateral internal iliac artery ligation. A B-Lynch compression suture can be performed to avoid hysterectomy, and this preserves future fertility. However, prompt recourse to hysterectomy is essential to reduce maternal morbidity and mortality. This management is summarized in Fig. 42.2.

Complications

Sheehan's syndrome

Severe PPH can lead to avascular necrosis of the pituitary gland, resulting in hypopituitarism. This can present as secondary amenorrhea or failure of lactation.

Treatment of early postpartum hemorrhage secondary to uterine atony

- Intravenous access/cross-match blood
- Induce uterine contractions by massaging the uterine fundus
- Give intravenous oxytocin or ergometrine
- Start oxytocic infusion
- Give intramuscular or intramyometrial prostaglandin
- Consider surgical options or uterine artery embolization

Fig. 42.2 Treatment of early PPH secondary to uterine atony.

Placenta accreta

With routine active management of the third stage of labor, the placenta is usually delivered within minutes of the infant. If the patient is not bleeding, up to 30 min can be left before undertaking manual removal under anesthesia. Rarely, the placenta is found to be morbidly adherent to the uterine wall, known as a placenta accreta. This condition is associated with paucity of underlying decidua:
- Placenta previa.
- Uterine scar, such as previous cesarean section.
- Multiparity.

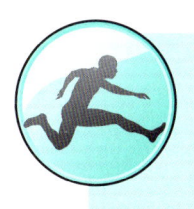

> The potential morbidity and mortality associated with PPH are so significant that earlier rather than delayed recourse to hysterectomy is important.

If the patient is not bleeding, then conservative management includes observation and antibiotics. However, more commonly, the patient has significant bleeding and surgery is necessary, including hysterectomy.

Uterine inversion

This rare complication of labor can be complete, when the uterine fundus passes through the cervix, or incomplete, when the fundus is still above the cervix. It can occur spontaneously, e.g. in association with a fundal placental site or a unicornuate uterus, or be the result of mismanagement of the third stage.

The more serious presentation is of severe lower abdominal pain followed by collapse and hemorrhage. The pain is secondary to tension on the infundibulopelvic ligaments. Treatment involves resuscitation of the patient, replacement of the uterus, either manually or hydrostatically, and oxytocin infusion.

Uterine rupture

This is seen very rarely in the US, except in association with a previous cesarean section. The incidence has fallen dramatically with the introduction of the LTCS (<1%), as opposed to the classical vertical incision of the uterus (up to 10%). Spontaneous rupture is much less common, seen in a patient of high parity, associated with the use of oxytocin to augment labor, and has a high maternal and fetal mortality.

Uterine rupture can present with an abnormal FHR tracing in labor (see Chapter 16), or with continuous abdominal pain and vaginal bleeding. Diagnosis is made at laparotomy and the treatment is surgical, either repair of the rupture or hysterectomy.

Late postpartum hemorrhage

This can be caused by:
- Retained products of conception.
- Endometritis.
- Molar pregnancy or choriocarcinoma.

Chapter 17 gives the relevant points in the history, examination, and work-up for the disorder, which most commonly presents with persistent vaginal bleeding.

Lactation

There are two main hormonal influences on breast tissue during pregnancy:
- Estrogen increases the number and the size of the ducts.
- Progesterone increases the number of alveoli.

Colostrum, which is rich in antibodies, is secreted in late pregnancy and production increases after delivery. The level of estrogen falls in the first 48 h after delivery so that prolactin can act on the alveoli and initiate lactation.

Suckling stimulates two reflexes:
1. The anterior lobe of the pituitary gland releases prolactin into the bloodstream, which induces the alveoli to secrete milk.
2. The posterior lobe of the pituitary gland releases oxytocin into the bloodstream, which causes contraction of the myoepithelial cells surrounding the alveoli so that the milk is ejected.

Postpartum infection

Definition
Also known as puerperal infection, this is defined as a maternal temperature of ≥38°C maintained for 24 h.

Incidence
Infection remains a major cause of maternal mortality (see Chapter 43). However, with improved hygiene and the use of antibiotics, the incidence has fallen to 1–3%.

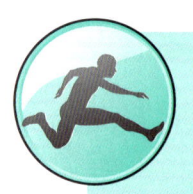

> Maternal sepsis is still one of the top five causes of maternal mortality and so must be investigated thoroughly and treated promptly.

Sites of infection
- Uterus.
- Abdominal incision.
- Perineum.
- Chest.
- Urinary tract.
- Breast.

History
The site of infection might be obvious from the patient's history. Dysuria and urine frequency would suggest a UTI. If there is also flank pain then there might be an ascending infection to the kidneys causing pyelonephritis. If the patient has a productive cough and complains of feeling short of breath, then she is likely to have a chest infection. This is typically a postoperative complication seen in the patient who has had a cesarean section.

A uterine infection is also more common after an operative intervention, such as a cesarean section or a manual removal of placenta. It typically presents with lower abdominal pain, sometimes with unpleasant-smelling vaginal discharge. Retained products of conception must be excluded. It is now routine practice to give prophylactic antibiotics at the time of a cesarean section. As well as protecting against a uterine infection, this also reduces the risk of a wound infection.

Infection in the perineum can also present with vaginal discharge, as well as localized discomfort. There is usually a history of a vaginal tear or an episiotomy. Acute mastitis, or infection of the breast, typically presents at the end of the first week after birth, as organisms that colonize the baby affect the breast. Infection presents with pain in one or both breasts associated with fever.

Examination
Check for pyrexia and tachycardia, which will be present with infection. Then examine the patient from head to toe, as suggested in Fig. 42.3.

Investigations
A WBC will be raised and a C-reactive protein level will also be high. Blood cultures are indicated if the temperature is ≥38°C.

Other investigations depend on the system that seems to be involved:
- Cervical cultures for uterine infection.
- Perineal swab.
- Wound swab for cesarean section patient.
- Mid-stream urine sample.
- Sputum sample.

Management
The antibiotic of choice will depend on local protocol, but usually involves a broad-spectrum antibiotic and anaerobic coverage with metronidazole for 5 to 7 days. Dicloxacillin might be more appropriate for mastitis or for a wound infection because the usual pathogen is a staphylococcus.

Postpartum mental illness

Incidence
Postpartum depression is one of the most common medical diseases of pregnancy, with 10% of women fulfilling the criteria for a depressive disorder. Psychosis is much rarer, affecting 0.2% of births.

These disorders should be distinguished from the "baby blues," which affects up to 70% of women, with a peak incidence on day 4 to 5. Tearfulness, anxiety, and irritability normally settle with reassurance and support from family and friends.

Postpartum mental illness

Fig. 42.3 Examination of the patient with a postpartum fever.

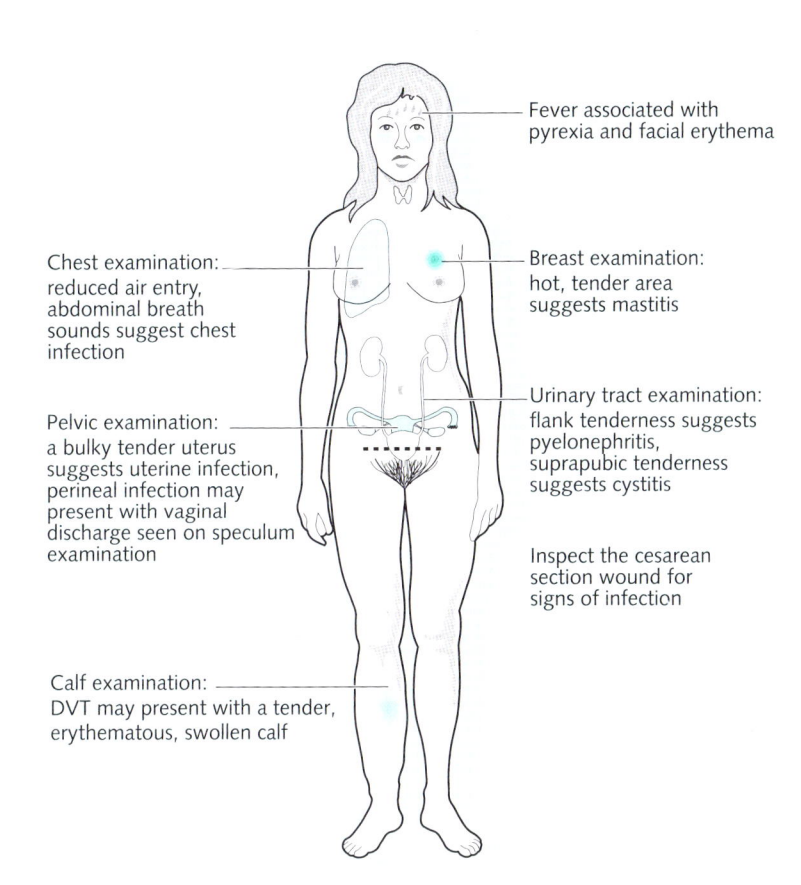

- Fever associated with pyrexia and facial erythema
- Chest examination: reduced air entry, abdominal breath sounds suggest chest infection
- Breast examination: hot, tender area suggests mastitis
- Pelvic examination: a bulky tender uterus suggests uterine infection, perineal infection may present with vaginal discharge seen on speculum examination
- Urinary tract examination: flank tenderness suggests pyelonephritis, suprapubic tenderness suggests cystitis
- Inspect the cesarean section wound for signs of infection
- Calf examination: DVT may present with a tender, erythematous, swollen calf

History

Chapter 36 lists the risk factors for postpartum depression and some of these should be sought at the time of the first prenatal visit. Puerperal psychosis in particular has associated risks: previous psychotic illness gives the woman a 50% chance of postpartum disease and a family history a 25% chance.

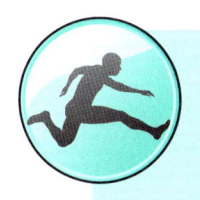

> Prediction from the antenatal history is one of the main factors in the early management of postpartum mental illness.

The common symptoms of postpartum depression and puerperal psychosis are shown in Figs 42.4 and 42.5 respectively. The peak time of

Symptoms of postpartum depression

- Anxiety
- Low mood
- Tiredness
- Irritability
- Feelings of inadequacy
- Ambivalence towards the baby
- Reduced or absent libido

Fig. 42.4 Symptoms of postpartum depression.

onset for postpartum depression is 4 to 6 weeks postpartum, whereas the onset of psychosis is usually very sudden.

Management

- Prevention.
- Pharmacological.
- Psychological/social.

255

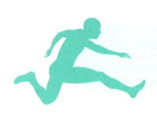

Symptoms of puerperal psychosis

- Insomnia or early morning wakening
- Lability of mood
- Overactivity
- Disorientation
- Lack of insight
- Hallucinations
- Persecutory beliefs

Fig. 42.5 Symptoms of puerperal psychosis.

The mainstay of management is prevention, which has improved recently as media interest increases public awareness. Early diagnosis and training of professionals to recognize the problems are also vital and have resulted in the development of the Edinburgh Postnatal Depression Scale, which is used successfully by health care providers across Europe, New Zealand, and Australia.

Drug treatment is described in Chapter 36. As with any drug in pregnancy, use should be considered if its benefits outweigh its risks. The tricyclic antidepressants can be given safely both antenatally and postnatally. The newer SSRI antidepressants are probably safe, although there is less evidence at this stage. Lithium is associated with cardiac anomalies, particularly Ebstein's anomaly, when used antenatally. It might also be toxic to the baby with breast-feeding. ECT is safe.

Health-care providers and support groups all have an important role in helping the mother with postpartum illness.

Thromboembolic disease

TED is one of the most common causes of pregnancy-related maternal mortality in the US (see Chapter 43). Chapter 36 describes the risk factors, diagnosis, and management in detail. Of particular importance are those women who are delivered by cesarean section. However, it is vital not to forget that a woman who has had a normal delivery might still have significant risk factors that necessitate thromboprophylaxis, such as obesity or hypertension.

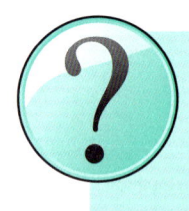

- What are the important factors in the etiology of early PPH?
- What are the first steps in the management of a patient who presents with an early PPH?
- What are the common sites of postpartum infection, and how would you investigate them?
- How prevalent is postpartum depression, and how can it be managed?
- What is the diagnosis and treatment of TED in the puerperium?

Further reading
Gabbe SG, et al. (2002) *Obstetrics: Normal and Problem Pregnancies*, 4th ed. (Churchill Livingstone, New York).

43. Maternal Death

Maternal mortality is defined as death of the mother during pregnancy, labor, and within 42 days of delivery or abortion, but recently deaths up to 1 year have been studied. Maternal deaths are divided into four categories: direct, indirect, coincidental (which used to be called fortuitous), and late (Fig. 43.1).

Pregnancy mortality surveillance system

Since 1987, the Centers for Disease Control, state health departments, and the American College of Obstetricians and Gynecologists Maternal Mortality Study Group have initiated The Pregnancy Mortality Surveillance System (PMSS). The most recent report summarizes pregnancy-related deaths from 1991 to 1999. The goals of the PMSS are to:
- Assess the main causes of death.
- Examine the trends, comparing rates of death with those in previous studies.
- Identify avoidable deaths and look at substandard care.
- Make recommendations about improving clinical care.
- Suggest areas for future research.

At a local level, hospitals can use the report to develop guidelines for the management of complications of pregnancy, and to review the care that their patients receive.

Definitions of the classes of maternal death

- Direct: resulting from obstetric complications
- Indirect: previous existing disease, or disease arising in pregnancy, aggravated by the physiologic effect of pregnancy (includes all asthma, cardiac disease, epilepsy, and suicide)
- Coincidental: unrelated cause, occurring in pregnancy or puerperium
- Late: >42 days, <12 months after termination/miscarriage/delivery

Fig. 43.1 Definitions of the classes of maternal death.

Figure 43.2 shows the maternal mortality rate since 1952. The fall in maternal mortality is thought to be due to a combination of improved obstetric and midwifery care and an improvement in the standards of living. The increasing rates seen in the last report are due to a change in the way that figures are collected; before 1991, the PMSS relied upon clinicians reporting deaths, so inevitably the data were incomplete.

> The maternal mortality rate for the US since 1982 has been approximately 7–8 in 100,000 maternities (only direct and indirect maternal deaths are included in this statistic).

Causes of maternal death

Figure 43.3 shows the main causes of maternal death in 1991–1999. The case studies below are derived from the most recent PMSS report.

Direct maternal deaths

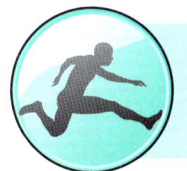

> Thromboembolism is the most common cause of direct maternal deaths.

Thromboembolic disease

TED is the most common cause of direct maternal death, accounting for more than 20% of deaths. Great effort has been made in recent years to improve prophylaxis for women at increased risk of thromboembolism in pregnancy, particularly those undergoing cesarean delivery, and national

257

Maternal Death

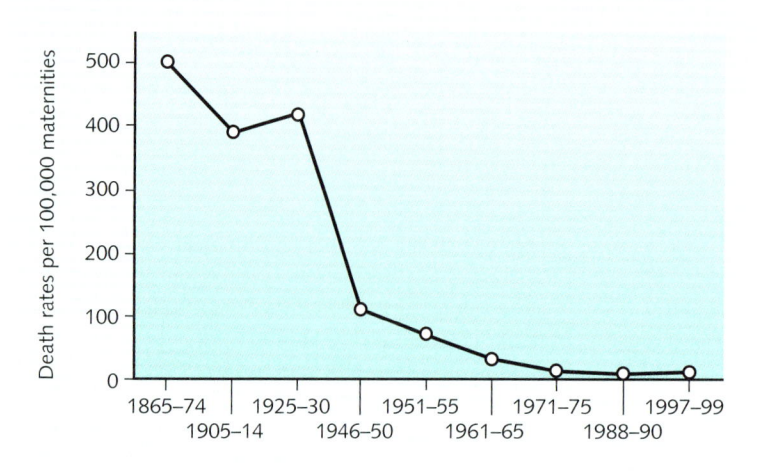

Fig. 43.2 Death rates from 1952 to the present.

Causes of maternal death, 1991–1999	
Cause	Percent of all deaths
Embolism	19.6
Hemorrhage	17.2
Hypertensive disorders	15.7
Sepsis	12.6
Cardiomyopathy	8.3
Cerebrovascular accident	5
Anesthesia	1.6
Other (majority includes cardiovascular, pulmonary, or neurologic problems)	19.2
Unknown	0.7

Fig. 43.3 Causes of maternal death, 1991–1999. (Adapted from http://www.cdc.gov/mmwr/preview/mmwrhtml/ss5202a1.HTM.)

guidelines exist recommending heparin and TED stockings as appropriate. However, all pregnant women are at risk (see Chapter 36) and women are still dying, often after the problem has been attributed to muscle strain, as illustrated in the case study below.

Case study: thromboembolic disease
An overweight woman aged over 30 with a strong family history of TED developed thrombophlebitis and was admitted to the hospital at 8 weeks' gestation with chest pain. Although the woman's general practitioner had suggested a diagnosis of PE, the medical registrar thought that chest X-ray and anticoagulation were contraindicated and the woman went home with a diagnosis of "musculoskeletal pain." Two days later she was readmitted and a V/Q scan was arranged to exclude PE; she died of PE before the scan was done.

Hypertensive disorders
Deaths from hypertensive disorders, including pre-eclampsia and eclampsia, are decreasing. The largest single cause of death of women in this group is intracranial hemorrhage, a complication of uncontrolled hypertension reflecting a failure to treat high blood pressure effectively. The need for monitoring to continue after delivery is vital, as illustrated in the following case study.

Case study: hypertension in pregnancy
A woman with a multiple pregnancy had a blood pressure of 90/60 mmHg at her initial prenatal visit. She was admitted to hospital during the pregnancy with pre-eclampsia and was subsequently delivered by cesarean section. Immediately prior to delivery her blood pressure was 140/80 mmHg and she had 3+ proteinuria. There was inadequate monitoring of her blood pressure after delivery, and 8h postnatally the reading was 260/140 mmHg. She developed neurological symptoms and was transferred to

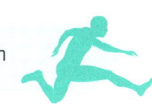

intensive care, where she died of a cerebral hemorrhage.

Hemorrhage

Hemorrhage-related deaths are also decreasing. Recommendations made by the PMSS emphasize the fact that the speed with which hemorrhage becomes life threatening means that any woman at increased risk should be identified antenatally and advised to deliver in a hospital with a blood-bank on site (see the following case study). Placenta previa poses a major risk, so consultant obstetricians and anesthesiologists should be involved in cesarean sections performed for this reason.

Case study: hemorrhage

A woman complained to her general practitioner of abdominal pain. Her period was late and a pregnancy test was positive. An appointment for a scan was arranged, but abdominal pain with diarrhea recurred before the date of the scan and the woman was taken to the hospital by ambulance. In transit she was noted to be pale, sweaty, and hypotensive. She then had a cardiac arrest with prolonged asystole. She was resuscitated and taken to the operating room, where laparotomy was performed. A ruptured tubal pregnancy was discovered. Unfortunately, major cerebral damage had resulted from prolonged asystole, and she died in the intensive care unit.

Sepsis

Deaths from septic abortion following illegal termination of pregnancy were, sadly, not uncommon before Roe vs. Wade in 1973. Sepsis declined as a major cause of maternal death thereafter, but has recently been increasing again. Deaths seen in 1991–1999 included those after miscarriage, after late intrauterine death, and following prolonged rupture of membranes, with septicemia associated with DIC.

Amniotic fluid embolism

AFE remains a significant cause of death, but, frustratingly, we still do not have any clear ideas of how to prevent or to treat this condition.

Ectopic pregnancy

Of the direct deaths associated with early pregnancy in 1991–1999, most were due to ectopic pregnancy, with the main problem being a failure to suspect the possibility of ectopic pregnancy in the first place. Presentation might be atypical with, for example, GI symptoms confusing the issue, but the diagnosis must be suspected in any woman who is unwell and has a positive pregnancy test (see Chapter 7).

Indirect maternal deaths

CNS disorders, cardiac disease, and psychiatric disease are the main categories in this section.

Central nervous system disorders

Cerebral hemorrhage and epilepsy are the most common cause of CNS deaths. Close monitoring of epilepsy in pregnancy is important, because anticonvulsant levels can change and women often feel ambivalent about continuing treatment due to the fetal side effects (see Chapter 36).

Cardiac disease

Heart disease is now as common as thromboembolism as a cause of maternal death. About 30% is due to congenital disease, including pulmonary hypertension, and 15% to ischemic heart disease. The remainder is due to other acquired heart disease. Rheumatic heart disease is uncommon in the US and when seen is usually in new immigrants.

Psychiatric disorders

Psychiatric disease is known to have caused or to have contributed to 12% of maternal deaths, 10% of which were due to suicide. Suicide often occurred later than 42 days after delivery, so is also counted as a "late" death and was often not reported as a maternal death. Alcohol and drug misuse are also covered in this category. The lack of specialist mental health teams and mother-and-baby units make it more difficult to treat these women optimally.

Case study: postpartum psychosis

A woman died in a road traffic accident after escaping from an inpatient psychiatric unit where she was being treated for postpartum psychosis. She had previously suffered from postpartum psychosis following the birth of a child some years earlier. There was no mention in her antenatal notes of her previous psychiatric history and she had midwifery-led care and a home delivery.

Shortly after this she became psychotic and required inpatient admission, during which time she expressed suicidal ideations.

Coincidental deaths

This section includes many different causes of death, but of particular concern are those due to domestic violence. Women suffering domestic violence are more likely to register late for prenatal care, to be poor attenders at prenatal clinic, and to have poor obstetric histories. Ideally, all women at the initial visit should be asked, directly but sensitively, about violence. A pregnant woman should be seen at least once on her own during pregnancy, and relatives should not be used as interpreters.

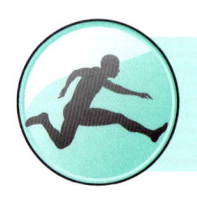

> About 30% of domestic violence starts in pregnancy.

Risk factors for maternal death

Maternal mortality increases with increasing maternal age and parity. Other factors include multiple pregnancy and IVF treatment, nonwhite ethnic origin, late registration, and lower social class.

> Women from the most deprived social class are 20 times more likely to die of direct or indirect causes than women in higher socioeconomic classes.

Substandard care was identified in 30% of cases of direct maternal deaths studied in the 1991–1999 report. The main causes were summarized as:
- Lack of communication and teamwork.
- Failure to appreciate the severity of illness.
- Suboptimal treatment.
- Wrong diagnosis.
- Failure of practitioners to refer-on to specialists in the hospital.
- Failure of consultants to attend, or inappropriate delegation of responsibility.
- Lack of clear policies for prevention and management of serious conditions.
- Failure to seek advice from other specialties when appropriate.

- What is the most common direct cause of maternal death?
- What is the longest period of time that can elapse between end of pregnancy and death for the case to be studied by the PMSS?
- What is the main direct cause of death in early pregnancy?

Further reading

MacKay AP, et al. (2005) An assessment of pregnancy-related mortality in the United States. *Paediatric and Perinatal Epidemiology* 19(3):206–14.

http://www.cdc.gov/mmwr/preview/mmwrhtml/ss5202a1.htm

HISTORY AND EXAMINATION

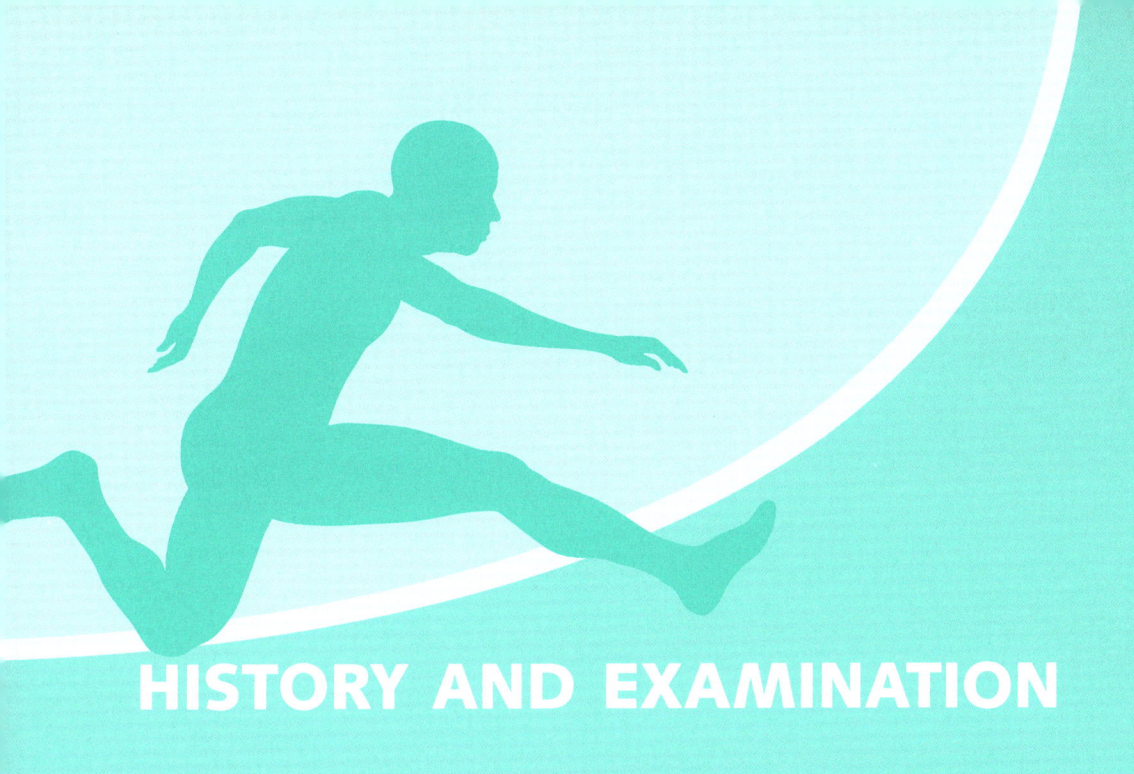

44.	Taking a History	263
45.	Prenatal Care	271
46.	Examination	279
47.	Common Investigations	293

44. Taking a History

The history plays a vital role in obstetrics and gynecology, often giving pointers to a diagnosis that is not always evident from examination and laboratory studies of the patient. Many women are embarrassed by having to discuss their gynecologic problems, especially to someone who is often younger than they are, so it is important to overcome this by developing a confident, friendly, and relaxed atmosphere. Always introduce and present yourself in an acceptable manner, be courteous and friendly without being overfamiliar, and always pay attention.

Patient details

It is surprising how often patient details are omitted from a history. Always record the following:
1. Name, date of birth, age, and address (sticky labels with this information are usually available).
2. Marital status, ethnic group, and occupation.
3. The date, time, and place of the consultation.
4. Source of referral, e.g. GP referral, self-admitted, labor floor.

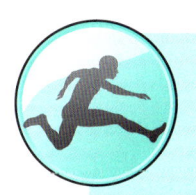

> It is useful to get into the habit of writing certain details in the top right-hand corner of the progress note, e.g.:
> - Age.
> - Parity.
> - Date of LMP.
> - Date of last Pap smear.

Chief complaint

The chief complaint documented in the referral letter does not always correlate to what the patient perceives as the main problem. Some patients have already been labeled with a diagnosis before you get to see them. Therefore, it is vital to ask the patient what she sees as her primary complaint and document this, preferably in her own words. If there are multiple symptoms, document each one and do so in order of severity.

During the examination, work-up, and treatment never lose track of the presenting complaint; management plans are not always appropriate. Conversely, the presenting complaint might be a cover for a different problem that the patient has difficulty discussing. Always ask if there is anything else bothering the patient that she wishes to discuss.

History of presenting illness

Details of the history of the presenting illness (HPI) should be ascertained. For instance:
- How long has the complaint been present or a problem? For example, a woman might complain that she has always had heavy periods but that they have only been a problem for the last 2 years.
- Was the onset of symptoms sudden or gradual? For example, severe hirsutism of rapid onset is likely to be due to an androgen-producing tumor.
- Was the onset associated with a previous obstetric or gynecologic event? For example, stress incontinence and childbirth.
- Are there any relieving or exacerbating factors? For example, symptoms of prolapse are often worse on standing and better on lying down.
- Are there any associated symptoms? For example, the painful periods of endometriosis are sometimes associated with frequent bowel movements.

If pain is the presenting complaint, then the following characteristics should be discussed and noted:
- Site: is the pain pelvic or abdominal? For example, ovarian pain can be felt quite high in the abdomen.

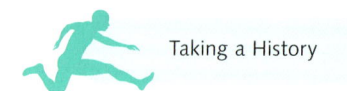

- Severity: how severe is the pain and to what extent does it disrupt everyday life? For example, the cyclical pain of endometriosis might necessitate regular time off work.
- Onset: sudden or gradual? For example, the pain from a torsed ovarian cyst is usually of very sudden onset.
- Character: is the pain sharp/knife-like, dull, heavy/dragging, colicky, stretching or twisting? Many adjectives have been used to describe pain or discomfort of gynecologic origin. For example, women with uterine prolapse might describe a pulling or a dragging pain/sensation; dysmenorrhea might be likened to labor pain.
- Duration: is the pain constant or intermittent. Frequency if intermittent? The pain of a degenerating fibroid in pregnancy will be constant, whereas the pain of threatened premature labor will be intermittent and frequent.
- Radiation: does the pain radiate? For example, endometriosis pain might radiate to the back or into the upper thighs.
- Relieving/exacerbating features: does anything make the pain better or worse, and this should include self-prescribed analgesia? For example, endometriosis symptoms are usually cyclical and associated with menstruation.
- Associated symptoms, e.g. symptoms of peritonitis or advanced malignancy.

Past gynecologic history

Menstrual history
The following characteristics of menstruation and the menstrual cycle should be noted:
- Age at menarche.
- LMP.
- Menstrual cycle: usually denoted as 5/28, where the numerator is the length of the period in days and the denominator is the length of the cycle in days. If period and cycle length are variable, then the shortest and longest are noted, e.g. 3–10/14–56.
- Menstrual flow: whether light, normal, or heavy. If heavy, the presence of clots, saturating pads, nighttime soiling, and the number of sanitary pads/towels used should be noted.
- Menstrual pain: is the pain mild, moderate, or severe? Has it been present since menarche, or is it of recent onset? Is the pain worse before or during the period?
- Associated symptoms, e.g. bowel or bladder dysfunction, nausea.
- Other bleeding: intermenstrual bleeding, postcoital bleeding, pre- or postmenstrual spotting.
- Age at menopause.

Sexual activity and contraception
Is the patient sexually active or in a relationship? Does the patient suffer from dyspareunia and, if so, is it superficial or deep? Is she or her partner using contraception and, if so, what? If she is on the pill, was it prescribed for contraceptive purposes or menstrual disorder?

Cervical screening
Has the patient undergone regular cervical screening? When was the last Pap smear taken? Have there ever been abnormal Pap smears?

Vaginal discharge
Is vaginal discharge present and, if so, is it normal or abnormal? If abnormal, what is the color and consistency and is it irritating? Was the onset associated with a change in sexual partner? Is there a history of sexually transmitted disease?

Past obstetric history

The parity and gravidity should be noted. Parity denotes the number of livebirths or stillbirths after 20 weeks' gestation, and gravidity is the number of pregnancies. Use of the terms 'parity' and 'gravidity' can become very complicated, especially with a history of multiple pregnancies. A more straightforward way of documenting previous pregnancies is to document the number of:
- Children.
- Miscarriages.
- Terminations.

Document the details of each pregnancy:
- The number of children with age and birth weight. Note any complications of pregnancy, labor, and the puerperium.
- The number of miscarriages, their gestation, and complications if any.
- The number of terminations of pregnancy, their gestation, method and indication, and complications if any.

Past medical history

This should include previous surgery, e.g. sterilization.

Review of systems

A brief review of systems should be made with special reference to the:
- GI tract: change in bowel habits, especially with menstruation.
- Genitourinary system: urinary frequency, nocturia, dysuria, incontinence.

Drug history

A careful drug history should be taken and should include hormonal contraception and HRT, which are often overlooked by the patient.

Family history

Inquire as to a family history of ovarian, uterine, and breast disease.

Social history

Occupation, smoking habits, and alcohol consumption should be noted. If surgery is contemplated, what is the support network at home?

Allergies

Document all known allergies.

Taking a History

Medical Record No. X349182
TURSICA, Stella   27 yr. old woman
4/29/79   Parity: 0
1/10/98   11:15   LMP: 5/15/97
                         Gestation: 34 + 2/40

CC: Vaginal bleeding at 34 weeks gestation
HPI: Onset: started spotting hours ago
         Gradually getting heavier since then
         Now bright red bleeding like a period
         Relieving/exacerbating factors: none
         Associated symptoms: none
PGH: Menarche, age 11 years
         Menstrual cycle: 5/28 regular. LMP: 5/15/97
         (Sure of dates), now 34 +2 weeks in
         First pregnancy
         Cervical cytology: regular Pap smears, all normal
         Last Pap smear at initial visit: normal
         Contraception: using the combined OCP
         Stopped 6 months before became pregnant
POH: Para or children: 0
         Gravida: Miscarriages: 0
                     Terminations: 0
         This pregnancy: dates confirmed by ultrasound scan
         Placenta said to be fundal
         Initial blood work: normal—rhesus negative
         Normal antenatal progress so far
PMH: Noncontributory
ROS: CVS: normal
         RS: normal
         GI: constipated since pregnant
         GUS: frequent micturition since pregnant
Meds: Iron for 6 weeks
Allergies: None known
Fam. Hx: Noncontributory

1. It is useful to write relevant details in the top right-hand corner of the progress note.

Referred by GP—seen on labor floor

2. Chief complaint should be brief, but it is helpful to mention relevant background information.

3. Mention only the pertinent negatives.

4. Always record the dose and frequency of any drugs. Always document that you have asked about drug allergies.

SHx: Housewife
Lives with husband
Smoking: 20 cigarettes/day
Alcohol: stopped when known to be pregnant

Fig. 44.1 Charting.

Charting

<u>PE:</u> Vitals: BP 100/60   P 90   RR 20
       General: Anxious
       HEENT: Trachea midline
       CVS: Regular rate + rhythm, 0 murmurs,
               regurgitation, or gallops
       Resp: CTAB*
               Breath sounds equal bilaterally
               Some rhonchi at L base
       Abd: Striae gravidarum, linea nigra
               Fundal height = 34 cm
       Soft, NT

*clear to auscultation bilaterally

       Leopolds: Singleton fetus
                   Longitudinal lie
                   Vertex, back on maternal left
       Toco: Quiet
       EFM: Baseline 130, mod. variability
                + accelerations, – decelerations
                Reactive
       Pelvic: Deferred until placenta previa excluded

<u>Summary</u>
27 year old female 34 weeks into first pregnancy
Presents with painless APH
In view of painless bleed and high presenting part placenta previa
needs to be excluded, even though early scan suggests placenta
not low lying

<u>Problem list:</u>
1. APH
   ? secondary to placenta previa
2. Rhesus negative (will require anti-D)
3. Smoking is a risk factor for APH
4. Need to exclude placenta previa

> 5. Record your initial observations—they are important. "Alert & chatty" or "Distressed & looks unwell" tell you a lot about the patient.

> 6. Always use diagrams to clarify your examination findings.

> 7. Always include a management plan—even when you are still a student. It might not be right, but you need to start training yourself to think like a doctor.

> 8. Sign your notes, including printed name and beeper number.

Signature
Printed name
Beeper number

Fig. 44.1—cont'd.

Taking a History

Medical Record No. X349182
BARNES, Joan   57 yr. old woman
4/29/47   Parity: 4024
1/10/98 11:15 LMP: Age 50 yrs
                Last Pap smear: 1 year ago—neg

CC: Referred by GP complaining of a lump in the vagina for 10 years

HPI: Onset: 10 years ago noticed a lump which has become bigger since menopause
Relieving/exacerbating factors: worse after standing and reduces on lying down.
Associated symptoms: dragging sensation in the pelvis, backache
Risk factors: multiparous, large babies, chronic bronchitis

PGH: Menarche, age 12 years
Menstrual cycle: 5/28, no menstrual problems. Menopause age 50 years
Cervical cytology: regular Pap smears, all normal; last Pap smear 1 year ago
Contraception: used condoms until sterilized

POH: Parity 4 + 2 or children: 4
 miscarriages: 2
 terminations: 0
1960: normal pregnancy, prolonged labor, forceps delivery, male infant 3.4 kg
1965: normal pregnancy, normal labor, spontaneous vaginal delivery (SVD), female infant 3.8 kg
1964: 12 week miscarriage, D&E (evacuation of retained products of conception)
1966: normal pregnancy, normal labor, SVD, male infant 4.8 kg
1968: normal pregnancy, normal labor, SVD, female infant 3.7 kg
1972: 8 week miscarriage, D&E

PMH: 1980: laparoscopic sterilization
1990: chronic bronchitis

ROS: CVS: normal
Resp: chronic cough, occasional green sputum
GI: no change in bowel habits
GUS: slight stress incontinence when coughing, does not want investigation, treatment

Meds: None
Allergies: None
Fam Hx: Mother had hysterectomy (not known why)
Father died age 74 years (chest problems)

SHx: Cashier
Lives with husband
Smoking: 20 cigarettes/day for 40 years
Alcohol: 20 drinks per week

1. It is useful to write relevant details in the top right-hand corner of the progress note.

Referred by GP

2. Chief complaint should be brief, but it is helpful to mention relevant background information.

3. Mention only the pertinent negatives.

4. Always record the dose and frequency of any drugs. Always document that you have asked about drug allergies.

Fig. 44.2 Charting.

PE: Vitals: BP 140/90
General: appears well; overweight
CVS: heart sounds normal no cardiac murmurs
RS: trachea midline equal expansion bilaterally
Abdomen: laparascopy scar
    soft
    nontender
    no masses
    normal bowel sounds
    rectal exam not done
Vulva: normal
Cervix: sitting at introitus
Bimanual: uterus 4-6 weeks size, mobile nontender,
    smooth outline
Speculum: cervix excoriated
Moderate cystocele
Moderate rectocele
Summary
57 year old multiparous woman complaining of symptoms of prolapse
Pelvic exam reveals second-degree prolapse of uterus associated with moderate pelvic floor prolapse

Problem list
1. Uterine and pelvic floor prolapse
2. Associated stress incontinence
3. Obesity and chronic bronchitis are exacerbating factors
4. Heavy smoker, moderate alcohol

5. Record your initial observations—they are important. "Alert & chatty" or "Distressed & looks unwell" tell you a lot about the patient.

6. Always use diagrams to clarify your examination findings.

7. Always include a management plan—even when you are still a student. It might not be right, but you need to start training yourself to think like a doctor.

8. Sign your notes, including printed name and beeper number.

Signature
Printed name
Beeper number

Fig. 44.2—cont'd.

45. Prenatal Care

Fundamental to the planning of prenatal care is the identification, at the initial visit, of factors that reveal the woman to be at risk of complications during her pregnancy, labor, and postpartum period (Fig. 45.1).

The history

History of the current pregnancy
First, ascertain the gestation of the present pregnancy. Ask for the date of the first day of the LMP and whether it was a normal period. Also check the usual cycle length and whether her periods are regular or irregular. Ask if she was on the OCP when she conceived (the baby will not suffer any ill effects, but the date of her LMP cannot be relied upon for estimation of gestation). Find out if she has had any problems so far, and if she has had any admissions or scans.

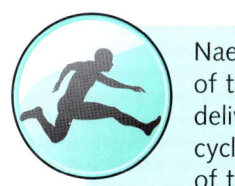

> Naegele's rule for calculation of the estimated date of delivery (assumes a 28-day cycle): add 7 to the first day of the LMP for the due date, and take 3 from the month of the LMP for the due month. For example, an LMP of March 1 gives a due date of December 8.

Past obstetric history
Past obstetric history records the outcome of all past pregnancies (Fig. 45.2). For pregnancies less than 20 weeks, document whether she had a miscarriage or a termination, and at what gestation. If the termination was for fetal abnormality, then this should be noted. For pregnancies lasting longer than 20 weeks, record:
- Mode of delivery and reason for cesarean/instrumental delivery.
- Gestation at delivery.
- Whether onset of labor was spontaneous or induced.
- Weight and sex of baby.
- Any significant prenatal problems.
- Problems experienced by the baby in the neonatal period.

Past gynecologic history
The date of the last Pap smear is recorded. If there have been abnormal Pap smears in the past, then the outcome of these, and treatment performed, must be noted. Most CIN in the US is treated by LEEP, which may not result in obstetric complications. Cone biopsy, which is used to treat a minority of cases, can result in significant cervical damage, resulting in cervical incompetence or stenosis (see Chapter 23).

Past medical history
Any admissions to the hospital, operations, or ongoing medical conditions should be documented. Particular attention should be paid to psychiatric history—not all psychiatric illness following childbirth is "simple" postpartum depression. Conditions that are likely to cause obstetric complications, or to worsen in pregnancy and the puerperium, include insulin-dependent diabetes, thromboembolism, thyroid disease, recurrent UTIs, depression, cardiac disease, anorexia nervosa, epilepsy, genital herpes infection, and (especially if the mother decides to discontinue her treatment) asthma (see Chapter 36).

Social history
This might need to be particularly sensitively elicited, and it might be appropriate to wait until the woman is alone before questioning. The key points to cover include:
- Smoking.
- Drug and alcohol use, documenting types of drug and amount used.
- Domestic violence: all women should be asked about this routinely (see Chapter 43).
- Support and social circumstances.

Factors in history and examination that make a pregnancy high risk		
History	Risk factors	Associated problems
Age	<18 years	Hypertensive disorders
		IUGR
	>35 years	Fetal chromosomal abnormality
		IUGR
		Stillbirth after 40 weeks
		Hypertensive disorders
Weight at initial visit	<45 kg	IUGR
	>100 kg	Hypertensive disorders
		Impaired glucose tolerance
		Shoulder dystocia
		Thromboembolism
Past obstetric history	Primaparous	Pre-eclampsia
	Grandmultiparous	Anemia
		IUGR
		Malpresentation
		Unstable lie
		PPH
	Previous manual removal of placenta	Recurrence of retained placenta
		Placenta previa
		PPH
	Previous cesarean section	Placenta previa
	Previous baby >4 kg	Shoulder dystocia
	Previous baby affected by medical or chromosomal abnormality	Recurrence: consider referral to neonatologist and/or genetic counselor
Past medical history	Hypertension	Hypertensive disorders
	Insulin-dependent diabetes	Miscarriage
		Stillbirth
		Congenital anomaly
		Macrosomia
		Shoulder dystocia
		Neonatal hypoglycemia
	Epilepsy	Cardiac abnormalities
		Palate abnormalities
		Neural tube defects
		Hemorrhagic disease of the newborn
		Labile drug levels

Fig. 45.1 Factors in history and examination that make a pregnancy high risk.

History	Risk factors	Associated problems
Past medical history (cont.)	Thromboembolism	DVT/PE in pregnancy and puerperium
	Thyroid disease	Maternal thyroid "storm"
		Neonatal hypo-/hyperthyroidism
	Recurrent UTIs	UTIs in pregnancy, leading to pyelonephritis, premature labor, or IUGR
	Psychiatric disorders	Exacerbation in postpartum period
	Anorexia nervosa	IUGR
Past gynecologic history	Cone biopsy	Cervical incompetence and mid-trimester miscarriage
	Genital herpes	Neonatal herpes encephalitis if lesions present at delivery
Family history	Diabetes	Impaired glucose tolerance
Social history	Domestic violence	Physical injury
		Depression and suicide
		Premature labor
		IUGR
	Cigarettes and cannabis	IUGR
		Neonatal respiratory distress syndrome
		Sudden infant death syndrome (SIDS)
		Childhood asthma and ear infections
	Alcohol	
	>4 drinks per day	Fetal alcohol syndrome
	>8 drinks/day	Cardiac defects
	Cocaine	Abruption
		IUGR
		Premature labor
		Microcephaly
		SIDS
	Amphetamines	Palate abnormalities
		Cardiac abnormalities
		IUGR
	Ecstasy (MMDA)	Musculoskeletal and cardiac abnormalities
	Barbiturates	Neonatal withdrawal
	Heroin	Miscarriage
		Stillbirth
		IUGR
		Neonatal withdrawal
		Hepatitis B and C, HIV (if injected)
	Methadone	Neonatal withdrawal

Fig. 45.1—cont'd.

History	Risk factors	Associated problems
Present pregnancy	Assisted conception	Multiple pregnancy
		Prematurity
		IUGR
	Recurrent APH	IUGR
	Multiple pregnancy	Miscarriage
		Chromosomal abnormality
		Hyperemesis
		Premature labor
		Anemia
		IUGR
		PPH
	Fibroids	PPH
		Unstable lie or obstructed labor in the lower segment of the uterus

Fig. 45.1—cont'd.

Past obstetric histories

Shorthand for the number and type of pregnancies includes referral to "primips" to denote women who have not had a >20-week pregnancy before and "multips" to denote women who have. Below is another shorthand method to refer to obstetric history, with examples to follow:

Gravida = total number of pregnancies

Parity = X/Y/Z/#
       X = number of full-term deliveries (>37 weeks)
       Y = number of preterm deliveries (20–36 weeks)
       Z = number of losses/terminations less than 20 weeks
       # = number of living children

Lynne is currently 22 weeks into this pregnancy and in the past has had two normal deliveries, one miscarriage at 8 weeks, and termination at 8 weeks. She is therefore gravida 5, para 2, or para 2022.

Hayley is currently at 12 weeks. She had a cesarean section last year and a stillbirth at 37 weeks 10 years ago. She is gravida 3, para 2, or para 2001.

Sonia is now 15 weeks. Her last pregnancy was twins who were delivered vaginally and prematurely at 25 weeks. Twins count as one delivery, so she is gravida 2, para 1, or para 0102.

Michelle is a late registrant at 30 weeks. She has had one previous pregnancy, an ectopic that was detected at 7 weeks, and was treated medically. She is gravida 2, para 0, or para 0010.

Fig. 45.2 Past obstetric histories.

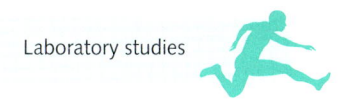

Laboratory studies

Family history
A family history of diabetes should prompt screening for gestational diabetes earlier than 28 weeks' gestation. Other conditions that have a strong familial inheritance and can affect the pregnancy include thromboembolism, pre-eclampsia, and cholestasis of pregnancy.

Examination

Examination should include:
- Weight and height, to calculate BMI.
- Blood pressure.
- Urinalysis.
- Uterine size (abdominally) and auscultation of fetal heart if >12 weeks.

Listening to the heart and lungs and performing breast and pelvic examinations are part of the initial prenatal visit.

Laboratory studies

These are summarized in Fig. 45.3.

Complete blood count
A CBC is performed at the initial visit and later in pregnancy to detect anemia (for treatment of anemia, see Chapter 36). This will also detect a low platelet count, i.e. idiopathic thrombocytopenia. If mild to moderate (platelets 50–100 × 10^9/L) then this poses little risk to the mother, but platelet levels must be monitored regularly. If severe, then the woman might require intravenous Ig. The risk of the fetus having thrombocytopenia is around 1 in 10, and is not predicted by the severity of the mother's condition.

Laboratory studies
- CBC
- Blood type and antibody screen
- Syphilis, rubella, hepatitis, and HIV serology
- Hemoglobin electrophoresis
- Midstream urine for culture
- Ultrasound screen for dating
- Cervical cultures for gonorrhea, chlamydia

Fig. 45.3 Laboratory studies.

Hemoglobin electrophoresis
Hemoglobinopathies can result in a mistaken diagnosis of anemia: carriers of the genes for sickle cell and thalassemia have a 'normal' hemoglobin that is lower than average. Diagnosis of hemoglobinopathy avoids unnecessary iron supplementation and allows identification of fetuses at risk of major thalassemia or sickle-cell disease. All women whose racial background predisposes them to hemoglobinopathy should be offered screening, and screening should be universal if the local population contains more than 15% of people of these races.

> Sickle-cell trait affects 1 in 10 people of African–American origin and 1 in 100 people originating from the Mediterranean and the Indian subcontinent. Alpha-thalassemia trait affects 1 in 15 people of Asian origin and 1 in 50 people of Mediterranean origin. Beta-thalassemia trait affects 1 in 7 people of Mediterranean origin, 1 in 30 of Asian origin, and 1 in 50 of African–American origin.

Blood type
If the woman is rhesus negative (dd) and her fetus is rhesus positive (DD or Dd) then she might form anti-D antibodies in the event of fetal and maternal blood mixing. As these can cross the placenta and attack the fetal blood cells, fetal anemia due to hemolysis can result in subsequent pregnancies. Giving therapeutic anti-D, which does not cross the placenta, after any incident where mixing of the fetal and maternal circulations is likely is known to reduce the mother's risk of developing her own anti-D, and reduces the risk of fetal hemolytic disease with subsequent pregnancies (Fig. 45.4). Prophylactic anti-D can also be administered, routinely, at 28 weeks' gestation.

Antibody screen
This is performed at the initial prenatal visit and on at least one other occasion later in pregnancy, usually around 28 weeks. Antibodies can occur in all women, not just those who are rhesus negative. A rising antibody titer raises worries of fetal

Prenatal Care

Events after which anti-D is given

- Delivery
- External cephalic version
- Termination of pregnancy
- Manual removal of placenta
- Bleeding in pregnancy at any gestational age
- Ectopic pregnancy
- Abdominal trauma in the third trimester
- Amniocentesis/CVS
- Evacuation of retained products of conception
- Abruption

Fig. 45.4 Events after which anti-D is given.

anemia, prompting ultrasound scans looking for signs of this, and, if indicated, FBS.

Rubella antibodies
Rubella acquired in pregnancy can have serious consequences, so the test is done to see whether a woman has immunity. If IgG is present then she has had the infection or has been vaccinated in the past. Exposure in the pregnancy should still be investigated if she develops symptoms, but the risk of reinfection is extremely low. If she is not immune, then she can be advised to avoid any contact with the infection and a vaccination can be given after the baby is born so that she will be protected in future pregnancies. As the vaccine is live it cannot be given during pregnancy.

Syphilis antibodies
Luckily, syphilis is rare, but because fetal infection can have devastating consequences and is easily treated by giving the mother penicillin, a case remains for screening in pregnancy.

Hepatitis antibodies
Detection of hepatitis B or C has implications for fetal health and for the long-term health of the woman and her partner. Hepatitis B can be transmitted to the fetus in utero, via transplacental hemorrhage, or at the time of delivery (vertical transmission). If infected, the baby will have a 90% chance of developing chronic hepatitis, with the possible sequelae of cirrhosis and primary hepatocellular carcinoma. Identifying a woman who is positive for hepatitis B antenatally allows the neonatal team the chance to try to prevent the baby from infection by administering vaccine neonatally. It also allows the woman to be monitored by the medical team; her partner and any other children can be screened.

Human immunodeficiency virus antibodies
All women should be encouraged to have HIV screening. Diagnosis of HIV in pregnancy can improve the outcome for the unborn child, the mother, her partner, and any other children (see Chapter 36). As this is now part of routine screening, there should be no stigma attached, and no penalty imposed by insurance companies.

Urinalysis and culture
The urine is dipped for protein, blood, and glucose and can also be analysed for leukocytes and nitrites. The urine is also sent for culture, as many pregnant women may have asymptomatic bacturia. This condition is treated during pregnancy due to the increased risk of pyelonephritis.

Proteinuria
If protein is detected on dipstick, then the first question should be whether the sample was contaminated with vaginal discharge and, if so, to ask for a repeat sample. If protein persists, then it must be investigated. Leukocytes and nitrites would add to the suspicion of a UTI, which can be excluded by sending a urine culture; do not be reassured by lack of symptoms, as pregnant women are often unaffected by "cystitis." If this is negative and proteinuria persists, then the possibility of renal disease or (later in pregnancy) pre-eclampsia should be considered (see Chapter 35). The first step is to obtain a 24-h urine collection to quantify the protein. Total protein excretion increases in pregnancy, so proteinuria should not be diagnosed until more than 0.3 g is excreted in 24 h.

Glycosuria
Finding glucose on dipstick is very common in pregnancy. In some cases it is due to impaired glucose tolerance or gestational diabetes, but in others a glucose tolerance test will not reveal this diagnosis. In the past it was thought that these women's glycosuria could be explained by an altered renal threshold for glucose, but physiological studies have not proven this. Instead, we must recognize that glycosuria is normal in some women in pregnancy.

Education at initial visit

Elements of quad screen*			
	Trisomy 21 (Down syndrome)	Trisomy 18	Neural tube defects
MSAFP (maternal serum AFP)	Decreases	Decreases	Increases
hCG (human chorionic gonadotropin)	Increases	Decreases	Not used
Estriol	Decreases	Decreases	Not used
Inhibin	Increases	Not used	Not used

*The triple screen uses only MSAFP, hCG, and estriol.

Fig. 45.5 Elements of quad screen.

Hematuria

Contamination with vaginal blood must be excluded. A urine culture should be sent to look for infection. If this is negative then consider a renal ultrasound for evidence of stones or renal disease.

Screening and prenatal diagnosis

Assessing the risk that the fetus is affected by some chromosomal abnormalities can be done by using a blood test (the quad screen or triple screen; see Figure 45.5) that looks at proteins in the maternal blood, or by using ultrasound, which measures the thickness of the fat pad in the nuchal fold of the fetal neck. Both types of test can give false-positive and false-negative results and are only risk assessments rather than diagnostic tests, but the result can help parents to decide whether they want more invasive tests, e.g. amniocentesis.

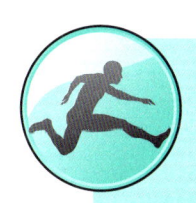

> Nuchal thickness is measured on ultrasound scan between 11 and 14 weeks' gestation. Serum screening is performed between 15 and 20 weeks' gestation.

Women who opt for diagnostic testing in the form of amniocentesis or chorionic villus sampling might be doing so for a variety of reasons (see Chapter 33). It is now recognized that ultrasound scanning at 18–20 weeks is the best method of screening for neural tube defects (e.g. spina bifida).

Planning prenatal care

A plan for the woman's prenatal care should be made at her initial visit after any risk factors affecting the pregnancy have been identified (see Fig. 45.1). The number of visits needed varies from woman to woman; most prenatal visits follow the pattern: initial visit (around 12 weeks), followed by visits every 4 weeks, i.e. 16, 20, 24, until 28 weeks, then every 2 weeks until 36 weeks, then weekly until delivery. If there is cause for concern at any time then this schedule will change to include extra visits, which may be in the community or at the hospital.

Education at initial visit

The initial visit is an opportunity for the woman to ask questions regarding her prenatal care and delivery, and for the midwife or doctor to ensure that advice about the following is given:
- Folic acid: taking folate supplements before conception and in the first trimester of pregnancy reduces the risk of fetal neural tube defects.
- Diet: certain foods are not advisable in pregnancy (Fig. 45.6).
- Exercise: it is safe to continue exercising in pregnancy, but sensible to modify the exercise routines as the pregnancy advances and to bear in mind that it is far easier to strain muscles because of increased progesterone levels.
- Seatbelts: it is illegal to go without a seatbelt, and pregnancy is not an exemption. The belt

should be worn above and below, not across, the abdomen.
- Smoking: smoking increases the risk of fetal and neonatal problems; it is also associated with SIDS and childhood illnesses.

Dietary advice in pregnancy

Food to avoid	Risk
Soft cheese	Listeria: fetal infection can lead to miscarriage or stillbirth
Unpasteurized milk and cheese	
Uncooked fish, e.g. sushi, smoked fish	
Unwashed salad/fruit/vegetables	Toxoplasma: fetal infection can lead to miscarriage, stillbirth, or long-term disability
Raw and rare meat	
Unpasteurized milk	
Shellfish	Can cause food poisoning, which can precipitate premature labor
Uncooked eggs	

Fig. 45.6 Dietary advice in pregnancy.

- Toxoplasma: infection is acquired from contact with cat feces, which can contaminate soil, so pregnant women are advised to wash fruit and salad carefully, not to handle cat litter, and to wear gloves if gardening. Animals can ingest infected soil, which can pass through the food chain unless meat is cooked through thoroughly, so women are advised against eating uncooked or "rare" meat in pregnancy.

Prenatal visits

At each visit, these points are covered:
- General health and well-being.
- Fetal movements.
- Urinalysis.
- Blood pressure.
- Abdominal palpation and fundal height measurement for fetal growth, lie, and presentation.
- Auscultation of the fetal heart.

Any worries or symptoms can be discussed. The so-called "minor" symptoms of pregnancy can cause major upset, yet some are simply treated. Common problems and suitable advice/treatment are shown in Fig. 45.7.

"Minor" symptoms of pregnancy

- Nausea: eating little and often, acupuncture, and anti-emetics. If severe vomiting develops, admission will be needed.
- Constipation: increase fruit in diet, drink plenty of water, and regular laxatives as necessary.
- Headache: often due to dehydration, but acetaminophen is safe in pregnancy.
- Pain due to ligament stretch and pubic symphysis separation: helped by regular acetaminophen and physiotherapy.
- Gastroesophageal reflux: avoid spicy foods, sleep in a more upright position, use liquid antacid preparations; sometimes use H_2 blockers (e.g. ranitidine).

Fig. 45.7 "Minor" symptoms of pregnancy: appropriate advice and treatment.

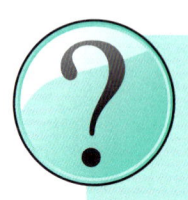

- What information will help you to estimate the gestation of pregnancy?
- Mrs Jones is in her fourth pregnancy. She has had two babies and a miscarriage. What is her gravidity and parity?
- Why screen for hepatitis and HIV in pregnancy?
- Which foods can transmit toxoplasmosis?
- What are the three main substances tested for at urinalysis?

46. Examination

General examination

General examination of the patient is extremely important and is often overlooked. Ensure that the patient is comfortable and not unduly exposed. Obstetric patients should not be examined flat on their backs because of the risk of postural supine hypotensive syndrome. The following general assessment should be made quickly:
- The patient's general well-being.
- The cardiovascular system, including pulse, blood pressure, cardiac murmurs, and clinical signs of anemia; edema can affect the hands, the periorbital region, the legs, and the sacral region.
- The respiratory system.

The urine should be tested for the presence of sugar and protein.

A chaperone should always be used when performing a gynecologic examination.

Abdominal examination

Inspection
Inspection of the abdomen is an important part of the abdominal examination.

Surgical scars
Surgical scars are often overlooked because of successful attempts to produce cosmetically pleasing scars. Transverse suprapubic and laparoscopy scars are commonly missed unless specifically looked for. Always check the umbilicus and pubic hairline for hidden scars. Multiple small scars might be present following minimally invasive surgical procedures.

Abdominal masses
Inspection for abdominal masses is important, although they might not be evident on inspection alone because of an increased BMI. The size and shape of the abdomen should be noted.

Stigmata of pregnancy
Striae gravidarum (stretch marks) caused by pregnancy hormones that stimulate the splitting of the dermis and can occur relatively early in pregnancy. New striae appear red and sometimes inflamed and can be sore and itchy; old striae, from previous pregnancies, are pale and silvery. They usually appear on the lower abdomen, upper thighs, buttocks, and breasts.

Increased skin pigmentation can occur in pregnancy and results in the linea nigra, a midline pigmentation from the xyphoid process to the pubic symphysis. Other areas that can undergo pigmentation in pregnancy include the nipples, the vulva, the umbilicus, and recent abdominal scars.

Palpation
Before palpating the abdomen, always inquire for areas of tenderness and palpate these areas last. Using the palm of the hand, gently palpate the four quadrants of the abdomen to elicit tenderness, guarding, and rebound.

On discovering an abdominal mass, the size, shape, position, mobility, and consistency should be assessed. If a mass is discovered then you should first ascertain whether it is arising from the pelvis. If you cannot palpate the lower aspect of the mass then it is probably arising from the pelvis. Pelvic tumors can generally be moved from side to side, but not up and down. Percussion can help outline the borders of a mass in an obese patient. Auscultation of the abdomen is important to assess bowel sounds, and in an obstetric patient the fetal heart should be auscultated using a fetal doptone.

Obstetric palpation
Uterine size
Uterine size is assessed by palpation and is a skill that is acquired through experience. A rough guide to the uterine size can be made from assessment of

Examination

the fundal height in relation to the topography of the abdomen, e.g. the pubic symphysis, umbilicus, and xyphoid process (Fig. 46.1). The fundus of the uterus should not be palpable abdominally until 12 weeks' gestation. By 36 weeks the fundus should be almost at the level of the xyphoid process, following which it drops as the fetal head engages into the maternal pelvis.

When palpating the uterine fundus, always start at the xyphoid process and work towards the umbilicus using the medial border of the hand or the fingertips. Percussing the fundus can be useful in obese women. Measuring the distance from the fundus to the pubic symphysis in centimeters (the fundal height) is a more objective method of assessing fundal height than using topography alone, but it is not a replacement for careful palpation. The fundal height measurement ±3 cm should equal the number of weeks amenorrhea after 20 weeks' gestation. Similarly, after 28 weeks' gestation the abdominal girth measured in inches at the level of the umbilicus should equal the number of weeks amenorrhea, although this is less reliable and not routinely performed.

Number of fetuses

The number of fetuses present can be calculated by assessing the number of fetal poles present. "Fetal pole" is the term used to denote the head or the breech. In a singleton pregnancy, two poles should be palpable unless the presenting part is deeply engaged in the pelvis. In multiple pregnancies, the number of poles present *minus one* should be palpable. For example, four poles are present in a twin pregnancy and only three should be palpable, as one is usually tucked away out of reach. In a triplet pregnancy, six poles are present and five should be palpable, and so on. This requires a high level of skill in abdominal palpation; but don't worry, the patient will usually tell you how many fetuses are present!

Fetal lie

This is the relationship between the long axis of the fetus and the long axis of the uterus. This can be longitudinal, transverse, or oblique (Fig. 46.2).

Fetal presentation

This is the part of the fetus that presents to the mother's pelvis. If the head is situated over the pelvis then this is termed a "cephalic presentation."

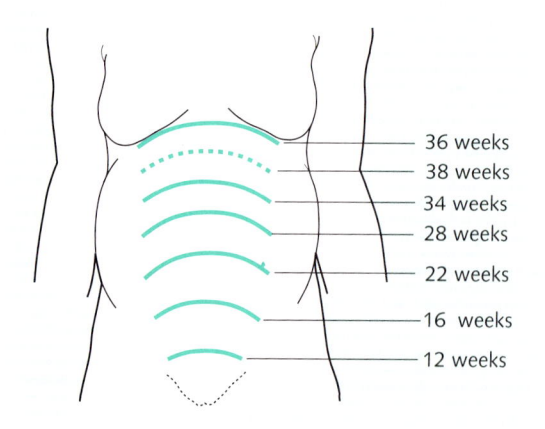

Fig. 46.1 Fundal height in relation to abdominal landmarks.

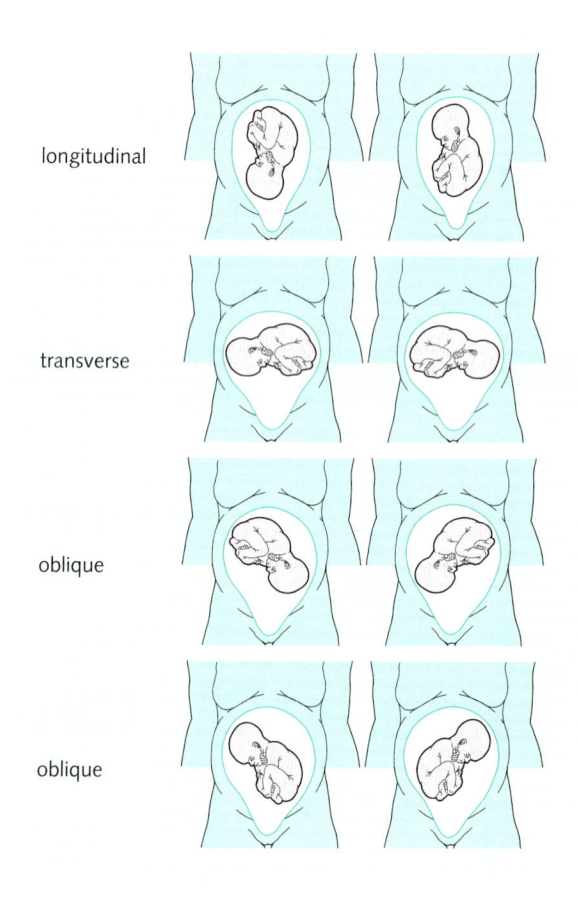

Fig. 46.2 The fetal lie. The relationship of the long axis of the fetus to the long axis of the uterus.

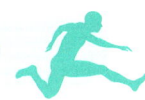

Three different types of cephalic presentation can occur, depending on the degree of flexion of the head on the fetal spine:
- A well flexed head will present by the vertex (the area bordered by the parietal bones and the anterior and posterior fontanelles).
- A partly extended head will present by the brow.
- A fully extended head will present by the face.

In a breech presentation the buttocks occupy the lower segment, and in an oblique lie the shoulder generally presents (Fig. 46.3). Any presentation other than a vertex presentation is called a malpresentation.

Engagement
The fetal head is said to be engaged when the widest diameter of the head (the BPD) has passed through the pelvic brim. Abdominal palpation of the head is assessed in fifths and is measured by palpating the angle between the head and the pubic symphysis (Fig. 46.4). The head is not engaged when three or more fifths of the head are palpable abdominally. The head is clinically engaged when two or fewer fifths of the head are palpable.

Position
The position of the presenting part is defined as the relationship of the denominator of the presenting part to the maternal pelvis. The denominator changes according to the presenting part, i.e. the occiput in a cephalic presentation, the mentum (chin) in a face presentation, and the sacrum in a breech presentation. An idea of the position can be gained at abdominal palpation by determining the position of the fetal back. If the back lies:
- On the maternal left, the position is likely to be left occiput transverse.
- On the maternal right, the position is likely to be right occiput transverse.
- More posteriorly (i.e. towards the mother's spine), the position is likely to be left or right OP.
- Anteriorly, the position is likely to be left or right occiput anterior (Fig. 46.5).

The position of the presenting part can be assessed accurately only by vaginal examination, because the head might not lie in the same axis as the fetal trunk.

Attitude
This term is no longer commonly used. It describes the relationship of the fetal parts to the fetus itself. For instance, when the head, back, and limbs of the fetus are flexed, as in the classic "fetal position," the fetus has a flexed attitude; conversely, it can be said to have an extended attitude.

Amniotic fluid volume
Clinical assessment of amniotic fluid volume is not as accurate as objective assessment using ultrasound. However, subjective assessment can alert the examiner to the possibility of reduced or increased amniotic fluid volume and instigation of the necessary investigations. Reduced amniotic fluid volume might be suggested when the uterus is small for dates with easily palpable fetal parts producing an irregular firm outline to the uterus. Increased amniotic fluid volume causes a large-for-dates uterus that is smooth and rounded and in which the fetal parts are almost impossible to distinguish. If suspected, an ultrasound scan should be ordered to assess objective measurements, such as depth of deepest pocket or AFI.

Difficulty palpating fetal parts
Many students worry that they will not be able to ascertain all the above information during an obstetric abdominal palpation. This is not always possible even in the most experienced hands, but it is important to understand why this might be so. Figure 46.6 shows some situations when palpation of the fetal parts might prove difficult.

Pelvic examination
Gynecologic pelvic examination
There are three important steps when performing a pelvic examination:
1. External inspection of the vulva.
2. Internal inspection of the vagina and cervix via a speculum.
3. Bimanual examination of the pelvis.

The most common position for carrying out a pelvic examination is the dorsal position with the woman lying on her back with her knees flexed. Make sure that the patient is as comfortable as possible and not too exposed.

Examination

Cephalic

Vertex   Brow   Face

Breech

Extended   Flexed   Footling

Shoulder

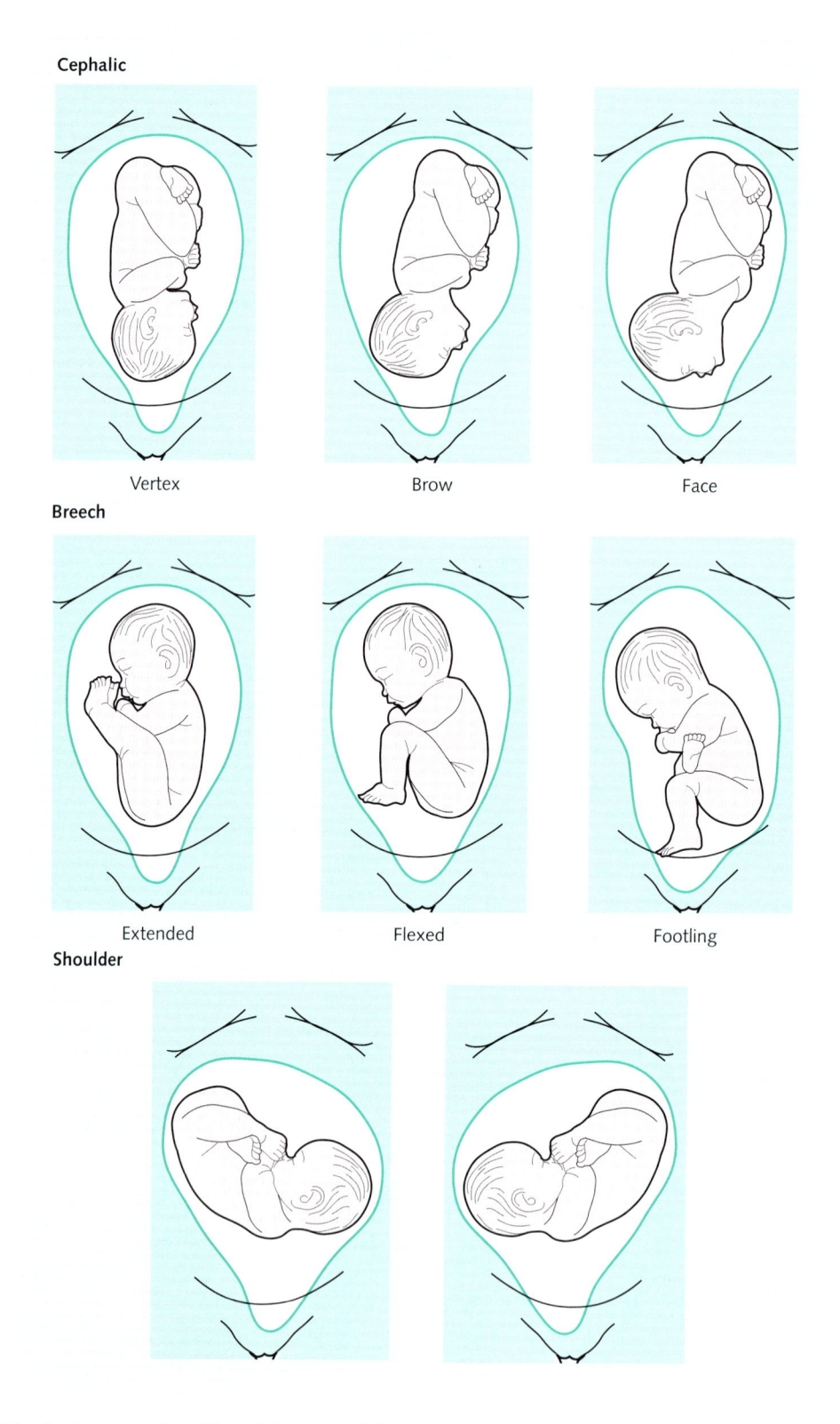

Fig. 46.3 The fetal presentation. The relationship of the presenting part of the fetus to the maternal pelvis.

Abdominal examination

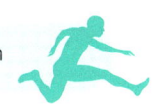

Fig. 46.4 Engagement of the fetal head.

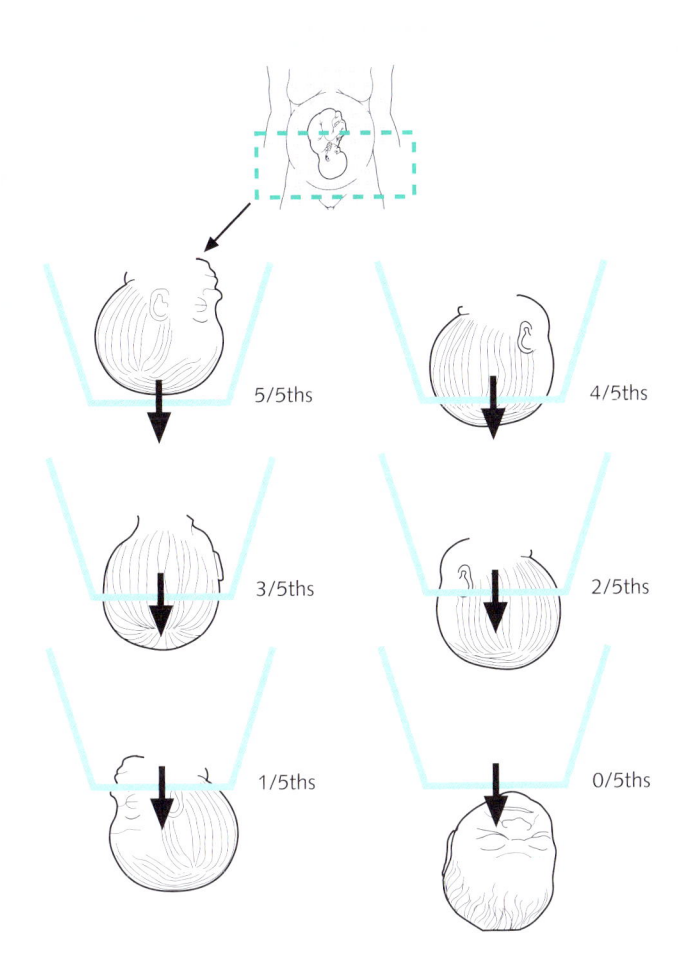

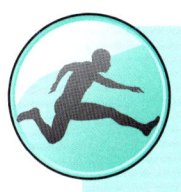

5/5ths   4/5ths
3/5ths   2/5ths
1/5ths   0/5ths

> During a gynecologic examination, the pelvic examination should always be preceded by inspection of the external genitalia and vaginal walls.

External examination of the vulva

The presence of abnormal discharge on the vulva should be noted, as should the anatomy of the external genitalia (Fig. 46.7). Parting the labia with the left hand, the entire area should be carefully inspected for inflammation, ulceration, swellings, atrophic changes, and leukoplakia (white plaques), and the clitoris and urethral orifice inspected. A deficient or scarred perineum are clues to previous trauma due to vaginal delivery. Vaginal or uterine prolapse through the introitus is assessed with and without the patient bearing down, and stress incontinence might be demonstrated when the patient coughs. Assessment of prolapse can only be adequately made with the patient in the left lateral position using a Sims' speculum.

Internal inspection of the vagina and cervix

To inspect the vagina and cervix, a speculum is used. Two types of speculum are used commonly: Cusco's (bivalve) and Sims' specula.

The Cusco speculum is used with the patient in the dorsal position and consists of two blades hinged outside the patient. When the blades are opened, the anterior and posterior walls of the vagina are separated allowing the vaginal fornices and cervix to be visualized. The main disadvantage

283

Examination

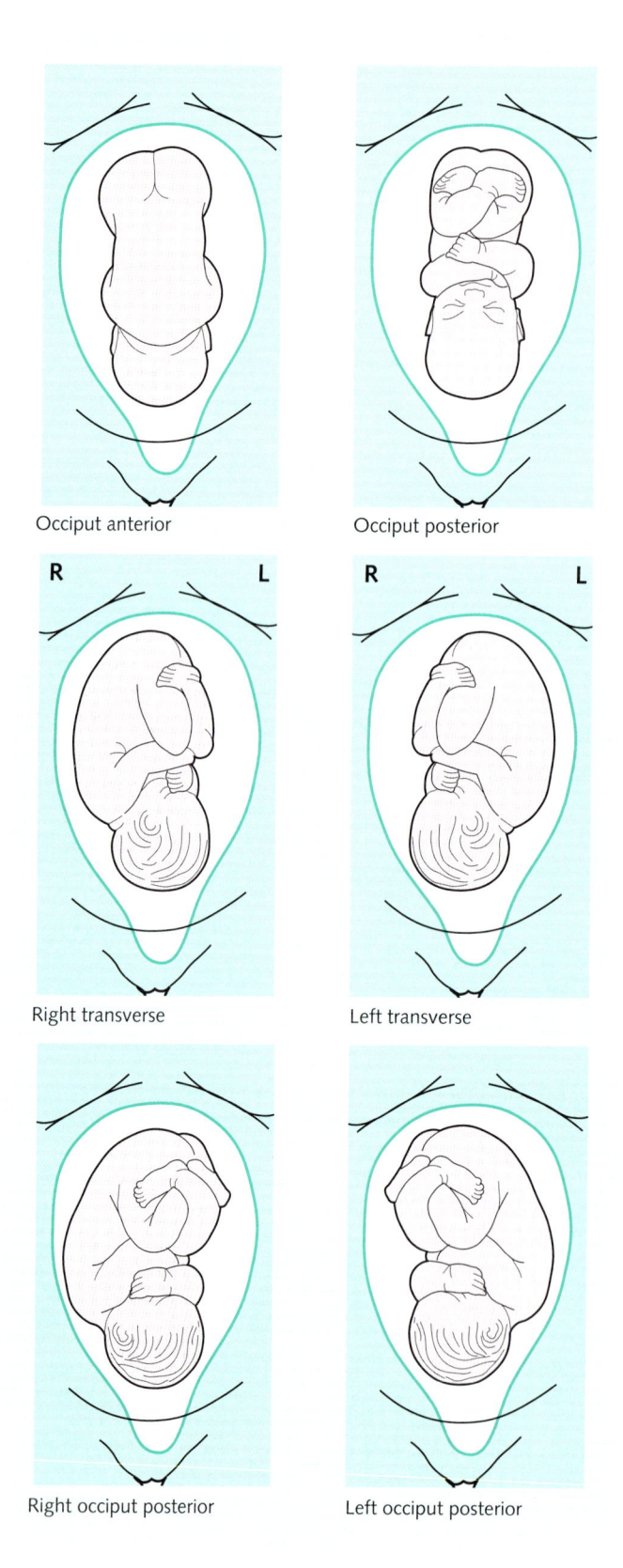

Occiput anterior

Occiput posterior

Right transverse

Left transverse

Right occiput posterior

Left occiput posterior

Fig. 46.5 The fetal position.

Abdominal examination

of the Cusco speculum is that the anterior and posterior walls of the vagina cannot be assessed adequately.

The Sims speculum is used to inspect the anterior and posterior walls of the vagina and is an excellent tool for assessing uterovaginal prolapse. It was originally developed to examine vaginal fistulas. With the patient in the left lateral, or Sims', position the blade of the speculum is inserted into the vagina and used to retract either the anterior or posterior walls. Uterovaginal prolapse can then be assessed with the patient bearing down.

Bimanual examination

It is usual to perform an internal examination using the lubricated index and middle fingers of the right hand, although in nulligravid and postmenopausal women it might be possible to use only the index finger. Palpation of the vaginal walls is important to exclude scarring, cysts, and tumors that can easily be missed on inspection. The vaginal fornices should be examined for scarring, thickening, and swellings that will suggest pelvic pathology. The size, shape, position, consistency, angle, and mobility of the cervix should be assessed. Moving the cervix from side to side might elicit cervical motion tenderness, and elevating the cervix anteriorly, thereby stretching the uterosacral ligaments, might cause pain in the presence of endometriosis.

The fingers of the right hand are then used to elevate or steady the uterus while the left hand palpates abdominally. An anteverted uterus is usually palpable between the two hands. A retroverted uterus is usually felt as a swelling in the posterior fornix and is not bimanually palpable unless it is flipped forward into an anteverted position and elevated into the anterior part of the pelvis. The different combinations of version and flexion of the uterus are shown in Fig. 46.8. The size, position, consistency, outline, and mobility of

Situations in which fetal parts might be difficult to palpate	
Types of reason	Description
Maternal reasons	Maternal obesity
	Muscular anterior abdominal wall
Uterine reasons	Anterior uterine wall fibroids
	Uterine contraction/Braxton Hicks contraction
Fetoplacental reasons	Anterior placenta
	Increased amniotic fluid volume

Fig. 46.6 Situations in which fetal parts might be difficult to palpate.

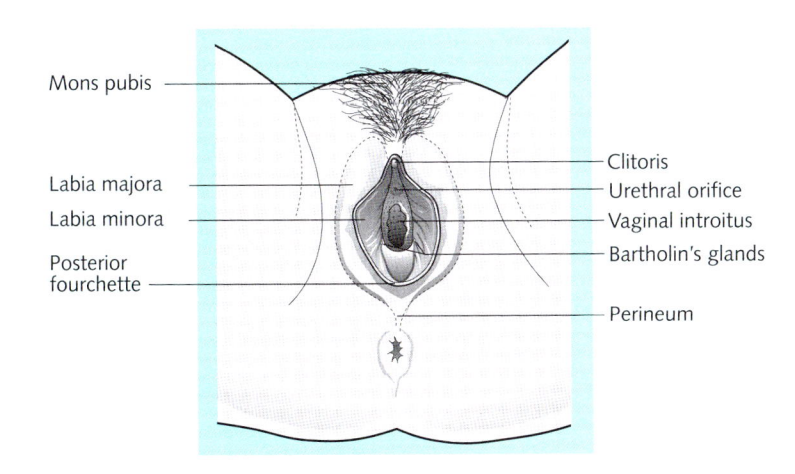

Fig. 46.7 The female external genitalia.

Examination

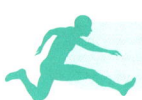

the uterus should all be noted. A pregnant uterus should feel soft and globular and roughly the size of an apple, large orange, and grapefruit at 6 weeks', 8 weeks', and 12 weeks' gestation respectively.

To examine the adnexa, the fingers of the right hand should be positioned in one of the lateral fornices and the adnexal region palpated between the two hands. Normal premenopausal ovaries are not always palpable, depending on the size of the patient. Fallopian tubes and postmenopausal ovaries should not be palpable. If an adnexal mass is discovered, then its size, shape, consistency, mobility, and whether it is fixed to the uterus or not should all be noted. The presence and degree of tenderness should be noted. In the presence of a suspected ectopic, pelvic examination should not be carried out prior to inserting a large intravenous cannula, as profound internal hemorrhage might occur if the ectopic pregnancy ruptures.

Obstetric pelvic examination

There are four components to the obstetric pelvic examination:
1. External inspection of the vulva.
2. Internal inspection of the vagina and cervix.
3. Vaginal examination.
4. Pelvic examination.

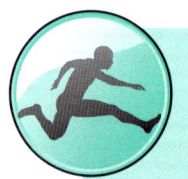

> An obstetric examination is incomplete without a blood pressure check, urinalysis, and auscultation of the fetus.

External examination of the vulva

The blood flow through the vulva and vagina increases dramatically in pregnancy, and due to engorgement the vulva might look swollen and edematous. The presence of vulvar varicosities should be noted. Note the presence of vaginal discharge or leaking amniotic fluid.

Internal inspection of the vagina and cervix

Examination of the vagina and cervix through a sterile Cusco's speculum should be performed using an aseptic technique. The vagina and cervix might take on a bluish tinge compared with the nonpregnant state. Increased vaginal and cervical secretions are normal in pregnancy. Inspection of the cervix might reveal amniotic fluid draining through the cervical os. Digital examination in the presence of ruptured membranes is likely to increase the risk of ascending infection. Exclusion of cervical pathology is important in the presence of APH, although care must be taken because, in the presence of placenta previa, bleeding might be exacerbated.

Vaginal examination

This should be performed under aseptic conditions in the presence of ruptured membranes. Once the cervix has been identified, the following characteristics should be determined:
- Dilatation.
- Length.

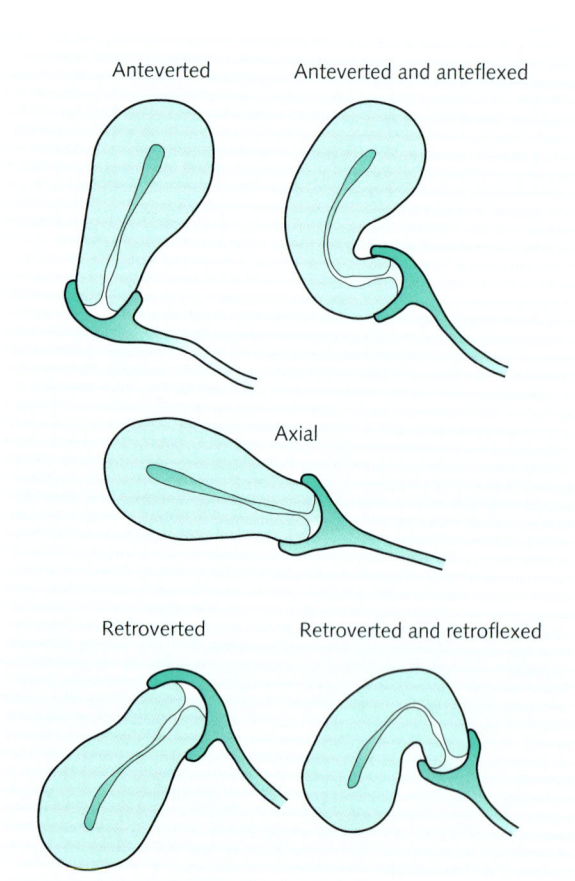

Fig. 46.8 Positions of the uterus.

Anteverted

Anteverted and anteflexed

Axial

Retroverted

Retroverted and retroflexed

- Station of presenting part.
- Consistency.
- Position.

Cervical dilatation
Cervical dilatation is assessed in centimeters using the examining fingers. One finger-breadth is roughly 1–1.5 cm. Full dilatation of the cervix is equivalent to 10 cm dilatation.

Cervical length
The normal length of the cervix is about 4 cm, and shortening occurs as the cervix effaces due to uterine contractions (Fig. 46.9).

Station of the presenting part
The station of the presenting part is determined by how much the presenting part has descended into the pelvis. The station is defined as the number of centimeters above or below a fixed point in the maternal pelvis, the ischial spines (Fig. 46.10).

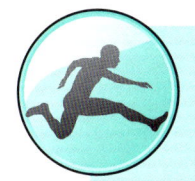

> When taking a Pap smear, a brush should always be used to sample the endocervix as well as a spatula.

Cervical consistency
Softening of the cervix occurs as pregnancy progresses, aiding cervical effacement and dilatation. The consistency of the cervix can be described as firm, mid-consistency, or soft.

Cervical position
This describes where the cervix is situated in the anteroposterior plane of the pelvis. As the cervix becomes effaced and dilated it tends to be pulled from a posterior to a more anterior position.

The Bishop score
Using the above characteristics, Bishop devised a scoring system to evaluate the "ripeness" or favorability of the cervix (Fig. 46.11). This system is often used when inducing labor to assess the likelihood of success. The higher the score, the more favorable the cervix and the more likely that induction of labor will be successful. It can also be used to assess cervical change in threatened premature labor.

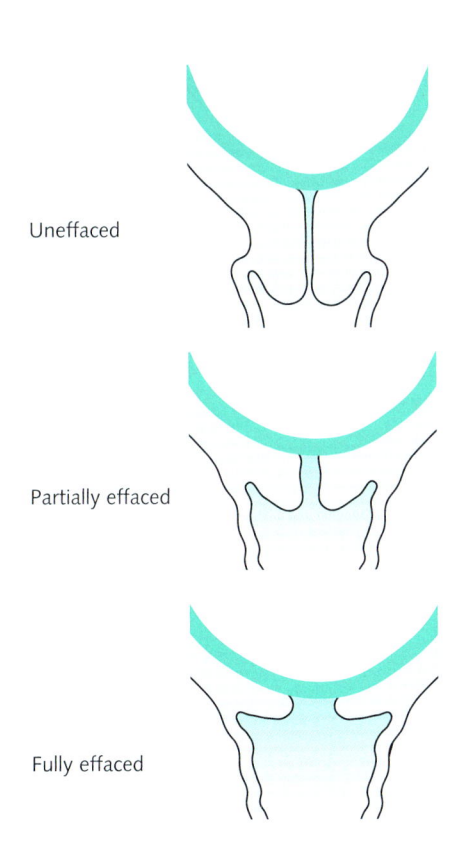

Fig. 46.9 Effacement of the cervix.

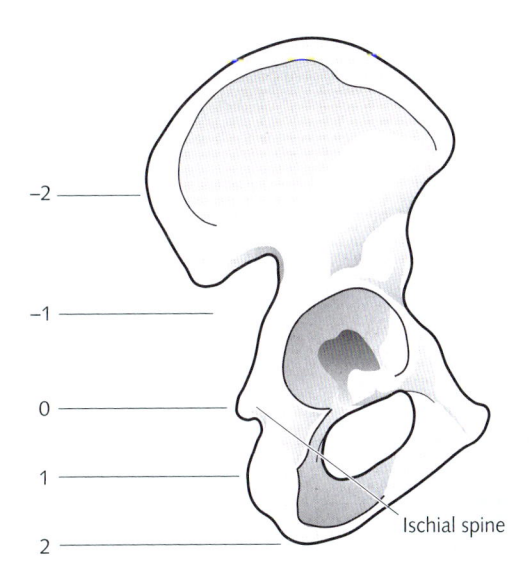

Fig. 46.10 The station of the presenting part.

Examination

The Bishop scoring system for the uterine cervix

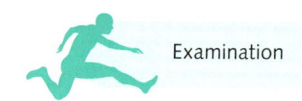

Cervical characteristic	Score 0	1	2	3
Dilatation (cm)	0	1–2	3–4	>5
Effacement (%)	0–30	40–50	60–70	>80
Station (cm)	−3	−2	−1 or 0	+1 or +2
Consistency	firm	medium	soft	
Position	posterior	mid	anterior	

Fig. 46.11 The Bishop scoring system for the uterine cervix.

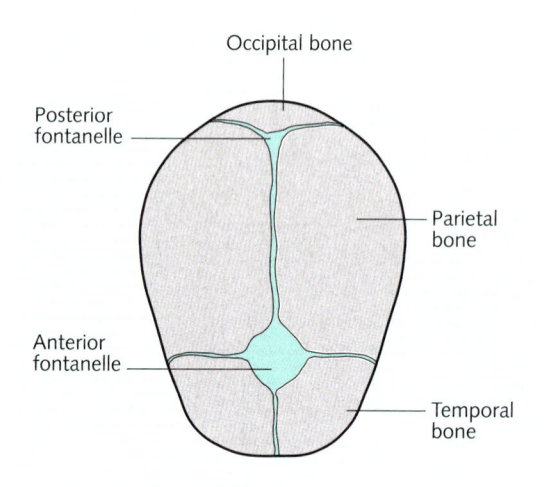

Fig. 46.12 The anterior and posterior fontanelles.

When assessing progress in labor one must always comment on engagement of head, cervical dilatation, cervical effacement, station of head in relation to ischial spines, position of head, molding, caput, and amniotic fluid color (e.g. meconium staining).

Pelvic examination

There are four basic pelvic types:
1. Gynecoid.
2. Android.
3. Anthropoid.
4. Platypoid.

Clinical assessment of the pelvis will reveal the characteristics of these pelvic types. Figure 46.14 summarizes the characteristics of the four basic pelvic types.

The pelvic inlet

The pelvic inlet is assessed clinically by measuring the diagonal conjugate (Fig. 46.15). This is the distance from the sacral promontory to the inferoposterior margin of the symphysis pubis (the true conjugate is measured to the anteroposterior margin of the symphysis pubis). In a normal gynecoid pelvis the sacral promontory cannot usually be reached. If it is, then the pelvic inlet is significantly reduced.

Defining the position of the presenting part

With a cephalic presentation, the anterior and posterior fontanelles and the sagittal sutures should be identified. The posterior fontanelle is Y-shaped and is formed when the three sutures between the occipital and parietal bones meet. The anterior fontanelle is larger, diamond-shaped, and formed by the four sutures between the parietal and temporal bones meeting (Fig. 46.12). The denominator for a cephalic presentation is the occiput, and for a breech presentation it is the sacrum. Having identified the denominator, the position of the presenting part can be defined (Fig. 46.13).

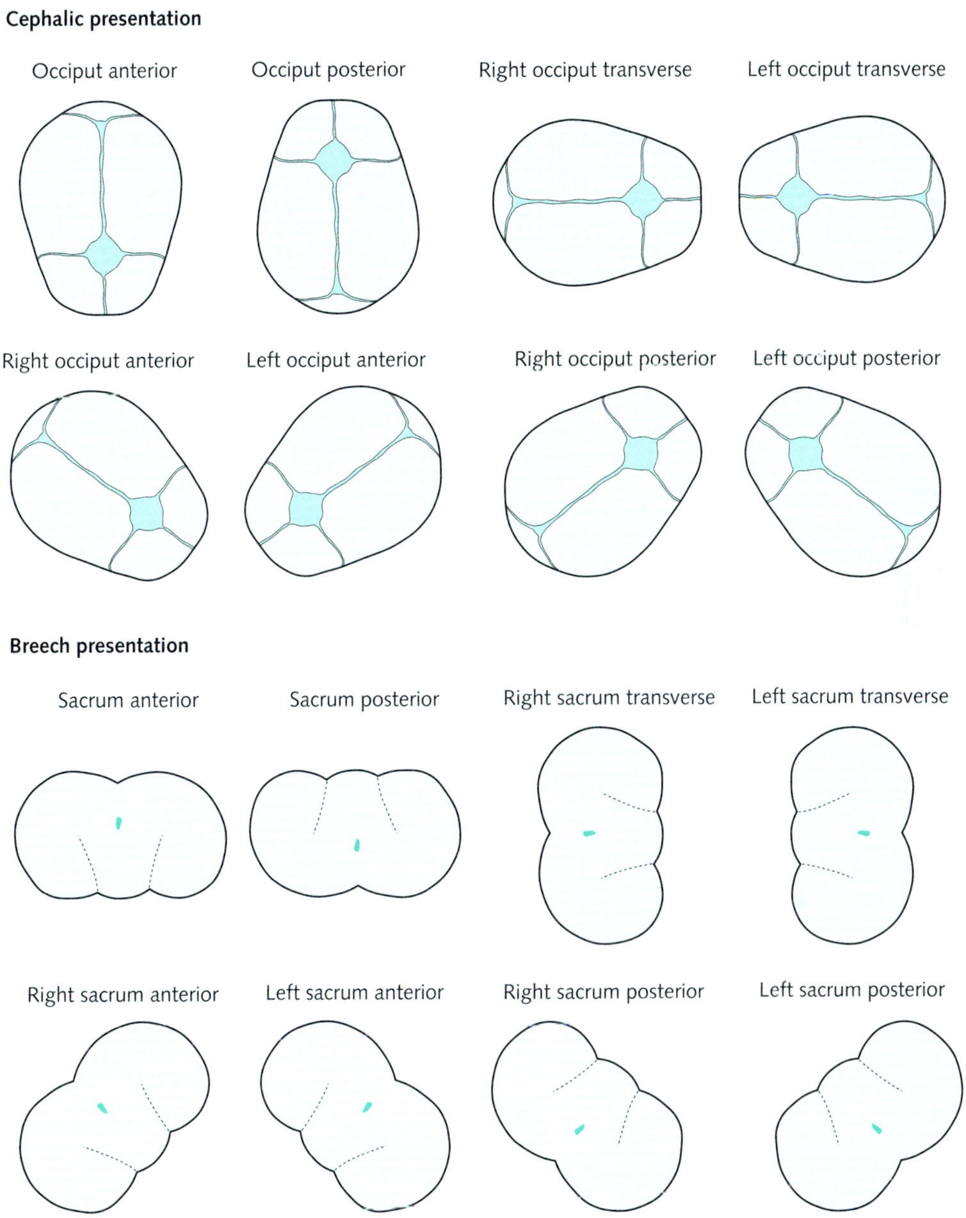

Abdominal examination

Cephalic presentation

Occiput anterior | Occiput posterior | Right occiput transverse | Left occiput transverse

Right occiput anterior | Left occiput anterior | Right occiput posterior | Left occiput posterior

Breech presentation

Sacrum anterior | Sacrum posterior | Right sacrum transverse | Left sacrum transverse

Right sacrum anterior | Left sacrum anterior | Right sacrum posterior | Left sacrum posterior

Fig. 46.13 Defining the position of the presenting part.

Examination

Pelvic type	Gynecoid	Anthropoid	Android	Platypoid
Incidence	50%	25%	20%	5%
Pelvic shape				
Pelvic inlet Obstetric Conjugate	Not reduced	Not reduced	Reduced	Reduced
Pelvic cavity Ischial spine Sacrospinous ligament	Not prominent > 3 cm	Not prominent > 3 cm	Prominent < 3 cm	Usually prominent > 3 cm
Pelvic outlet Intertuberous diameter	> 4 knuckles wide	< 4 knuckles wide	< 4 knuckles wide	> 4 knuckles wide
Pelvic walls	Parallel	Parallel	Convergent	Divergent

Fig. 46.14 Summary of the four basic pelvic-type characteristics.

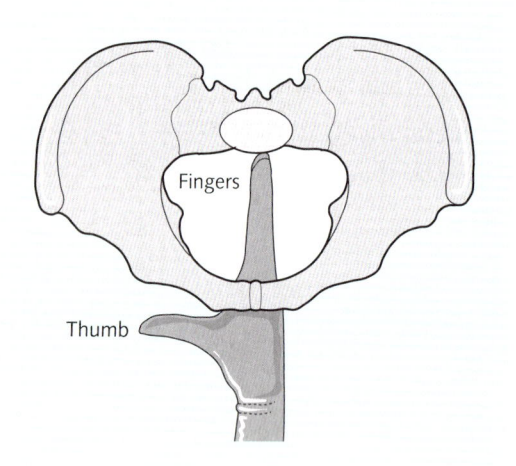

Fig. 46.15 Assessing the pelvic inlet.

The pelvic cavity

The pelvic cavity is assessed by palpating the sacral curve, which should be concave away from the examining fingers (Fig. 46.16). A straight sacrum indicates a reduced pelvic capacity. The sacrospinous ligament runs from the ischial spine to the sacrum and should be wide enough to accommodate more than two fingers (>3 cm). Prominent ischial spines suggest a shortened interspinous distance.

Abdominal examination

Fig. 46.16 Assessing the pelvic cavity.

Normal curve – convex away from examining fingers

Flat sacral curve

A

B

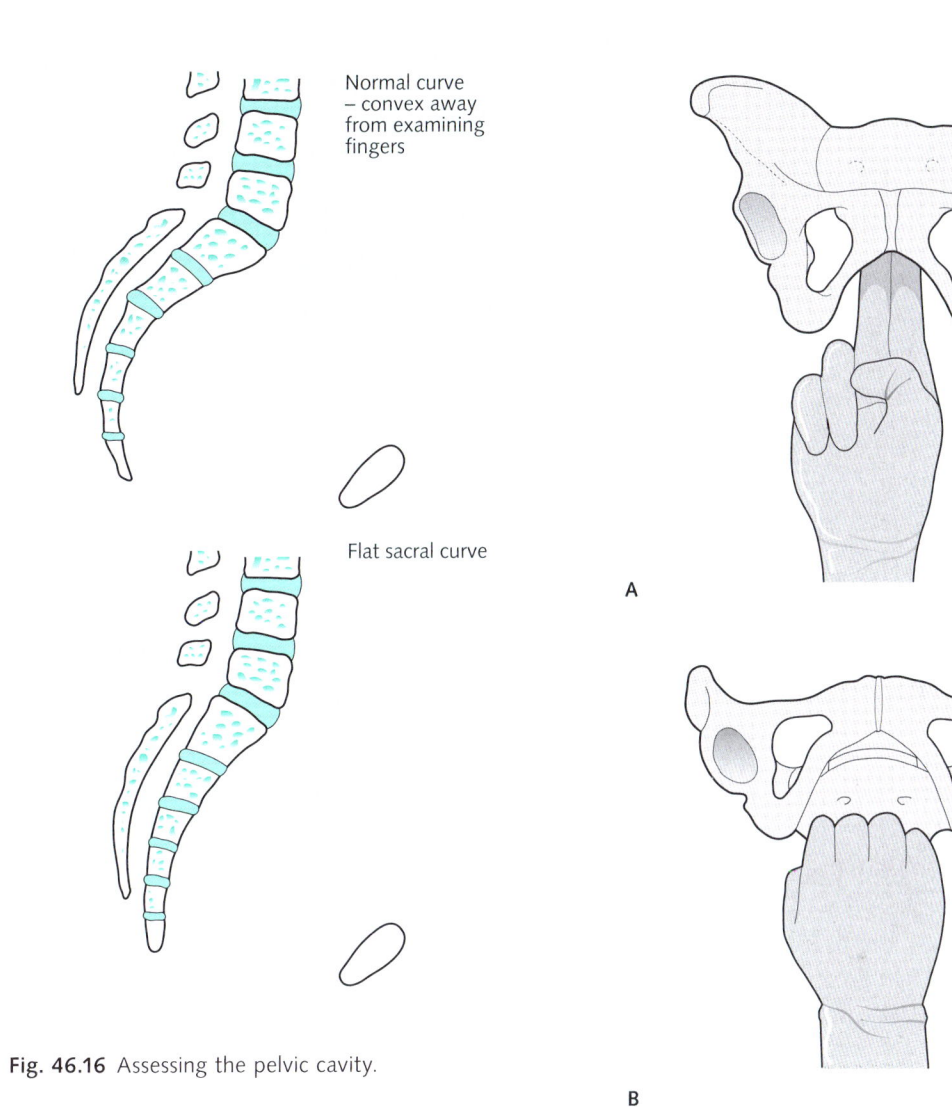

Fig. 46.17 Assessing the pelvic outlet.

The pelvic outlet

The pelvic outlet is assessed by the subpubic angle and the intertuberous distance. A subpubic angle of less than 90° and an intertuberous distance of less than four knuckles wide indicate the possibility of a reduced outlet (Fig. 46.17).

It has become increasingly recognized that the best test of a pelvis is the dynamic process of labor itself, so formal pelvic assessment is no longer performed as a routine. However, the Bishop score is used in the assessment of cervical favorability prior to induction of labor.

47. Common Investigations

Imaging techniques

Imaging techniques are used widely in both obstetrics and gynecology. Results of imaging tests should be interpreted carefully in the light of the history and clinical findings.

Ultrasound scanning

Ultrasound examination of the pregnant and nonpregnant pelvis is probably the most common investigation performed in obstetrics and gynecology. Ultrasound waves passing through the pelvis are reflected in varying degrees depending on the density of the tissues present. For instance, bone is very reflective (or echogenic) and appears white on the monitor, whereas fluid is less echogenic and appears dark on the monitor. Interpretation of these echoes is the mainstay of diagnosis in ultrasound.

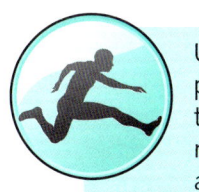

> Ultrasound examination of the pelvis (particularly transvaginal) is almost a mandatory part of the assessment of most gynecologic problems.

The nonpregnant pelvis
To examine the nonpregnant pelvis, a full bladder is required. This lifts the uterus from under the pubic bone, allows a "window" through which to view the pelvic contents, and helps push the bowel out of the pelvis.

The uterus
The dimensions of the uterus can be measured and the position noted. Abnormal textures in the myometrium can suggest the presence of fibroids or adenomyosis. The midline echo corresponds to the endometrial thickness and will vary depending on the menstrual cycle. Pathology of the endometrial cavity, such as endometrial hyperplasia, endometrial polyps, or submucous fibroids, might be detected. IUDs will show up as very bright echoes.

The ovaries
The size and position of the ovaries can be assessed. In PCOS (see Chapter 32), the polycystic ovary is, on average, twice the normal volume with thickened central stroma and 10 or more peripherally sited follicles. Follicular tracking is possible in women trying to conceive. Ovarian tumors can be identified ultrasonographically, but differentiation between benign and malignant tumors cannot be made with certainty. Figure 47.1 shows some of the ultrasound characteristics of benign and malignant ovarian tumors.

The fallopian tubes
The fallopian tubes are not normally visible by ultrasound. However, when they are blocked and distended with fluid (hydrosalpinx) they will appear as cystic structures that might be mistaken for ovarian cysts.

Ultrasound and pregnancy
A gestational sac can be seen in the uterine cavity from as early as 5 weeks' amenorrhea (Fig. 47.2), especially when using a transvaginal probe. The fetal heart is detectable with ultrasound by 6 weeks' amenorrhea. Crown–rump length (CRL) is a useful measurement with which to date the fetus up to 12 weeks' amenorrhea, by which time CRL measurement becomes inaccurate due to flexion of the fetus. After the first trimester, the BPD is a more accurate measurement with which to date the pregnancy.

Early pregnancy complications
A blighted ovum or anembryonic pregnancy occurs when the embryo fails to develop; "missed abortion" is the term used when an embryo has died in utero. In the presence of an ectopic pregnancy, the usual ultrasonic finding is that of a thickened endometrium in the presence of an

Common Investigations

Ultrasound characteristics of benign and malignant tumors

	Benign	Malignant
Size	<5 cm	>5 cm
Laterality	Unilateral	Bilateral
Cyst walls	Thin	Thick
Septa	Absent	Thick, incomplete
Solid areas	Absent	Present
Ascites	Absent	Present

Fig. 47.1 Ultrasound characteristics of benign and malignant tumors.

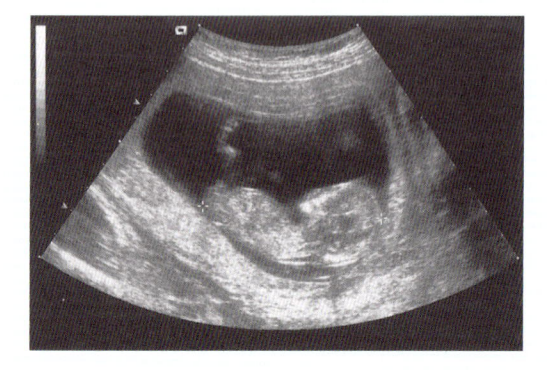

Fig. 47.2 Ultrasound in early pregnancy.

adnexal mass. In only about 5% of ectopic pregnancies can a viable pregnancy be seen outside the uterus with ultrasound. The most important role of ultrasound in the management of a suspected ectopic pregnancy is to confirm a viable intrauterine pregnancy.

Anatomy scans
Most obstetric units offer routine anatomy scans between 18 and 20 weeks' gestation. Different fetal anomalies are best detected at different times throughout the pregnancy, but 18–20 weeks appears to be the optimum time for a screening anatomy scan. Apart from gross anatomical defects, certain "markers," such as choroid plexus cysts, renal pyelectasis, and echogenic bowel, might be identified and can be associated with chromosomal abnormalities.

Fetal growth
Fetal growth is assessed clinically in a normal singleton pregnancy. In situations when the uterine size is not compatible with dates or a clinical assessment is difficult, e.g. in the presence of obesity or multiple pregnancy, objective measurements of fetal head circumference, BPD, and abdominal circumference can be measured using ultrasound and plotted on fetal growth charts. Scanning at regular intervals allows the growth of the fetus to be monitored.

Assessment of amniotic fluid volume
This is useful in the management of IUGR and postdates pregnancy. Reduced amniotic fluid volume can indicate the presence of placental insufficiency and might be an indication for delivery of the fetus, depending on the clinical background. Reduced amniotic fluid volume might also be due to spontaneous rupture of the membranes.

Doppler studies
Doppler ultrasound assessment of the uteroplacental blood flow can be useful in the presence of fetal growth restriction due to placental insufficiency. Dilatation of middle cerebral vessels and absent or reversed end diastolic flow in the umbilical artery suggest a compromised fetus that is diverting its blood flow to essential organs, such as the brain and kidneys, and is an indication for delivery. Doppler studies need to be interpreted carefully in the light of the clinical picture.

Safety of ultrasound scanning
Experimental evidence has not shown any harmful effects of ultrasound when used as a diagnostic test.

X-ray
Two X-ray procedures that were more commonly used in the past but still have clinical significance are:
1. Erect lateral pelvimetry: can be used in situations where a contracted pelvis needs to be excluded, e.g. in the management of a breech presentation. The inlet and outlet of the pelvis can be measured objectively, as can the curve of the sacrum. This procedure can be performed using CT scanning, but for reasons already

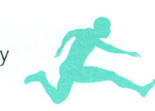

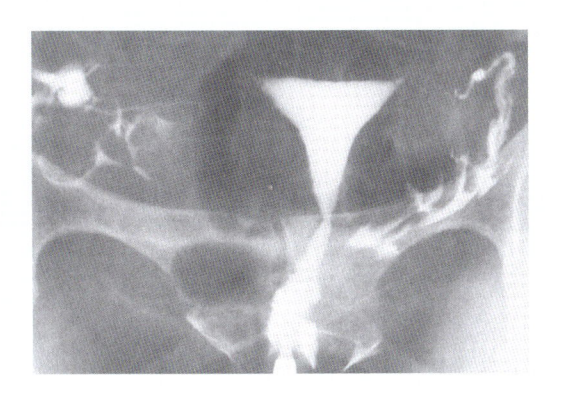

Fig. 47.3 An HSG.

discussed (see Chapter 39) is less commonly used these days.
2. Hysterosalpingography: can be used to assess the uterine cavity and the patency of the fallopian tubes (Fig. 47.3). A catheter is inserted into the cervix and radiocontrast medium injected into the uterine cavity while X-rays are taken. It does not allow the exclusion of pelvic pathology as does laparoscopic assessment of the pelvic organs, but is still useful in the presence of tubal blockage to assess whether the blockage is distal or proximal; it also allows excellent delineation of the uterine cavity.

Laparoscopy

Laparoscopy is the mainstay of diagnosing pelvic disease and has effectively replaced exploratory laparotomies. The advantage of laparoscopy over imaging techniques is that the pelvic and other intra-abdominal organs can be visualized directly through endoscopes.

Technique
The vast majority of procedures are performed under general anesthesia. Having emptied the bladder, a veress needle is inserted into the lower abdomen through a subumbilical incision. Carbon dioxide is pumped into the peritoneal cavity to produce a pneumoperitoneum (to a pressure of approximately 18 mmHg) and then a trocar and cannula are inserted through the same incision into the pneumoperitoneum. A laparoscope can then be passed down the cannula and the pelvic organs visualized (Fig. 47.4). Complications include perforation of bladder, bowel, or blood vessels, and gas embolism.

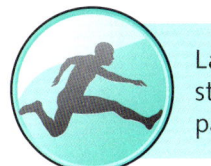

> Laparoscopy is the gold-standard investigation of pelvic pain.

Hysteroscopy

A hysteroscope is an endoscope that is inserted transcervically into the uterus to inspect the uterine cavity (Fig. 47.5). It is the best way of identifying intrauterine pathology, such as endometrial polyps, submucous fibroids, and endometrial carcinoma, and has replaced the conventional D&C for this purpose. It can be performed under either general or local anesthesia. A distention medium is required to separate the uterine walls, normal saline and carbon dioxide being the most commonly used. It is a relatively safe procedure, but complications include perforation of the uterus, gas embolism, and infection.

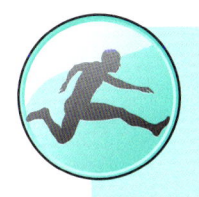

> Hysteroscopy is now the gold-standard investigation of abnormal uterine bleeding and can be performed as an outpatient investigation.

Cervical cytology/colposcopy

Squamous carcinoma of the cervix is amenable to screening because it exhibits a pre-invasive phase. Screening is carried out by cytological examination of the cervix by obtaining a Pap smear. Using a bivalve speculum, the visible cervix is gently scraped through 360°, first to the left and then to the right, using a cervical sampler (Fig. 47.6). A cytobrush can be used to sample the lower endocervical region. The specimens are placed on a

295

Common Investigations

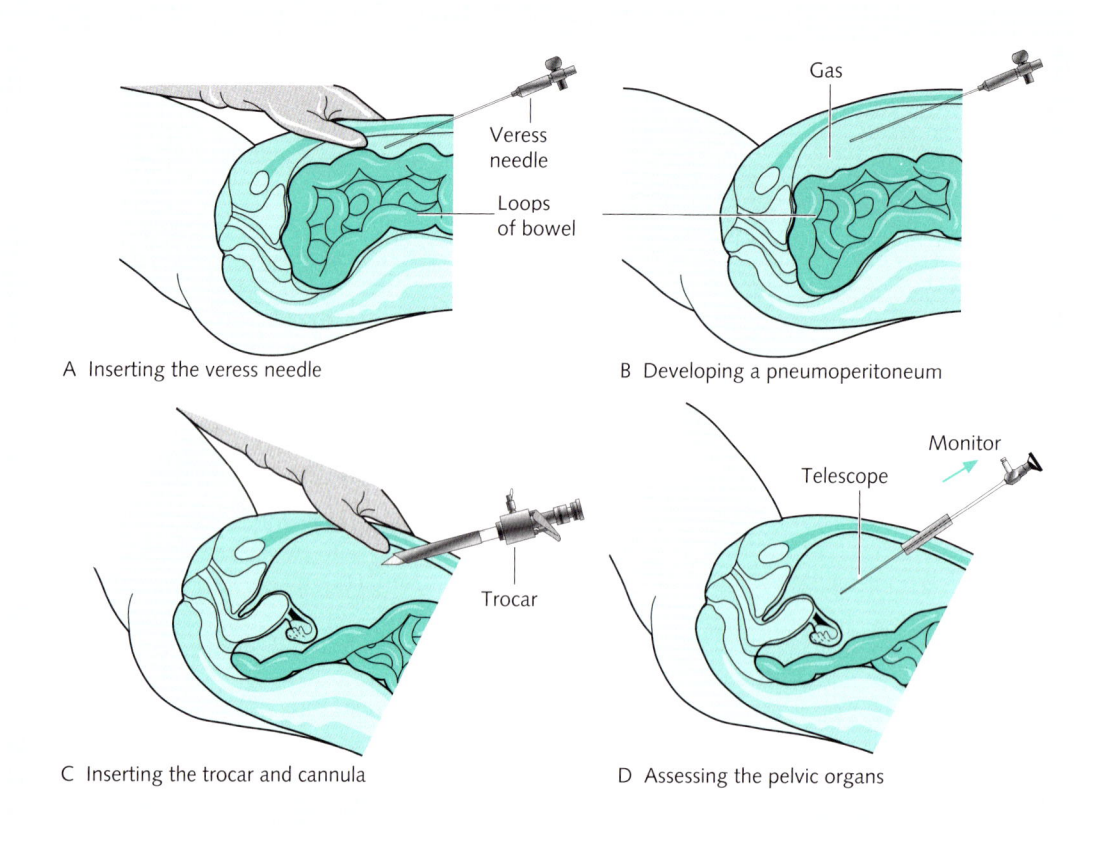

Fig. 47.4 Laparoscopic technique.

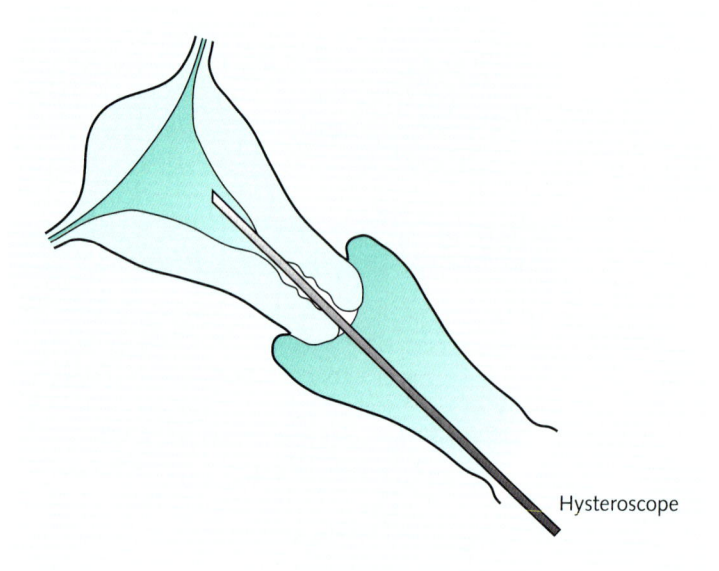

A Inserting the veress needle

B Developing a pneumoperitoneum

C Inserting the trocar and cannula

D Assessing the pelvic organs

Fig. 47.5 Hysteroscopic technique.

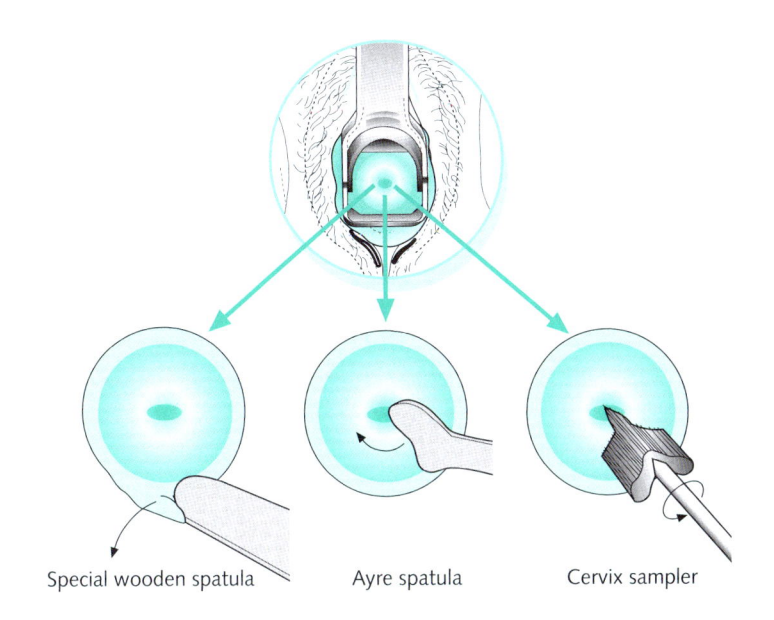

Fig. 47.6 Cervical Pap smear technique.

glass slide and fixed immediately with an alcohol solution. Women with cytology suggestive of CIN or women with an abnormal-looking cervix are then referred for colposcopy.

The colposcope is a binocular microscope enabling the surface epithelium of the cervix to be assessed under magnification and is usually performed in the outpatient setting. The patient is positioned in a modified lithotomy position and the cervix exposed using a bivalve speculum. The cervix is then viewed through the colposcope to identify any lesions, such as leukoplakia or frank invasion. Acetic acid solution (5%) is then gently but liberally applied to the entire surface of the cervix. Coagulation of proteins by the acetic acid in abnormal epithelial areas produces white changes, so called acetowhite changes.

Areas of CIN appear as distinct acetowhite lesions with clearly demarcated edges, and the associated abnormal vessel formation produces the typical mosaic and punctate patterns. The extent of the lesion should be noted, with particular regard paid to extension into the cervical canal. All abnormal-looking areas should be biopsied for histologic assessment.

Urodynamics

This term includes all the tests that assess the function of the lower urinary tract disorders, which include incontinence and voiding difficulties.

Flow studies
Using a flowmeter, the flow rate of urine can be measured. This should be above 15 mL/s, and a low flow rate suggests either outflow obstruction or poor detrusor contraction.

Cystometry
The bladder is a reservoir designed to increase in volume at low pressure. Cystometry measures bladder pressure during filling or voiding. Pressure catheters are inserted into the bladder via the urethra and also the rectum. The rectal catheter represents intra-abdominal pressure and is subtracted from the intravesical pressure to give the detrusor pressure. Detrusor pressure is measured during rapid filling of the bladder to detect the presence of detrusor instability. During voiding, detrusor contractility can be measured and outflow resistance and detrusor function assessed.

Videocystourethrography

VCU is the most informative of urodynamic studies and involves radiologically monitoring the bladder and urethra during cystometry. Congenital anomalies, diverticulum, fistulas, and ureteric reflux can all be identified during the filling phase. On coughing, bladder neck descent and GSI might be seen; and on voiding, ureteric reflux, urethral fistulas, and outflow pathology may be identified.

Glossary

ABC	airway, breathing, circulation	ICSI	intracytoplasmic sperm injection
AFE	amniotic fluid embolism	Ig	immunoglobulin
AFI	amniotic fluid index	IUGR	intrauterine growth restriction
ALT	alanine transaminase	IUI	intrauterine insemination
APH	antepartum hemorrhage	IVF	in vitro fertilization
AROM	artificial rupture of the membranes	IVP	intravenous pyelogram
AST	aspartate transaminase	LEEP	loop electrosurgical excision procedure
AZT	zidovudine	LH	luteinizing hormone
BMI	body mass index	LMP	last menstrual period
BPD	biparietal diameter	LMWH	low molecular weight heparin
bpm	beats per minute	LTCS	low transverse cesarean section
BSO	bilateral salpingo-oophorectomy	MAP	mean arterial pressure
CAH	congenital adrenal hyperplasia	MBL	menstrual blood loss
CBC	Complete blood count	MI	myocardial infarction
CIN	cervical intraepithelial neoplasia	MRI	magnetic resonance imaging
CMV	cytomegalovirus	MS	multiple sclerosis
CNS	central nervous system	NSAID	nonsteroidal anti-inflammatory drug
CPD	cephalopelvic disproportion	NST	nonstress test
CRL	crown–rump length	OCP	oral contraceptive pill
CT	computed tomography	OHSS	ovarian hyperstimulation syndrome
CVS	chorionic villus sampling	OP	occiput posterior
D&C	dilatation and curettage	PCOS	polycystic ovary syndrome
D&E	dilatation and evacuation	PCR	polymerase chain reaction
DI	donor insemination	PE	pulmonary embolism
DIC	disseminated intravascular coagulation	PGD	pre-implantation genetic diagnosis
DO	detrusor overactivity	PID	pelvic inflammatory disease
DUB	dysfunctional uterine bleeding	PIH	pregnancy-induced hypertension
DVT	deep vein thrombosis	PMB	postmenopausal bleeding
ECG	electrocardiogram	PMSS	Pregnancy Mortality Surveillance System
ECT	electroconvulsive therapy		
ECV	external cephalic version	PPH	postpartum hemorrhage
EFW	estimated fetal weight	SGA	small for gestational age
FBS	fetal blood sampling	SHBG	sex hormone binding globulin
FHR	fetal heart rate	SSRI	selective serotonin reuptake inhibitor
FISH	fluorescent in situ hybridization	T&S	type and screen
FSH	follicle stimulating hormone	TAH	total abdominal hysterectomy
GnRH	gonadotrophin-releasing hormone	TED	thromboembolic disease
GSI	genuine stress incontinence	TSH	thyroid-stimulating hormone
HbA1c	glycosylated hemoglobin	TTTS	twin-to-twin transfusion syndrome
hCG	human chorionic gonadotrophin	UTI	urinary tract infection
HELLP	hemolysis, elevated liver enzymes, low platelets	VCU	videocystourethrography
		VIN	vulvar intraepithelial neoplasia
HPV	human papilloma virus	V/Q	ventilation perfusion isotope (scan)
HRT	hormone replacement therapy	WBC	white blood cell count
HSG	hysterosalpingogram		

Index

A

ABC *see* airways, breathing, circulation (ABC)
abdominal examination, 279–280 *see also* abdominal palpation
  early pregnancy bleeding/pain, 34
  infertility, 41
  postpartum hemorrhage, 80
abdominal inspection, 279
abdominal masses, 279
abdominal pain
  algorithm, 60f
  antepartum hemorrhage, 49
  endometriosis, 108
  lab studies, 59f
  in second and third trimester pregnancy, 57–60
    diagnosis, 58f
    differential diagnosis, 57
    history, 57–58
    physical examination, 58–59
abdominal palpation
  abnormal FHR tracing in labor, 76
  APH, 50
  hypertension in pregnancy, 62
  pelvic pain, 13
  prolapse, 30
  vaginal discharge, 18
abdominopelvic mass
  uterine fibroids, 103
acanthosis nigricans
  infertility, 41
activities of daily living
  pelvic pain, 16
acute fatty liver of pregnancy, 58t, 200–201
adrenal androgens, 176
α-adrenergic agonists
  voiding disorders, 138
age
  early pregnancy failure, 157
  pregnancy risk, 272f
  vulvar symptoms, 21
airways, breathing, circulation (ABC)
  postpartum hemorrhage, 80
albuterol
  nebulized
    maternal collapse, 86
alcohol
  dependence, 203–204
  pregnancy risk, 273f
allergies, 265
  vaginal discharge, 17
amenorrhea, 3–6, 91–94, 173
  abnormal bleeding, 3–6
  algorithm, 91f
  causes, 4t
  chromosomal analysis, 5
  complications, 92
  examination, 4–5
  gynecologic history, 3
  history, 3–4

  hormone profiles, 5
  hypothalamic, 92
  imaging studies, 5–6
  post-pill, 3
  treatment, 92–93
  work-up, 5–6, 91–92
amniocentesis, 180, 181f
  prenatal diagnosis, 179–180
amniotic fluid embolism
  direct maternal deaths, 259
  maternal collapse, 84
amniotic fluid volume, 281
  ultrasound scan, 294
amniotomy
  labor induction, 240, 241f
amphetamines
  pregnancy risk, 273f
anabolic steroids
  retrograde ejaculation, 40
analgesia
  labor
    pharmacologic methods, 238f
  maternal collapse, 86
androgens
  adrenal, 176
  amenorrhea, 92
  exogenous, 176–177
  ovarian, 176
  PCOS, 176f
anemia
  iron-deficiency
    menstruation, 6
anencephaly, 70
anesthesia
  epidural
    labor, 238f
  local
    maternal collapse, 86
  spinal
    labor, 238f
angiotensin-converting enzyme inhibitors
  pregnancy-induced hypertension, 192
anorexia nervosa
  pregnancy risk, 273f
anosmia
  Kallmann's syndrome, 4
antenatal bleeding, 83
antepartum hemorrhage (APH), 186, 207–211
    see also placental abruption; placenta previa
  algorithm, 50f
  circumvallate placenta, 210
  defined, 49
  differential diagnosis, 49f
  etiology, 208f
  incidence, 207
  management, 210f
  placental abruption, 208–210
  placenta previa, 207–208

Index

antepartum hemorrhage (APH) (*Continued*)
  recurrent
    pregnancy risk, 274f
    stillbirth, 65
  unexplained, 210
  vasa previa, 210
anterior colporrhaphy
  prolapse, 147
antibiotic therapy
  premature labor, 215
antibody screening
  pregnancy, 275–276
anticholinergic agents
  detrusor overactivity, 140
  voiding disorders, 138
anticonvulsant therapy
  complications, 199f
anti-D, 276f
antidepressants
  tricyclic
    depression, 202
    detrusor overactivity, 140
    voiding disorders, 138
antimuscarinic drugs
  detrusor overactivity, 140
antiphospholipid antibodies
  early pregnancy failure, 157
  miscarriage, 154
antiphospholipid antibodies assay
  early pregnancy bleeding/pain, 36
antisperm antibodies
  infertility, 43
APH *see* antepartum hemorrhage (APH)
appendectomy
  pelvic pain, 12
appendicitis
  second and third trimester pregnancy abdominal pain, 58t
AROM *see* artificial rupture of the membranes (AROM)
artificial rupture of the membranes (AROM), 72, 226
Asherman's syndrome, 94, 99
aspirin
  pregnancy-induced hypertension, 189–190
asthma, 195
asymptomatic cysts
  ovarian, 115–116
    management, 115f
atosiban
  premature labor, 216f
atropine
  side effects, 140f
atypical myometrial tumors, 120

B

baby blues, 202
backache
  prolapse, 29
bacterial vaginalis
  fishy odor, 21
bacterial vaginosis
  early pregnancy bleeding/pain, 36
  miscarriage, 155
  vaginal discharge, 17
barbiturates
  pregnancy risk, 273f
barrier methods, 167–168

baseline fetal heart rate, 73
baseline variability
  FHR tracing, 73
benign and malignant tumors
  ultrasound scan, 294f
benign epithelial tumors
  ovaries, 113
benign germ cell tumors
  ovaries, 113
benign ovarian tumors, 113–116
  classification, 113f
  diagnosis, 114
  differential diagnosis, 114f
  etiology, 113–114
  history, 114
  incidence, 113
  management, 115–116
  physical examination, 114–115
  work-up, 115
benign sex cord stromal tumors
  ovaries, 114
beta agonists
  premature labor, 216f
bethanechol
  voiding difficulties, 141
bilateral salpingo-oophorectomy (BSO), 112
bimanual examination, 285–286
bimanual pelvic examination
  pelvic pain, 13–14
biopsy
  cone
    CIN, 122
    pregnancy risk, 273f
  endometrial
    heavy bleeding, 7
    menorrhagia, 96
  pelvic pain, 16
bipolar disorder, 203
Bishop score, 287, 288f
bisphosphonates
  menopause, 165
bleeding *see also* early pregnancy; hemorrhage; postmenopausal bleeding (PMB)
  abnormal, 3–10
    absent periods, 3–6
    algorithm, 9f
    drugs, 4
    heavy periods, 6–7
    history, 7–8
    intermenstrual and postcoital bleeding, 7
    painful periods, 7–8
    postmenopausal bleeding, 9–10
  antenatal, 83
  intermenstrual and postcoital, 7
    causes, 7t
  pictorial assessment chart, 95f
α-blockers
  ejaculation, 41
β-blockers
  impotence, 41
  pregnancy-induced hypertension, 192
blood pressure *see also* hypertension
  abnormal FHR tracing in labor, 76
  in pregnancy, 62
blood sampling
  fetal, 76, 181–182
    contraindications, 77f

Index

blood tests
  APH, 50
  early pregnancy bleeding/pain, 35
  hypertension in pregnancy, 64
  infertility, 41
  second and third trimester pregnancy abdominal pain, 59
  stillbirth, 67
blood type
  early pregnancy bleeding/pain, 35
  pregnancy, 275
body mass index (BMI)
  amenorrhea, 3
  hypothalamic amenorrhea, 92
  infertility, 41
bony passages
  failure to progress in labor, 69
bony pelvis
  abnormalities, 241f
  labor, 231
    failure to progress, 241
bowel
  symptoms in prolapse, 30
bradycardia
  fetal
    abnormal FHR tracing in labor, 76
breastfeeding
  epilepsy, 199
breech delivery
  cesarean section, 225
  vaginal, 222f–224f
    fetal injuries, 221f
breech presentation, 219–224
  classification, 219
  complications, 219–220
  diagnosis, 219
  management, 221
  transverse lie, 225–226
  unstable lie, 225–226
  vaginal
    antenatal assessment, 221
Brenner tumors
  ovaries, 114
bromocriptine
  hyperprolactinemia, 94
brow presentation, 228
  labor, 228
BSO see bilateral salpingo-oophorectomy (BSO)

C

cabergoline
  hyperprolactinemia, 94
CAH see congenital adrenal hyperplasia (CAH)
calcium
  dietary
    menopause, 165
calcium antagonists
  pregnancy-induced hypertension, 192
calcium channel blockers
  premature labor, 216f
candidal infection
  vaginal discharge, 17, 18
cannabis
  infertility, 40
  pregnancy risk, 273f
carbachol
  voiding difficulties, 141
carboprost (Hemabate)
  placenta previa, 83

cardiac disease
  indirect maternal deaths, 259
  menopause, 163
cardiotocograph (CTG), 73
CBC see complete blood count (CBC)
celomic metaplasia
  endometriosis, 107
central nervous system
  absent periods, 3
central nervous system disorders
  indirect maternal deaths, 259
cephalopelvic disproportion (CPD)
  labor
    failure to progress, 241
cerebral vein thrombosis
  maternal collapse, 87
cervical canal
  transvaginal scan, 215f
cervical carcinoma, 123
  colposcopy, 123f
  management, 123, 124f
  pathology, 123
  presentation, 123
  risk factors, 123f
  staging, 123, 123f
  work-up, 123
cervical cerclage
  miscarriage, 155
  premature labor, 215–216
cervical colposcopy, 295–297
cervical consistency, 287
cervical cytology, 295–297
cervical dilatation, 287
  abnormal patterns, 69f
  cervical fibroid, 69
  premature labor, 214
cervical examination
  pelvic pain, 13
cervical insufficiency
  early pregnancy bleeding/pain, 36
  miscarriage, 154
cervical intraepithelial neoplasia (CIN), 120–121
  etiology, 121
  grades, 121f
  management, 121
  vulvar symptoms, 21
cervical length, 287
cervical Pap smear
  technique, 297f
cervical screening, 264
cervical surgery
  cervical dilatation, 69
cervix
  effacement, 287f
  internal inspection, 283–285, 286
  labor
    failure to progress, 241–242
cesarean section, 248–249
  breech delivery, 225
  indications, 248
  low transverse
    complications, 250
    indications, 250f
    technique, 249–250
  premature labor, 216
Chandelier sign
  PID, 13
charting, 266f–269f

Index

Chlamydia trachomatis
   infertility, 40
   PID, 133
cholecystitis
   second and third trimester pregnancy abdominal pain, 58t
cholestasis of pregnancy, 66, 200–201, 201f
cholestyramine
   cholestasis of pregnancy, 201
chorioamnionitis
   stillbirth, 65
choriocarcinoma
   postpartum hemorrhage, 80
chorionicity
   diagnosis, 184–185, 185f
chorionic villus sampling, 181
chromosomal analysis
   absent periods, 5
cigarettes
   pregnancy risk, 273f
CIN *see* cervical intraepithelial neoplasia (CIN)
circumcision
   female, 69–70
circumvallate placenta, 210
cisplatin
   ovarian carcinoma, 118
clean catch urine sample
   second and third trimester pregnancy abdominal pain, 59
clear cell leiomyoma, 120
climacteric, 161
clomiphene
   anovulation, 149
clonidine
   menopause, 164
cocaine
   maternal collapse, 86
   pregnancy risk, 273f
   retrograde ejaculation, 40
coincidental death
   indirect maternal deaths, 260
coitus interruptus, 167
colchicine
   retrograde ejaculation, 40
colic
   renal
      second and third trimester pregnancy abdominal pain, 58t
colorrhaphy
   SUI, 140
colpopexy
   sacral
      prolapse, 147
colposcopy
   cervix, 122, 295–297
   vulva, 22
colposuspension
   enterocele, 145
coma
   diabetic
      management, 84
      hyperosmolar nonketotic, 84
combined oral contraceptive pill
   contraindications, 168f
complete blood count (CBC)
   early pregnancy bleeding/pain, 35
   heavy periods, 6
   menorrhagia, 96

   pelvic pain, 14
   postpartum hemorrhage, 81
   pregnancy, 275
   second and third trimester pregnancy abdominal pain, 59
composite theories
   endometriosis, 108
cone biopsy
   CIN, 122
   pregnancy risk, 273f
congenital adrenal hyperplasia (CAH), 175
   amenorrhea, 3, 92
constipation
   second and third trimester pregnancy abdominal pain, 58t
contraception, 6, 167–171, 168f, 264 *see also* oral contraceptive pill (OCP)
   hormonal, 168–169
   pelvic pain, 12
   postcoital, 169
Coombs' test
   stillbirth, 67
cord prolapse
   abnormal FHR tracing in labor, 76
   fetal presentation, 221f
counseling
   cholestasis of pregnancy, 201
couple history
   infertility, 40
CPD *see* cephalopelvic disproportion (CPD)
CTG *see* cardiotocograph (CTG)
Cusco's speculum examination
   early pregnancy bleeding/pain, 34–35
Cushing syndrome, 175, 176
   infertility, 41
cyclical pain
   endometriosis, 108
cystadenomas
   serous
      ovaries, 113
cystic teratoma
   mature
      ovaries, 113
cystitis
   second and third trimester pregnancy abdominal pain, 58t
   sensory urgency, 138
cystocele
   prolapse, 29
cystometry, 297
   definition, 25f
   urinary incontinence, 27
cystoscopy
   urinary incontinence, 27, 139
cystourethrocele
   prolapse, 29

D

danazol
   endometriosis, 111
   menorrhagia, 98
death *see also* maternal death
   coincidental
      indirect maternal deaths, 260
   perinatal
      breech presentation, 219–220
debulking surgery
   uterine endometrial tumors, 120

decelerations
  FHR tracing, 73–74, 74f
deep transverse arrest, 229–230
deep vein thrombosis (DVT), 203
defining position of presenting part, 288, 289f
delayed puberty, 174f
delivery
  breech
    cesarean section, 225
  fetus, 235–236
  forceps, 247–248, 249f
    technique, 248
  instrumental
    complications, 247f
  mechanisms, 235
  mode of, 79–80
  postpartum, 79–80
  uterus, 235
  vacuum, 246–247
    indications, 247, 247f
    instrumentation, 247f
    technique, 247
  vaginal breech, 222f–224f
    fetal injuries, 221f
depression
  menopause, 46
  postpartum, 202
    symptoms, 254f
  pregnancy, 201–202
    risk factors, 202f
dermoid cysts
  ovaries, 113
detrusor overactivity (DO), 25, 26
  definition, 25f
DI see donor insemination (DI)
diabetes
  gestational, 197–198
diabetes mellitus, 195–198
  amenorrhea, 3
  anemia, 196f
  failure to progress in labor, 70
  preexisting, 196–197, 197f
  pregnancy risk, 272f, 273f
  retrograde ejaculation, 40
  vaginal discharge, 18
  vulva, 21
diabetic coma
  management, 84
diazepam
  maternal collapse, 86
DIC see disseminated intravascular coagulation (DIC)
dietary calcium
  menopause, 165
digital examination
  APH, 50
dilatation
  cervical
    abnormal patterns, 69f
disseminated intravascular coagulation (DIC)
  maternal collapse, 84, 86
  stillbirth, 67
distigmine
  voiding difficulties, 141
dizygotic twins, 183–184, 185f
DO see detrusor overactivity (DO)
domestic violence
  pregnancy risk, 273f
donor insemination (DI), 151

Doppler studies, 294
Down syndrome
  stillbirth, 65
drospirenone, 177
  endometrial hyperplasia, 93
  endometriosis, 110
  menorrhagia, 97
drug and alcohol dependence, 203–204
drug history, 265
  hypertension in pregnancy, 62
  infertility, 40
DUB see dysfunctional uterine bleeding (DUB)
DVT see deep vein thrombosis (DVT)
dysfunctional uterine bleeding (DUB)
  menorrhagia, 95
dysgenesis
  gonadal
    amenorrhea, 92
dysgerminoma
  amenorrhea, 92
dysmenorrhea, 6, 7–8
  causes, 8t
  endometriosis, 110
  examination, 8
  treatment, 8
  work-up, 8
dyspareunia
  algorithm, 15f
  differential diagnosis, 12f
  drug history, 12
  infertility, 40
  menopause, 161
  past gynecologic history, 12
  past medical/surgical history, 12
  pelvic pain, 11
  sexual history, 12–13

E
early pregnancy
  bleeding/pain in
    algorithm, 36f
    differential diagnosis, 33f
    history, 33–34
    intrauterine, 36
    physical examination, 34–35
    recurrent miscarriage, 35–37
    second and third trimester, 49–51
      differential diagnosis, 49
      history, 49–50
      management, 51
      physical examination, 50
      work-up, 50–51
    trophoblastic disease, 37
    work-up, 35
  ultrasound scan, 294f
early pregnancy failure, 153–155
  ectopic pregnancy, 155–157
  miscarriage, 153–155
  trophoblastic disease, 157–159
eclampsia, 191–192
  complications, 192
  management, 192
Ecstasy (MMDA)
  maternal collapse, 86
  pregnancy risk, 273f
ectopic pregnancy, 155–157
  clinical evaluation, 156
  direct maternal deaths, 259

ectopic pregnancy (*Continued*)
  early pregnancy failure, 155–157
  etiology, 156
  follow-up, 157
  implantation sites, 155f
  predisposing factors, 34f
  prognosis, 157
  tubal, 34
eczema
  vulva, 21, 132
edema
  facial
    hypertension in pregnancy, 62
egg collection, 150f
electrolyte test
  second and third trimester pregnancy abdominal pain, 59
embolism *see also* pulmonary embolism
  amniotic fluid
    direct maternal deaths, 259
    maternal collapse, 84
embryo transfer, 151f
emergency contraception, 169
endocrine disorders
  absent periods, 3
endometrial ablation
  menorrhagia, 99
endometrial biopsy
  heavy bleeding, 7
  menorrhagia, 96
endometrial carcinoma
  amenorrhea, 92
  postmenopausal bleeding, 100
endometrial hyperplasia, 119
  amenorrhea, 92, 93
  treatment, 93
endometrial polyps
  postmenopausal bleeding, 100
endometrial tumors *see* uterine endometrial tumors
endometrioid tumors
  ovaries, 114
endometriosis, 107–112
  classification, 109f
  clinical evaluation, 110
  complications, 110
  differential diagnosis, 110
  etiology, 107–108, 107f
  infertility, 40, 108–110
  pelvic pain, 12
  sites, 108, 108f
  surgery, 111–112
  symptoms, 108, 109f
  treatment, 110–112, 111f
enterocele
  prolapse, 29
enuresis
  nocturnal
    definition, 25f
epididymoorchitis
  infertility, 40
epidural anesthesia
  labor, 238f
epilepsy, 198–199
  pregnancy risk, 272f
episiotomy, 245–246
  incisions, 245f
  indications, 245f
  repair, 246b

epithelial tumors
  ovaries, 113
epithelioid leiomyoma, 120
estrogen deficiency
  menopause, 46
Evista
  menopause, 165
examination, 279–291 *see also* speculum examination
  abdominal, 279–280
    early pregnancy bleeding/pain, 34
    infertility, 41
    postpartum hemorrhage, 80
  bimanual, 285–286
  bimanual pelvic
    pelvic pain, 13–14
  Cusco's speculum
    early pregnancy bleeding/pain, 34–35
  digital
    APH, 50
  general, 279
  gynecologic, 281
  maternal vaginal
    abnormal FHR tracing in labor, 76
  obstetric pelvic, 286
  pelvic, 281, 288
    endometriosis, 110
    prolapse, 31
  pregnancy risk, 272f–274f
  Sims' speculum
    prolapse, 30, 31, 146
  vaginal, 286–287
    early pregnancy bleeding/pain, 35
    infertility, 41
    second and third trimester pregnancy abdominal pain, 59
exophytic tumor
  vulva, 22
external rotation, 237f

F
face presentation, 226–227
  labor, 226–227
  vaginal delivery, 228f
  vaginal examination, 227f
facial edema
  hypertension in pregnancy, 62
fallopian tubes
  ultrasound scan, 293
Falope rings, 170
family history, 265
  hypertension in pregnancy, 62
  pregnancy risk, 273f
family planning
  natural, 167
fatty liver of pregnancy
  acute, 58t, 200–201
FBS *see* fetal blood sampling (FBS)
febrile morbidity
  hysterectomy, 99
female circumcision, 69–70
female external genitalia, 285f
female genital mutilation, 69–70
female sterilization, 170–171
  counseling, 170–171
female urinary incontinence, 25f
feminization
  testicular
    amenorrhea, 92

fertility
  physical examination, 41
fertilization
  in vitro, 150
fertilization in vitro, 149
fetal abnormality
  early pregnancy failure, 157
  labor failure to progress, 242
fetal blood sampling (FBS), 76, 181–182
  contraindications, 77f
fetal bradycardia
  abnormal FHR tracing in labor, 76
fetal growth
  ultrasound scan, 294
fetal heart rate (FHR), 73–77
  accelerations, 73
  baseline, 73
  continuous, 75–76, 75f
  features, 73–74, 74f
  history, 76
  investigating, 76
  monitoring algorithm, 77f
  physical examination, 76
  physiology, 75
  pregnancy, 35
  uterine contraction monitoring, 75
fetal hypoxia
  acute, 75
  chronic, 75
fetal lie, 280, 280f
fetal malformations, 186
fetal malposition
  labor failure to progress, 242
fetal malpresentation
  labor failure to progress, 242
fetal monitoring
  APH, 51
fetal position, 281, 284f
fetal presentation, 280–281, 282f
  stillbirth, 66
fetal reduction, 188
fetal size
  labor failure to progress, 242
fetal skull
  diameter, 234f
  landmarks, 234f
fetocide
  selective, 188
fetus
  antenatal assessment, 186
  attitude, 281
  difficulty palpating, 281, 285f
  engagement, 281, 283f
  number, 280
FHR see fetal heart rate (FHR)
fibroids
  menorrhagia, 95
  postmenopausal bleeding, 100
  pregnancy risk, 274f
fibromas
  ovaries, 114
Filshie clips, 170
FISH see fluorescent in situ hybridization (FISH)
fishy odor, 21
fistulas
  urinary incontinence, 26
flow studies, 297

fluid overload
  endometrial ablation, 99
fluorescent in situ hybridization (FISH), 180
Fluoxetine (Prozac)
  depression, 202
follicle-stimulating hormone (FSH), 5
follicular cysts
  ovaries, 113
fontanelles, 288f
forceps
  types, 248f
forceps delivery, 247–248, 249f
  indications, 247–248
  technique, 248
Fothergill procedure
  prolapse, 147
found ligament pain
  second and third trimester pregnancy abdominal pain, 58t
free thyroxine, 5
FSH see follicle-stimulating hormone (FSH)
fundal height
  abdominal landmarks, 280f
fundoscopy
  hypertension in pregnancy, 62

G
gabapentin
  epilepsy, 199
gallstones
  second and third trimester pregnancy abdominal pain, 58t
ganglion blockers
  voiding disorders, 138
genetic diagnosis
  pre-implantation, 182
genetic factors
  endometriosis, 107–108
  miscarriage, 154
genital herpes
  pregnancy risk, 273f
genitalia
  female external, 285f
genital mutilation
  female, 69–70
genital tract anomaly
  amenorrhea, 92
genital tract trauma
  early postpartum hemorrhage, 251
genuine stress incontinence (GSI), 25, 26, 137
  definition, 25f
germ cell tumors
  ovaries, 113
gestational diabetes, 197–198
glucose test
  second and third trimester pregnancy abdominal pain, 59
glyceryl trinitrate patches
  premature labor, 216f
glycosuria
  pregnancy, 276
glycosylated hemoglobin (HbA1c)
  stillbirth, 67
gonadal dysgenesis
  amenorrhea, 92
gonadoblastoma
  amenorrhea, 92
gonadotrophin-releasing hormone agonists
  menorrhagia, 98

Index

gonadotrophin-releasing hormone analogs
    endometriosis, 111
    uterine fibroids, 104–105
gonadotrophins
    amenorrhea, 92
grandmultiparous
    pregnancy risk, 272f
growth
    fetal
        ultrasound scan, 294
GSI *see* genuine stress incontinence (GSI)
gynecologic endocrinology, 173–178
    amenorrhea, 173
    hirsutism, 173–174
    virilism, 173–174
gynecologic examination, 281
gynecologic history
    absent periods, 3
    hypertension in pregnancy, 62
    infertility, 40
    past, 271
        pregnancy risk, 273f
gynecologic malignancy, 117–127
    cervical carcinoma, 123
    cervix, 120–121
    etiology, 117–118
    ovarian, 117–118
    uterine endometrial tumors, 119–120
    uterine sarcoma, 120
    vaginal tumors, 126–127
    vulvar tumors, 124–125

H

Hashimoto's thyroiditis, 205
HbA1c
    stillbirth, 67
hCG *see* human chorionic gonadotrophin (hCG)
head
    delivery, 236f
    station, 71f
heart rate *see* fetal heart rate (FHR)
HELLP *see* hemolysis, elevated liver enzymes, low platelets (HELLP)
Hemabate
    placenta previa, 83
hematocolpos
    amenorrhea, 92
hematuria
    pregnancy, 277
hemoglobin
    APH, 50
hemoglobin electrophoresis
    pregnancy, 275
hemolysis, elevated liver enzymes, low platelets (HELLP), 57f
    second and third trimester pregnancy abdominal pain, 58t, 59
hemorrhage *see also* antepartum hemorrhage (APH); bleeding
    direct maternal deaths, 259
    endometrial ablation, 99
    ruptured ectopic pregnancy, 34
heparin
    thromboembolism, 204
hepatitis antibodies
    pregnancy, 276
heroin
    pregnancy risk, 273f

heterotopic pregnancy, 157
hirsutism, 173–177, 175f
    amenorrhea, 3
    complications, 177
    etiology, 176–177
    idiopathic, 177
    infertility, 41
    treatment, 177
    work-up, 177
history *see also* gynecologic history; obstetric history; social history
    chief complaint, 263
    couple
        infertility, 40
    drug, 265
        hypertension in pregnancy, 62
        infertility, 40
    family, 265
        hypertension in pregnancy, 62
        pregnancy risk, 273f
    medical
        infertility, 40
        past, 265, 271
        pregnancy risk, 272f–273f
    menstrual, 264
        infertility, 40
    past gynecologic, 264
    patient deaths, 263
    pregnancy risk, 272f–274f
    presenting illness, 263–264
    sexual
        dyspareunia, 12–13
    taking, 263–269
HIV *see* human immunodeficiency virus (HIV)
hormonal contraception, 168–169
hormone profiles
    absent periods, 5
hormone replacement therapy (HRT)
    contraindications, 164f
    menopause, 163–165
    pelvic pain, 12
    prolapse, 146–147
    routes of administration, 164f
hormone-secreting tumors, 94
HPV *see* human papilloma virus (HPV)
HRT *see* hormone replacement therapy (HRT)
HSG *see* hysterosalpingogram (HSG)
human chorionic gonadotrophin (hCG), 5
    serum
        early pregnancy bleeding/pain, 35
        pelvic pain, 14
β-human chorionic gonadotrophin (β-hCG)
    early pregnancy bleeding/pain, 35
human immunodeficiency virus (HIV), 199–200, 200f
    antibodies
        pregnancy, 276
    complications, 199
    management, 199–200
    screening, 200
    vaginal discharge, 18
human papilloma virus (HPV), 121, 122f
hydralazine
    pregnancy-induced hypertension, 192
hydrocortisone
    intravenous
        maternal collapse, 86
hydrosalpinges, 149

hyperemesis
    early pregnancy bleeding/pain, 37
hyperglycemia
    maternal collapse, 86
hypermagnesemia
    calcium gluconate, 86
hyperosmolar nonketotic coma, 84
hyperprolactinemia
    amenorrhea, 93
    bromocriptine, 94
    treatment, 94f
hypertension *see also* preeclampsia; pregnancy-induced hypertension
    in pregnancy, 61–64
        algorithm, 63f
        differential diagnosis, 61
        direct maternal deaths, 258–259
        history, 61
        physical examination, 61–62
        work-up, 62–64
    pregnancy risk, 272f
hyperthyroidism, 205
hypoglycemia, 84
    maternal collapse, 86
hypothalamic amenorrhea, 92
hypothyroidism, 205–206
    menorrhagia, 95
    signs, 205f
hysterectomy
    long-term complications, 99
    menorrhagia, 99–100
    prolapse, 145
    total abdominal, 112
        bilateral salpingo-oophorectomy, 120
    uterine fibroids, 105
    vaginal
        prolapse, 147
hysterosalpingogram (HSG), 42f, 149
    early pregnancy bleeding/pain, 36
hysteroscopy, 295
    heavy bleeding, 7
    infertility, 43
    painful periods, 8
    postmenopausal bleeding, 10
    technique, 296f

I

ICSI *see* intracytoplasmic sperm injection (ICSI)
idiopathic hirsutism, 177
imaging techniques, 293–294
immunologic factors
    endometriosis, 107–108
implantation theory
    endometriosis, 107
incomplete placenta
    early postpartum hemorrhage, 252
indomethacin
    premature labor, 216f
infection *see also* postpartum infection
    early pregnancy failure, 157
    endometrial ablation, 99
    urinary tract
        recurrent, 273f
        second and third trimester pregnancy abdominal pain, 57
        urinary incontinence, 26–27
    vulva, 22

infection screening
    pelvic pain, 14
    stillbirth, 67
infertility, 39–43, 149–152
    anovulation, 149
    causes, 39f
    epididymoorchitis, 40
    history, 39–41
    male, 150–151
    OHSS, 151–152
    pie chart, 39f
    prognosis, 152
    tubal problems, 149–150
    unexplained, 151
    uterine and pelvic problems, 149
    uterine fibroids, 103
    work-up, 41–42
injectable progestins, 169
insemination
    intrauterine, 150–151
instrumental delivery
    complications, 247f
intercourse
    antepartum hemorrhage, 49
intermenstrual bleeding
    abnormal bleeding, 7
    causes, 7t
interstitial laser photocoagulation
    uterine fibroids, 105
intra-abdominal pressure
    chronically raised
        prolapse, 145
intracytoplasmic sperm injection (ICSI), 151f
intrauterine devices (IUD), 169–170, 170f
    advantages, 169
    disadvantages, 170
    menorrhagia, 97–98
intrauterine fetal demise *see* stillbirth
intrauterine insemination (IUI), 150–151, 151
intrauterine pregnancy
    ultrasound, 36f
intrauterine pressure catheter (IUPC), 72
intravenous hydrocortisone
    maternal collapse, 86
investigations, 293–298
in vitro fertilization (IVF), 149, 150
iron-deficiency anemia
    menstruation, 6
ischemic heart disease
    amenorrhea, 92
IUD *see* intrauterine devices (IUD)
IUI *see* intrauterine insemination (IUI)
IUPC *see* intrauterine pressure catheter (IUPC)
IVF *see* in vitro fertilization (IVF)

K

Kallmann's syndrome
    anosmia, 4
karyotyping
    early pregnancy bleeding/pain, 36
    infertility, 42
KB *see* Kleihauer–Betke (KB) test
Kegel exercises
    SUI, 139
ketorolac
    maternal collapse, 86

Index

kidney stones
  second and third trimester pregnancy abdominal pain, 58t
Kleihauer–Betke (KB) test
  stillbirth, 67

L
labetalol
  pregnancy-induced hypertension, 192
labia majora
  medial aspect, 125f
labor, 231–243 *see also* premature labor
  analgesia
    pharmacologic methods, 238f
  cervical dilatation
    abnormal patterns, 69f
  early, 236f
  failure to progress in, 69–72, 241–243
    algorithm, 71f
    causes, 70f
    examination, 71f
    history, 69–70
    management, 72
    physical examination, 70–71
    work-up, 71–72
  first stage, 237–239
    fetal monitoring, 237–239
    maternal monitoring, 237
  induction, 240–241
    complications, 240
    indications, 240, 240f
  onset, 231
  preterm, 186
  progress, 231–235
  second and third trimester pregnancy abdominal pain, 58t
  second stage, 236f
    management, 239
  third stage
    complications, 251–256
    management, 239–240
  trial, 250
labor curve, 69f
lactation
  third stage of labor, 253
lamotrigine
  epilepsy, 199
laparoscopy, 295
  painful periods, 8
  technique, 295, 296f
last menstrual period (LMP)
  early pregnancy bleeding/pain, 33
  pelvic pain, 12
LEEP *see* loop electrosurgical excision procedure (LEEP)
leiomyoma
  clear cell, 120
  epithelioid, 120
leiomyosarcoma, 120
LH *see* luteinizing hormone (LH)
lichen sclerosis, 129, 129f
  characteristics, 131f
  vulva, 22
ligament pain
  found
    second and third trimester pregnancy abdominal pain, 58t

liver disorders
  pregnancy, 200–201
liver function test
  second and third trimester pregnancy abdominal pain, 59
LMP *see* last menstrual period (LMP)
LMSH
  thromboembolism, 204
local anesthesia
  maternal collapse, 86
locked twins, 188
loop electrosurgical excision procedure (LEEP), 69
  CIN, 122
Loveset's maneuver
  breech presentation, 221–222
luteal cysts
  ovaries, 113
luteinizing hormone (LH), 5
lymphatic embolization
  endometriosis, 107

M
MacDonald suture
  premature labor, 216, 217f
magnesium
  maternal collapse, 86
  pregnancy-induced hypertension, 192
  premature labor, 216f
male sterilization, 171
malignant tumors
  ultrasound scan, 294f
malposition, 228–229
  deep transverse arrest, 229–230
  occiput posterior position, 228–229
malpresentation, 219–226
  breech presentation, 219–224
  brow presentation, 228
  causes, 220f
  classification, 220f
  external cephalic version, 220–221
  face presentation, 226–227
  fetal
    labor failure to progress, 242
  management, 220
Manchester repair (Fothergill procedure)
  prolapse, 147
MAP *see* mean arterial pressure (MAP)
maternal age
  early pregnancy failure, 157
maternal blood pressure
  abnormal FHR tracing in labor, 76
maternal collapse, 83–87
  acute myocardial infarction, 84
  amniotic fluid embolism, 84
  diabetic emergency, 84–86
  drug toxicity, 86
  eclampsia, 84
  hemorrhage, 83–84
  puerperal sepsis, 86
  resuscitation, 85f
  thromboembolism, 87
maternal death, 257–260
  causes, 257–260, 258f
  classes
    definitions, 257
  direct, 257–258
    ectopic pregnancy, 259

Index

hypertensive disorders, 258–259
  indirect, 259–260
  risk factors, 260
maternal illness
  early pregnancy failure, 157
maternal observations
  abnormal FHR tracing in labor, 76
maternal pulse
  abnormal FHR tracing in labor, 76
Mauriceau–Smellie–Veit maneuver
  breech delivery, 225
McBurney's point
  second and third trimester pregnancy abdominal pain, 59
mean arterial pressure (MAP), 84
medical history
  infertility, 40
  past, 265, 271
    pregnancy risk, 272f–273f
menopause, 45–47, 161–165
  algorithm, 47f
  bleeding disturbances, 45
  cardiovascular disease, 163
  clinical features, 161–165, 162f
  definitions, 161
  differential diagnosis, 45
  end-organ atrophy, 161
  evaluation, 163
  examination, 163
  immediate effects, 162f
  long-term symptoms, 46–47
  nonhormonal drug treatment, 164–165
  osteoporosis, 162–163, 163f
  pathophysiology, 161
  presentation, 45
  psychologic symptoms, 45–46, 162
    differential diagnosis, 46f
  systemic symptoms, 46
    differential diagnosis, 46f
  treatment, 163–165
  vasomotor symptoms, 45, 161
menorrhagia, 94–100
  causes, 6t
  complications, 97
  diagnosis, 94–95
  etiology, 95, 95f
  iatrogenic causes, 96
  incidence, 94
  intrauterine devices, 170
  investigating, 96–97, 96f
  pathology, 95 96
  systemic conditions, 95
  treatment, 97–98, 97f
menstrual abnormalities
  uterine fibroids, 103
menstrual history, 264
  infertility, 40
menstrual periods *see* periods
menstruation
  iron-deficiency anemia, 6
  pattern, 6
  retrograde
    endometriosis, 107
mental illness *see* postpartum mental illness; psychiatric disorders
meperidine
  labor, 238f

metformin
  endometrial hyperplasia, 93
methadone
  pregnancy risk, 273f
methergine
  placenta previa, 83
methotrexate
  tubal pregnancy, 157
microbiology
  infertility, 41–42
micturition
  frequency of, 26
    definition, 25f
  urgency of, 26
    definition, 25f
miscarriage, 34
  early pregnancy failure, 153–155
  etiology, 154f, 157
  management, 157–158
  recurrent, 154–155
    etiology, 154–155
    treatment, 155
  shock, 34
  types, 33f
Mittelschmerz
  pelvic pain, 12
mixed mullerian tumors, 120
MMDA
  maternal collapse, 86
  pregnancy risk, 273f
modified Pomeroy tubal ligation, 170
molar pregnancy, 37f, 82, 158f
  clinical evaluation, 158
  diagnosis, 158
  incidence, 158
  management, 158–159
  postpartum hemorrhage, 80
monozygotic twins, 184, 185f
montevideo units (MVU), 72
morbidity
  febrile
    hysterectomy, 99
  perinatal
    malpresentation, 220
mortality
  perinatal
    breech presentation, 219–220
    pregnancy surveillance system, 257
motor vehicle accident
  antepartum hemorrhage, 49
mucinous cystadenoma
  ovaries, 114
Mullerian tumors
  mixed, 120
multiple pregnancy, 183–188, 186f
  complications, 186
  diagnosis, 183
  etiology, 183–187
  high order, 188
  incidence, 183
  pregnancy risk, 274f
multiple sclerosis
  pregnancy, 201
mumps orchitis
  postpubertal
    infertility, 40
MVU *see* montevideo units (MVU)

Index

myomectomy
  uterine fibroids, 105
myometrial sarcoma, 120

N

naloxone
  maternal collapse, 86
natural family planning, 167
nebulized albuterol
  maternal collapse, 86
Neisseria gonorrhoeae
  PID, 133
nifedipine
  pregnancy-induced hypertension, 192
  premature labor, 216f
nitric oxide donors
  premature labor, 216f
nitrofurantoin
  retrograde ejaculation, 40
nitrous oxide
  labor, 238f
nocturia
  definition, 25f
nocturnal enuresis
  definition, 25f
nonpregnant pelvis
  ultrasound scan, 293
nonsteroidal anti-inflammatory drugs (NSAID)
  infertility, 40
  maternal collapse, 86
  menorrhagia, 97
  premature labor, 216f
nonstress test (NST)
  APH, 51
  second and third trimester pregnancy abdominal pain, 59–60
NSAID *see* nonsteroidal anti-inflammatory drugs (NSAID)
NST *see* nonstress test (NST)
nuchal thickness, 277

O

obesity
  infertility, 41
obstetric history
  hypertension in pregnancy, 62
  infertility, 40
  past, 264, 271, 274f
    pregnancy risk, 272f
  second and third trimester pregnancy abdominal pain, 57
obstetric palpation, 279–280
obstetric pelvic examination, 286
obstetrics
  operative intervention, 245–250
occiput posterior position, 228–229
  labor, 229
OCP *see* oral contraceptive pill (OCP)
odor
  fishy, 21
OHSS *see* ovarian hyperstimulation syndrome (OHSS)
oligomenorrhea, 3
opiates
  maternal collapse, 86
oral contraceptive pill (OCP), 6, 168
  absent periods, 3
  combined
    contraindications, 168f

endometriosis, 111
  menorrhagia, 98
osteopenia
  menopause, 47
osteoporosis
  amenorrhea, 92
  menopause, 46–47, 47, 162–163, 163f
ovarian androgens, 176
ovarian carcinoma
  CA125, 118
  chemotherapy, 118
  management, 118
  postmenopausal bleeding, 100
  presentation, 117
  risk factors, 118f
  screening, 118
  staging, 117f
  studies, 117–118
  surgery, 118
  ultrasound, 117–118
ovarian cyst
  pelvic pain, 12
  second and third trimester pregnancy abdominal pain, 58t
  torsion
    second and third trimester pregnancy abdominal pain, 59
ovarian failure
  amenorrhea, 92
ovarian hyperstimulation syndrome (OHSS), 151–152
ovarian tumors, 113–116
  classification, 113f
  diagnosis, 114
  differential diagnosis, 114f
  etiology, 113–114
  history, 114
  incidence, 113
  management, 115–116
  physical examination, 114–115
  work-up, 115
ovaries
  Brenner tumors, 114
  endometrioid tumors, 114
  fibromas, 114
  follicular cysts, 113
  labor failure to progress, 242
  ultrasound scan, 293
oxybutynin
  detrusor overactivity, 140
oxytocin, 72
  labor induction, 240
  placenta previa, 83
  stillbirth, 67
oxytocin receptor antagonists
  premature labor, 216f

P

Paget's disease
  vulva, 22, 125, 132
    characteristics, 131f
pain *see also* abdominal pain; dysmenorrhea; dyspareunia; early pregnancy; pelvic pain
  cyclical
    endometriosis, 108
  found ligament
    second and third trimester pregnancy abdominal pain, 58t
  uterine fibroids, 103

Index

palpation *see also* abdominal palpation
  abdomen, 279
  obstetric, 279–280
  pelvic
    benign ovarian tumors, 115
pancreatitis
  second and third trimester pregnancy abdominal pain, 58t
papilledema
  hypertension in pregnancy, 62
Pap smear, 120–121, 287
  algorithm, 122f
  cervical
    technique, 297f
paroxetine (Paxil)
  depression, 202
passages
  bony
    failure to progress in labor, 69
  labor, 231–233
passenger
  failure to progress in labor, 70
  labor, 233–234
    failure to progress, 242
Paxil
  depression, 202
PCOS *see* polycystic ovary syndrome (PCOS)
PCR *see* polymerase chain reaction (PCR)
pelvic cavity, 290
  assessing, 291f
pelvic dyspareunia, 11–16
pelvic examination, 281, 288
  bimanual
    pelvic pain, 13–14
  endometriosis, 110
  obstetric, 286
  prolapse, 31
pelvic floor, 144
  exercises
    prolapse, 146
  muscles
    anatomy, 144f
pelvic inflammatory disease (PID), 133–135
  antibiotic therapy, 135f
  complications, 134, 134f
  definition, 133
  development, 134f
  diagnosis, 133
  etiology, 133
  examination, 133–134
  history, 133
  incidence, 133
  pelvic pain, 12
  prevention, 135
  risk factors, 134f
  treatment, 135
  vaginal discharge, 17
  work-up, 134
pelvic inlet, 233f, 288
  assessing, 290f
pelvic ligaments, 144
pelvic masses
  pelvic pain, 14
pelvic organ prolapse, 143–148
  clinical features, 145–146
  definition, 143–144
  etiology, 145
  incidence, 144
  management, 146–147
  pelvic anatomy, 144
  predisposing factors, 145f
  types, 143f
pelvic outlet, 233f, 291
  assessing, 291f
pelvic pain, 11–16, 11t
  abdominal palpation, 13
  algorithm, 15f
  bimanual pelvic examination, 13–14
  biopsy, 16
  blood tests, 14
  chief complaint, 11–12
  differential diagnosis, 11
  dyspareunia, 11
  endometriosis, 12
  history, 11–12
  infection screen, 14
  laparoscopy, 16
  pelvic masses, 14
  physical exam, 13–14
  radiological investigations, 14–16
  social history, 13
  vulvar/vaginal/cervical inspection, 13, 13t
  work-up, 14–16, 14f
pelvic palpation
  benign ovarian tumors, 115
pelvic-type characteristics, 290f
pelvic ultrasound scan
  absent periods, 5
  amenorrhea, 92
  heavy periods, 6
  menorrhagia, 96
  painful periods, 8
  pelvic pain, 14
  postmenopausal bleeding, 10
pelvis
  bony
    abnormalities, 241f
    failure to progress in labor, 241
    labor, 231
  nonpregnant
    ultrasound scan, 293
peptic ulcer
  second and third trimester pregnancy abdominal pain, 58t
perinatal morbidity
  malpresentation, 220
perinatal mortality
  breech presentation, 219–220
perineal infiltration
  labor, 238f
perineal repair, 246
periods *see also* amenorrhea; dysmenorrhea
  heavy, 6–7
    CBC, 6
    examination, 6
    history, 6
    work-up, 6
  last
    early pregnancy bleeding/pain, 33
    pelvic pain, 12
pessaries
  vaginal
    prolapse, 147
photocoagulation
  interstitial laser
    uterine fibroids, 105

Index

physiologic cysts
  ovaries, 113
PID *see* pelvic inflammatory disease (PID)
PIH *see* pregnancy-induced hypertension (PIH)
pinworms
  vulva, 23
pipelle sampling
  uterine endometrial tumors, 120
pituitary macroadenoma
  transphenoidal removal
    diabetes insipidus, 94
pituitary microadenoma
  osteoporosis, 93
placenta
  circumvallate, 210
  delivery, 239f
  incomplete
    early postpartum hemorrhage, 252
  retained
    early postpartum hemorrhage, 252
placenta accreta
  placenta previa, 208
  third stage of labor, 253
placental abruption, 208–210
  antepartum hemorrhage, 49
  APH, 51
  complications, 210
  defined, 208–209
  examination, 209
  history, 209
  incidence, 209
  management, 210
  second and third trimester pregnancy abdominal pain, 57, 58t
  types, 209f
  work-up, 209–210
placenta previa, 207–208
  antepartum hemorrhage, 49
  APH, 51
  complications, 208
  defined, 207
  diagnosis, 207
  examination, 207
  history, 207
  incidence, 207
  investigations, 208
  management, 208
  painless vaginal bleeding, 207
  vs. placental abruption, 83, 83f
  ultrasound, 208f
PMB *see* postmenopausal bleeding (PMB)
polycystic ovary syndrome (PCOS), 3, 175
  amenorrhea, 3, 92
  androgens, 176f
  hypothalamic amenorrhea, 92–93
  infertility, 41
  miscarriage, 154
polymerase chain reaction (PCR), 180
Pomeroy tubal ligation
  modified, 170
postcoital bleeding
  abnormal bleeding, 7
  causes, 7t
postcoital contraception, 169
postcoital test
  infertility, 42
posterior colporrhaphy
  prolapse, 147

postmenopausal atrophy
  prolapse, 145
postmenopausal bleeding (PMB), 9, 100–102
  abnormal bleeding, 9–10
  algorithm, 101f
  causes, 8t, 100–101, 100f
  examination, 10
  history, 9–10
  work-up, 10
postpartum delivery, 79–80
postpartum depression, 202
  symptoms, 254f
postpartum hemorrhage (PPH), 79–82, 187–188
  causes, 84f
  defined, 251
  differential diagnosis, 79–80, 79f
  early, 80, 80f, 81, 251
    complications, 252–253
    etiology, 251
    incidence, 251
    management, 252, 252f
    prevention, 251
  history, 79–80
  late, 80–81, 81
    third stage of labor, 253
  management
    algorithm, 81f, 82f
    physical examination, 80–81
  pituitary failure, 3
  placenta previa, 208
  work-up, 81
postpartum infection, 254
  definition, 254
  examination, 254
  history, 254
  incidence, 254
  investigations, 254
  management, 254
  sites, 254
postpartum mental illness, 254–256
  examination, 254f
  history, 255
  incidence, 254
  management, 255
postpartum psychosis, 202–203
  indirect maternal deaths, 259–260
postpartum thyroiditis, 206
post-pill amenorrhea, 3
postpubertal mumps orchitis
  infertility, 40
power
  failure to progress in labor, 70, 71
  labor, 235
    failure to progress, 242–243
PPH *see* postpartum hemorrhage (PPH)
precocious puberty, 173, 174f
preeclampsia, 190–191
  changed parameters, 64
  complications, 191, 191f
  hypertension in pregnancy, 62
  management, 190
  pathology, 190
  second and third trimester pregnancy abdominal pain, 57, 58t, 59
  signs, 62f
pregnancy *see also* early pregnancy; ectopic pregnancy; molar pregnancy; multiple pregnancy; tubal pregnancy

acute fatty liver of, 58t, 200–201
amenorrhea, 92
cholestasis of, 66, 200–201, 201f
current
   history, 271
dietary advice, 278f
early
   bleeding in, 33–37
early complications
   ultrasound scan, 293–294
examination, 275
family history, 275
fatty liver of
   acute, 58t, 200–201
heterotopic, 157
intrauterine
   ultrasound, 36f
laboratory studies, 275, 275f
medical disorders, 195–206
minor symptoms, 278f
mortality surveillance system, 257
present
   pregnancy risk, 274f
second and third trimester
   abdominal palpation, 58–59
termination, 171
twin
   complications, 187–188
   delivery, 187
   intrapartum management, 187–188, 187f
   presentation, 184f
ultrasound scan, 293
uncomplicated
   uterine contraction, 75
unwanted, 167–171
pregnancy-induced hypertension (PIH), 186, 189–193
   drug therapy, 192
   nonproteinuric, 189–190
   second and third trimester pregnancy abdominal pain, 57
pregnancy test, 5
   pelvic pain, 14
pre-implantation genetic diagnosis (PGD), 182
premature labor, 213–217
   causes, 213f
   cesarean section, 216
   clinical evaluation, 214–215
   drug therapy, 216f
   future pregnancies, 217
   incidence, 213–214
   management, 214f
   mode of delivery, 216
   pathogens, 214f
   risk, 213f
   treatment, 215
prenatal care, 271–278
   history, 271–272
   initial visit education, 277–278
   planning, 277
prenatal diagnosis, 179–182, 180f, 277
   suitable conditions, 180f
   techniques, 179–182
prenatal visits, 278
presentation *see also* breech presentation; malpresentation
   brow, 228
      labor, 228

face, 226–227
   labor, 226–227
   vaginal delivery, 228f
   vaginal examination, 227f
fetal, 280–281, 282f
   stillbirth, 66
pressure catheter
   intrauterine, 72
pressure symptoms
   uterine fibroids, 103
preterm labor, 186
primaparous
   pregnancy risk, 272f
progesterone
   infertility, 41
progesterone-only pill, 168–169
progestin (drospirenone)
   endometrial hyperplasia, 93
   endometriosis, 110
   menorrhagia, 97
progestins
   injectable, 169
prolactin
   amenorrhea, 92
   infertility, 42
   serum, 5
prolapse, 29–31 *see also* pelvic organ prolapse
   algorithm, 31f
   cord
      abnormal FHR tracing in labor, 76
      fetal presentation, 221f
   differential diagnosis, 29f
   enterocele, 29
   history, 29–30
   physical examination, 30–31
   predisposing factors, 30f
   SUI, 137
   work-up, 31
prostaglandins
   inhibitors
      menorrhagia, 97
   labor induction, 240
   stillbirth, 67
proteinuria
   hypertension in pregnancy, 62
   pregnancy, 276
Prozac
   depression, 202
pruritus
   vulvar, 21
      algorithm, 22f
      differential diagnosis, 21f
psoriasis
   vulva, 21, 23, 132
psychiatric disorders
   indirect maternal deaths, 259
   pregnancy, 201–203
   pregnancy risk, 273f
psychosis
   postpartum, 202–203
      indirect maternal deaths, 259–260
   puerperal
      symptoms, 256f
puberty
   delayed, 174f
   precocious, 173
   Tanner's system, 4, 5t

pudendal block
  labor, 238f
puerperal psychosis
  symptoms, 256f
pulmonary embolism, 203
  maternal collapse, 87
  streptokinase, 87
pulse
  maternal
    abnormal FHR tracing in labor, 76
pyelonephritis
  second and third trimester pregnancy abdominal pain, 58t

Q
quad screening, 277f

R
radical vulvectomy, 126
radiotherapy
  complications, 126f
Raloxifene (Evista)
  menopause, 165
rectocele, 145
  prolapse, 29
recurrent urinary tract infection
  pregnancy risk, 273f
renal colic
  second and third trimester pregnancy abdominal pain, 58t
renal stones
  second and third trimester pregnancy abdominal pain, 58t
restitution, 237f
retained placenta
  early postpartum hemorrhage, 252
retinopathy
  hypertension in pregnancy, 62
retrograde menstruation
  endometriosis, 107
review of systems, 265
rhesus group
  stillbirth, 65, 66
rhythm method, 167
ring pessary
  vaginal discharge, 18
ritodrine
  premature labor, 216f
rubella antibodies
  pregnancy, 276
rubella immunity
  infertility, 41

S
sacral colpopexy
  prolapse, 147
sacrospinous fixation
  prolapse, 147
salbutamol
  premature labor, 216f
saline wet prep
  yeast infection, 23
salpingectomy
  tubal pregnancy, 156
salpingostomy
  tubal pregnancy, 156
salpingotomy
  tubal pregnancy, 156

sarcoma
  myometrial, 120
  stromal, 120
  uterine, 120
schizophrenia, 203
screening
  antibody
    pregnancy, 275–276
  cervical, 264
  infection
    pelvic pain, 14
    stillbirth, 67
  pregnancy, 277
  quad, 277f
selective fetocide, 188
selective serotonin reuptake inhibitors (SSRI)
  depression, 202
semen analysis
  infertility, 42
  normal parameters, 43f
sensory urgency
  urinary incontinence, 26
sepsis
  direct maternal deaths, 259
septic shock
  maternal collapse, 86
serous cystadenomas
  ovaries, 113
sertraline (Zoloft)
  depression, 202
serum β-human chorionic gonadotrophin
  early pregnancy bleeding/pain, 35
serum human chorionic gonadotrophin
  pelvic pain, 14
serum prolactin, 5
serum testosterone, 5
sex cord stromal tumors
  ovaries, 114
sexual activity, 264
sexual history
  dyspareunia, 12–13
sexual intercourse
  antepartum hemorrhage, 49
sexually transmitted disease
  vulva, 23
Sheehan's syndrome, 3, 94
  early postpartum hemorrhage, 252
Shirodkar suture
  premature labor, 216
shock
  septic
    maternal collapse, 86
shoulders
  delivery, 237f
Sims' speculum examination
  prolapse, 30, 31, 146
skull
  fetal
    diameter, 234f
    landmarks, 234f
slings
  SUI, 139
smoking
  CIN, 121
  infertility, 40

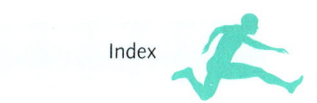

social history, 265, 271
  infertility, 40
  pelvic pain, 13
  pregnancy risk, 273f–274f
soft passages
  failure to progress in labor, 69–70
soft tissue
  labor, 231–233
soft tissue of pelvis
  labor failure to progress, 241–242
solid teratomas
  mature
    ovaries, 113
sonohysterogram
  infertility, 42
speculum examination
  APH, 50
  Cusco's
    early pregnancy bleeding/pain, 34–35
    postpartum hemorrhage, 80
    second and third trimester pregnancy abdominal pain, 59
  Sims'
    prolapse, 30, 31, 146
    vaginal discharge, 18
sperm
  injection into egg, 151f
  intracytoplasmic injection, 151f
spinal anesthesia
  labor, 238f
squamous carcinoma
  cervical, 123
  vulva, 22, 132
SSRI see selective serotonin reuptake inhibitors (SSRI)
station of presenting part, 287, 287f
sterilization, 167–171
  female, 170–171
    counseling, 170–171
  male, 171
steroids
  anabolic
    retrograde ejaculation, 40
stigmata
  pregnancy, 279
stillbirth, 65–67
  causes, 65f
  Down syndrome, 65
  follow-up, 67
  history, 65–66
  management, 67
  rate, 65, 66f
  work-up, 66–67
streptokinase
  pulmonary embolism, 87
stress incontinence
  definition, 25f
  detrusor instability, 25
  genuine, 25, 26, 137
    definition, 25f
stress urinary incontinence (SUI), 137, 139–140
  mechanism, 138f
stretch marks, 279
striae gravidarum, 279
stromal sarcoma, 120
stromal tumors
  ovaries, 114
SUI see stress urinary incontinence (SUi)
sulfasalazine
  retrograde ejaculation, 40

symphysis pubis dysfunction
  second and third trimester pregnancy abdominal pain, 58t
symptomatic cysts
  ovarian, 116
syphilis antibodies
  pregnancy, 276
systems
  review of, 265

T

TAH see total abdominal hysterectomy (TAH)
TAH-BSO see total abdominal hysterectomy-bilateral salpingo-oophorectomy (TAH-BSO)
Tanner's system
  puberty, 4, 5t
taxol
  ovarian carcinoma, 118
teratomas
  mature
    ovaries, 113
    solid, 113
terazosin
  voiding difficulties, 141
terbutaline
  premature labor, 216f
testicular atrophy
  infertility, 40
testicular feminization
  amenorrhea, 92
testosterone
  serum, 5
theca cell tumors
  ovaries, 114
thrombocytopenia, 205
thromboembolism, 203
  direct maternal deaths, 257–258
  pregnancy, 204f
  pregnancy risk, 273f
  third stage of labor, 256
thrombophilic defects
  miscarriage, 154
thyroid disease
  amenorrhea, 3
  infertility, 42
  pregnancy, 205–206
  pregnancy risk, 273f
thyroiditis
  Hashimoto's, 205
  postpartum, 206
thyroid nodules, 206–207
thyroid-stimulating hormone (TSH), 5
thyroxine
  free, 5
thyroxine replacement, 206
tocolysis
  premature labor, 215
tolterodine
  detrusor overactivity, 140
Toradol (ketorolac)
  maternal collapse, 86
total abdominal hysterectomy (TAH), 112
total abdominal hysterectomy-bilateral salpingo-oophorectomy (TAH-BSO)
  uterine endometrial tumors, 120
transphenoidal pituitary macroadenoma removal
  diabetes insipidus, 94

trichomonas vaginalis
  fishy odor, 21
tricyclic antidepressants
  depression, 202
  detrusor overactivity, 140
  voiding disorders, 138
triplets, 184
trophoblastic disease, 157–159
  early pregnancy failure, 157–159
TSH see thyroid-stimulating hormone (TSH)
T&S sample
  APH, 50
  pelvic pain, 14
  second and third trimester pregnancy abdominal pain, 59
TTTS see twin-to-twin transfusion syndrome (TTTS)
tubal ectopic pregnancy, 34
tubal ligation
  modified Pomeroy, 170
tubal patency
  test, 42
tubal pregnancy, 156–157
  medical treatment, 157
  surgery, 156–157, 157f
  treatment, 156–157
Turner's syndrome, 4
  infertility, 41
twin pregnancy
  complications, 187–188
  delivery, 187
  intrapartum management, 187–188, 187f
  presentation, 184f
twins, 183–184
  locked, 188
  monozygotic, 184
twin-to-twin transfusion syndrome (TTTS), 186–187
  stillbirth, 66

U

ultrasound scan, 293–294 see also pelvic ultrasound scan
  anatomy, 294
  APH, 51
  early pregnancy bleeding/pain, 35
  hypertension in pregnancy, 64
  infertility, 41
  miscarriage, 157
  postpartum hemorrhage, 81
  prenatal diagnosis, 179
  safety, 294
  second and third trimester pregnancy abdominal pain, 60
  stillbirth, 65, 67
uncomplicated pregnancy
  uterine contraction, 75
unwanted pregnancy, 167–171
urea test
  second and third trimester pregnancy abdominal pain, 59
ureterovaginal fistula
  urinary incontinence, 26
urge incontinence, 26
  definition, 25f
urgency of micturition, 26
  definition, 25f
urinalysis
  hypertension in pregnancy, 62–63
  pregnancy, 276
  second and third trimester pregnancy abdominal pain, 59
  stillbirth, 66
urinary incontinence, 25–28, 137–141 see also stress urinary incontinence (SUI)
  algorithm, 27f
  complications, 139
  definition, 25f
  detrusor overactivity, 140
  etiology, 137–139
  female, 25f
  fistulas, 141
  history, 25–26
  incidence, 137
  laboratory studies, 26–27
  physical examination, 26
  sensory urgency, 140
  treatment, 139
  urodynamics, 27
  voiding difficulties, 140–141
  work-up, 139
urinary tract infection (UTI)
  recurrent
    pregnancy risk, 273f
  second and third trimester pregnancy abdominal pain, 57
  urinary incontinence, 26–27
urine culture
  pregnancy, 276
urine pregnancy test, 5
  pelvic pain, 14
urine sample
  clean catch
    second and third trimester pregnancy abdominal pain, 59
urodynamics, 297–298
uroflowmetry
  definition, 25f
  urinary incontinence, 27
urogynecologic terms
  definitions, 25f
uterine abnormalities
  miscarriage, 154
uterine atony, 79
  early postpartum hemorrhage, 251, 252
    treatment, 252f
  maternal collapse, 84
uterine bleeding
  abnormal, 91–102
    amenorrhea, 91–94
    menorrhagia, 94–100
    postmenopausal, 100–102
  dysfunctional
    menorrhagia, 95
uterine cavity
  abnormal
    early pregnancy failure, 157
uterine contraction
  fetal heart rate acceleration, 73f
uterine descent
  classification, 30f
  prolapse, 30
uterine endometrial tumors, 119–120
  incidence, 119
  investigation, 120
  MRI, 120
  pathology, 119
  presentation, 119
  prognosis, 120
  radiotherapy, 120

318

risk factors, 119, 119f
spread, 119
staging, 119f
treatment, 120
uterine fibroids, 103–110
  categorization, 104f
  clinical evaluation, 104
  complications, 103–104
  factors influencing incidence, 104f
  medical therapy, 104–105
  second and third trimester pregnancy abdominal pain, 58t
  surgical treatment, 105
  symptoms, 103, 104f
  treatment advances, 105–106
  treatment indications, 104
uterine inversion
  postpartum hemorrhage, 80
  third stage of labor, 253
uterine perforation
  endometrial ablation, 99
uterine rupture
  maternal collapse, 83–84
  third stage of labor, 253
uterine sarcoma, 120
uterine size, 279–280
  stillbirth, 66
uterus
  labor
    failure to progress, 241
  positions, 286f
  rudimentary horn, 7f
  ultrasound scan, 293
UTI see urinary tract infection (UTI)

V
vacuum delivery, 246–247
  indications, 247, 247f
  instrumentation, 247f
  technique, 247
vacuum extractor, 246–247
vagina
  internal inspection, 283–284, 286
  labor
    failure to progress, 242
vaginal bleeding, 9
vaginal breech delivery, 222f–224f
  fetal injuries, 221f
vaginal breech presentation
  antenatal assessment, 221
vaginal cancer
  staging, 126f
vaginal discharge, 17–19, 264
  algorithm, 19f
  differential diagnosis, 17, 17f
  drug history, 18
  gynecologic history, 17–18
  history, 17–18
  past medical history, 18
  physical exam, 18–19
  sexual history, 18
  work-up, 18f, 19
vaginal dryness
  menopause, 161
vaginal examination, 286–287
  abnormal FHR tracing in labor, 76
  early pregnancy bleeding/pain, 35
  infertility, 41

maternal
  abnormal FHR tracing in labor, 76
  pelvic pain, 13
  second and third trimester pregnancy abdominal pain, 59
vaginal hysterectomy
  prolapse, 147
vaginalis
  trichomonas
    fishy odor, 21
vaginal pessaries
  prolapse, 147
vaginal tape
  SUI, 139
vaginal tumors, 126–127
  etiology, 126
  investigation, 126
  management, 127
  presentation, 126
  prognosis, 127
vasa previa, 210
vasectomy, 171
VCU see videocystourethrography (VCU)
venous embolization
  endometriosis, 107
vesicovaginal fistula
  urinary incontinence, 26
videocystourethrography (VCU), 298
  definition, 25f
  urinary incontinence, 27
VIN see vulvar intraepithelial neoplasia (VIN)
violence
  domestic
    pregnancy risk, 273f
virilism, 173–177
  amenorrhea, 3
  complications, 177
  etiology, 176–177
  treatment, 177
  work-up, 177
visits
  prenatal, 278
vitamin D
  menopause, 165
voiding disorders
  neurologic causes, 138f
  urinary incontinence, 26
vulva
  anatomy, 131f
  examination, 146
  external examination, 283, 286
  history, 129
  labor
    failure to progress, 242
vulvar cancer
  stages, 125f
vulvar disease, 129–132
  characteristics, 131f
  dermatologic conditions, 132
vulvar dystrophy, 22, 129
  hyperplastic, 129
  nomenclature, 129f
vulvar inspection
  pelvic pain, 13
vulvar intraepithelial neoplasia (VIN), 124–125, 129–132
  characteristics, 131f
  etiology, 124
  incidence, 124

319

Index

vulvar intraepithelial neoplasia (VIN) (*Continued*)
  management, 125–126
  pathology, 124–125
  presentation, 125
  prognosis, 126
  radiotherapy, 126
  spread, 125
  staging, 125
  vulva, 22
  work-up, 125
vulvar neoplasia, 129–132
vulvar pruritus, 21
  algorithm, 22f
  differential diagnosis, 21f
vulvar symptoms, 21–23
  age, 21
  dermatologic, 23
  examination, 22–23
  history, 21–22
  psychosomatics, 22
  work-up, 23
vulvar tumors, 124–125
  VIN, 124–125

vulvectomy
  complications, 126f
  radical, 126

W
warfarin
  thromboembolism, 204
WBC *see* white blood count (WBC)
weight
  pregnancy risk, 272f
white blood count (WBC)
  pelvic pain, 14

X
X-ray, 294–295

Y
Yasmin, 177
  endometrial hyperplasia, 93

Z
Zoloft
  depression, 202